T0264161

Clinical Heart Failure Scenarios: From Prevention to Overt Disease and Rehabilitation

Editor

FRANCESCO ANTONINI-CANTERIN

HEART FAILURE CLINICS

www.heartfailure.theclinics.com

Consulting Editor
EDUARDO BOSSONE

Founding Editor
JAGAT NARULA

April 2021 • Volume 17 • Number 2

ELSEVIER

1600 John F. Kennedy Boulevard • Suite 1800 • Philadelphia, Pennsylvania, 19103-2899

http://www.theclinics.com

HEART FAILURE CLINICS Volume 17, Number 2
April 2021 ISSN 1551-7136, ISBN-13: 978-0-323-79586-9

Editor: Joanna Collett
Developmental Editor: Jessica Cañaberal

Heart Failure Clinics (ISSN 1551-7136) is published quarterly by Elsevier Inc., 360 Park Avenue South, New York, NY 10010-1710. Months of publication are January, April, July, and October. Business and editorial offices: 1600 John F. Kennedy Boulevard, Suite 1800, Philadelphia, PA 19103-2899. Periodicals postage paid at New York, NY, and additional mailing offices. Subscription prices are USD 277.00 per year for US individuals, USD 661.00 per year for US institutions, USD 100.00 per year for US students and residents, USD 300.00 per year for Canadian individuals, USD 684.00 per year for Canadian institutions, USD 315.00 per year for international individuals, USD 684.00 per year for international institutions, and USD 100.00 per year for Canadian and foreign students/residents. To receive student and resident rate, orders must be accompanied by name of affiliated institution, date of term, and the *signature* of program/residency coordinator on institution letterhead. Orders will be billed at individual rate until proof of status is received. Foreign air speed delivery is included in all *Clinics* subscription prices. All prices are subject to change without notice. **POSTMASTER:** Send address changes to *Heart Failure Clinics*, Elsevier Health Sciences Division, Subscription Customer Service, 3251 Riverport Lane, Maryland Heights, MO 63043. **Customer Service: 1-800-654-2452 (US and Canada). From outside of the US and Canada, call 314-447-8871. Fax: 314-447-8029. For print support, E-mail: JournalsCustomerService-usa@elsevier.com. For online support, E-mail: JournalsOnlineSupport-usa@elsevier.com.**

Reprints. For copies of 100 or more of articles in this publication, please contact the Commercial Reprints Department, Elsevier Inc., 360 Park Avenue South, New York, NY 10010-1710. Tel.: 212-633-3874; Fax: 212-633-3820; E-mail: reprints@elsevier.com.

Heart Failure Clinics is covered in *MEDLINE/PubMed (Index Medicus).*

Contributors

CONSULTING EDITOR

EDUARDO BOSSONE, MD, PhD, FCCP, FESC, FACC
Division of Cardiology, AORN Antonio Cardarelli Hospital, Naples, Italy

EDITOR

FRANCESCO ANTONINI-CANTERIN, MD
Division of Cardiology, High Specialization Rehabilitative Hospital, Motta di Livenza, Treviso, Italy

AUTHORS

DI NARO AGNESE, MD
Cardiology Unit, High Specialization Rehabilitation Hospital Motta di Livenza, Treviso, Italy

MARCO AMBROSETTI, MD
Specialist in Internal Medicine and Cardiology, Cardiological Rehabilitation Unit, ASST Crema, Italy

FRANCESCO ANTONINI-CANTERIN, MD
Division of Cardiology, High Specialization Rehabilitative Hospital, Motta di Livenza, Treviso, Italy

CARMEN C. BELADAN, MD, PhD
University of Medicine and Pharmacy "Carol Davila," Euroecolab, Emergency Institute for Cardiovascular Diseases "Prof. Dr. C. C. Iliescu," Bucharest, Romania

NICOLA BERNARDI, MD
Cardiology Division, Spedali Civili, University of Brescia, Brescia, Italy

DENNIS BERNIEH, PhD
Department of Cardiovascular Sciences, University of Leicester, Leicester, United Kingdom

ANDREA BONELLI, MD
Cardiology Division, Spedali Civili, University of Brescia, Brescia, Italy

MARCO BOSISIO, MD
Cardiology Division, Spedali Civili, University of Brescia, Brescia, Italy

EDUARDO BOSSONE, MD, PhD, FCCP, FESC, FACC
Division of Cardiology, AORN Antonio Cardarelli Hospital, Naples, Italy

SIMONA B. BOTEZATU, MD
University of Medicine and Pharmacy "Carol Davila," Euroecolab

FRANCESCA BURSI, MD, PhD, MSc
Division of Cardiology, Heart and Lung Department, San Paolo Hospital, ASST Santi Paolo and Carlo, University of Milan, Milano, Italy

FILIPPO CADEMARTIRI, MD, PhD, FESC
IRCCS SDN, Naples, Italy

MARTINA CAIAZZA, MD
Department of Translational Medical Sciences, University of Campania "Luigi Vanvitelli," Naples, Italy

PAOLO CALABRO', MD, PhD
Department of Translational Medical Sciences, University of Campania "Luigi Vanvitelli," Naples, Italy

EMILIANO CALVI, MD
Cardiology Division, Spedali Civili, University of Brescia, Brescia, Italy

MARIA LUDOVICA CARERJ, MD
Departments of Biomedical and Dental Sciences and Morphological and Functional Images, AOU Polclinico G. Martino, University of Messina, Messina, Italy

SCIPIONE CARERJ, MD
Department of Clinical and Experimental Medicine – Cardiology Unit, AOU Policlinico G. Martino, University of Messina, Messina, Italy

SALVATORE LA CARRUBBA, MD, PhD
Villa Sofia Hospital, Palermo, Italy

ANTONIO CITTADINI, MD
Department of Translational Medical Sciences, Federico II University of Naples, Naples, Italy

CARLA CONTALDI, MD, PhD
Department of Cardiology, University Hospital of Salerno, Cava de' Tirreni, Salerno, Italy

ANNA D'AGOSTINO, PhD
IRCCS SDN Nuclear and Diagnostic Research Institute, Naples, Italy

ANTONELLO D'APONTE, MD
Department of Experimental Medicine, Section of Human Physiology and Unit of Dietetics and Sports Medicine, University of Campania "Luigi Vanvitelli," Naples, Italy

ROBERTA D'ASSANTE, PhD
Department of Translational Medical Sciences, Federico II University, Naples, Italy

SHARLENE M. DAY, MD, PhD
Department of Internal Medicine, University of Michigan, Ann Arbor, Michigan, USA

MARIAROSARIA DE LUCA, MD
Department of Translational Medical Sciences, Federico II University, Naples, Italy

SANTO DELLEGROTTAGLIE, MD, PhD
Division of Cardiology, Ospedale Accreditato Villa Dei Fiori, Acerra, Naples, Italy; Zena and Michael A. Wiener Cardiovascular Institute/ Marie-Josee and Henry R. Kravis Center for Cardiovascular Health, Icahn School of Medicine at Mount Sinai, New York, USA

GIANLUCA DI BELLA, MD, PhD
Department of Clinical and Experimental Medicine – Cardiology Unit, AOU Policlinico G. Martino, University of Messina, Messina, Italy

CONCETTA DI NORA, MD
Department of Cardiothoracic Science, Azienda Sanitaria Universitaria Integrata di Udine, Italy

SARA DOIMO, MD
Cardio-Cerebro-Vascular Pathophysiology Department, Cardiology Unit, Azienda Sanitaria "Friuli Occidentale," Pordenone, Italy

RIVABEN DANTE EDUARDO, MD
Cardiology Unit, High Specialization Rehabilitation Hospital Motta di Livenza, Treviso, Italy

NICOLOSI ELISA, MD
Cardiology Unit, High Specialization Rehabilitation Hospital Motta di Livenza, Treviso, Italy

MOHAMED ELTAYEB, MRCP (UK)
Department of Cardiovascular Sciences, University of Leicester, Leicester, United Kingdom

AUGUSTO ESPOSITO, MD
Department of Translational Medical Sciences, University of Campania "Luigi Vanvitelli," Naples, Italy

FADL-ELMULA M. FADL ELMULA, MD
Heart Centre, King Faisal Specialist Hospital and Research Centre, Riyadh, Saudi Arabia

ANDREA FAGGIANO, MD
Fondazione IRCCS Ca' Granda Ospedale Maggiore Policlinico, University of Milan, Milan, Italy

POMPILIO FAGGIANO, MD
Cardiology University of Brescia and Fondazione Poliambulanza, Brescia, Italy

FRANCESCO FERRARA, MD, PhD
Department of Cardiology, University Hospital of Salerno, Cava de' Tirreni, Salerno, Italy

MARIA TERESA FLORIO, MD
Division of Internal Medicine, University of Campania “Luigi Vanvitelli,” Naples, Italy

MICHELE FUSARO, MD
Department of Radiology, Santa Maria di Ca’ Foncello Hospital, Treviso, Italy

FEDERICA GUIDETTI, MD
Department of Cardiology, University Heart Center, University Hospital Zurich, Zurich, Switzerland

MUHAMMAD ZUBAIR ISRAR, PhD
Department of Cardiovascular Sciences, University of Leicester, Leicester, United Kingdom

GIUSEPPE LIMONGELLI, MD, PhD, FESC
Department of Translational Medical Sciences, University of Campania “Luigi Vanvitelli,” Naples, Italy; Member of ERN GUARD-HEART; Institute of Cardiovascular Sciences, University College of London, St. Bartholomew’s Hospital, London, United Kingdom

UGOLINO LIVI, MD
Department of Cardiothoracic Science, Azienda Sanitaria Universitaria Integrata di Udine, Italy

LUCA LONGOBARDO, MD
Department of Clinical and Experimental Medicine, AOU Policlinico G. Martino, University of Messina, Messina, Italy

DAL CORSO LORENZA, MD
Cardiology Unit, High Specialization Rehabilitation Hospital Motta di Livenza, Treviso, Italy

ROBERTA MANGANARO, MD, PhD
Department of Clinical and Experimental Medicine – Cardiology Unit, AOU Policlinico G. Martino, University of Messina, Messina, Italy

MICHAL MARCHEL, MD, PhD
1st Department of Cardiology, Medical University of Warsaw, Warsaw, Poland

ALBERTO M. MARRA, MD, PhD
Department of Translational Medical Sciences, Federico II University of Naples, Naples, Italy

CIRO MAURO, MD
AORN A Cardarelli, Cardiac Rehabilitation Unit, Cardiology Division, A Cardarelli Hospital, Naples, Italy

LAURA MERLO, MD
Specialist in Sports and Exercise Medicine, Sports Medicine Unit, AULSS 2, Treviso, Italy

GIOVANNI MESSINA, MD, PhD
Department of Experimental Medicine, Section of Human Physiology and Unit of Dietetics and Sports Medicine, University of Campania "Luigi Vanvitelli," Naples, Italy

ANTONIO MICARI, MD, PhD
Departments of Biomedical and Dental Sciences and Morphological and Functional Images, AOU Polclinico G. Martino, University of Messina, Messina, Italy

EMANUELE MONDA, MD
Department of Translational Medical Sciences, University of Campania “Luigi Vanvitelli,” Naples, Italy

MARCELLINO MONDA, MD, PhD
Department of Experimental Medicine, Section of Human Physiology and Unit of Dietetics and Sports Medicine, University of Campania "Luigi Vanvitelli," Naples, Italy

ELISABETTA MOSCARELLA, MD
Department of Translational Medical Sciences, University of Campania “Luigi Vanvitelli,” Naples, Italy

MARTINA NESTI, MD
Cardiovascular and Neurology Department, Ospedale San Donato, Arezzo, Italy

IACOPO OLIVOTTO, MD, PhD
Cardiomyopathy Unit and Genetic Unit, Careggi University Hospital, Florence, Italy

GIUSEPPE PACILEO, MD
Department of Translational Medical Sciences, University of Campania “Luigi Vanvitelli,” Naples, Italy

LEOPOLDO PAGLIANI, MD, PhD
Cardiology Unit, High Specialization Rehabilitation Hospital Motta di Livenza, Treviso, Italy

GIUSEPPE PALMIERO, MD
Department of Cardiology, AORN Ospedali dei Colli - Monaldi Hospital, Inherited and Rare Cardiovascular Diseases Unit, Department of Translational Medical Sciences, University of Campania "Luigi Vanvitelli," Naples, Italy

ALESSANDRO PATTI, MD
Specialist in Sports and Exercise Medicine, Sports Medicine Unit, AULSS 2, Treviso, Italy

DANIELA PAVAN, MD
Cardio-Cerebro-Vascular Pathophysiology Department, Cardiology Unit, Azienda Sanitaria "Friuli Occidentale," Pordenone, Italy

MAURIZIO CUSMÀ PICCIONE, MD, PhD
Department of Clinical and Experimental Medicine – Cardiology Unit, AOU Policlinico G. Martino, University of Messina, Messina, Italy

BRIGIDA RANIERI, PhD
IRCCS SDN Nuclear and Diagnostic Research Institute, Naples, Italy

SALVATORE REGA
Department of Translational Medical Sciences, Federico II University of Naples, Naples, Italy

LUIGIA ROMANO, MD
Department of General and Emergency Radiology, A Cardarelli Hospital, Naples, Italy

MARTA RUBINO, MD
Inherited and Rare Cardiovascular Diseases Unit, Department of Translational Medical Sciences, University of Campania "Luigi Vanvitelli," Naples, Italy

VINCENZO RUSSO, MD, PhD
Chair of Cardiology, Department of Translational Medical Sciences, University of Campania "Luigi Vanvitelli," Naples, Italy

ANDREA SALZANO, MD, PhD, MRCP (London)
IRCCS SDN Nuclear and Diagnostic Research Institute, Naples, Italy

PATRIZIO SARTO, MD
Specialist in Sports and Exercise Medicine, Specialist in Cardiology, Sports Medicine Unit, AULSS 2, Treviso, Italy

ALESSANDRA SCATTEIA, MD
Division of Cardiology, Ospedale Accreditato Villa Dei Fiori, Acerra, Naples, Italy

OLGA SCUDIERO, MD, PhD
Department of Molecular Medicine and Medical Biotechnology, CEINGE Advanced Biotechnologies, Task Force on Microbiome Studies, University of Naples "Federico II," Naples, Italy

IAIN B. SQUIRE, MD, FRCP
Department of Cardiovascular Sciences, University of Leicester, Leicester, United Kingdom

TORU SUZUKI, MD, PhD, FRCP
Department of Cardiovascular Sciences, University of Leicester, Leicester, United Kingdom

GIOVANNI TESSARIN, MD
Department of Medicine-DIMED, Institute of Radiology, University of Padova, Padua, Italy

OLGA VRIZ, MD
Heart Centre, King Faisal Specialist Hospital and Research Centre, Alfaisal University, School of Medicine, Riyadh, Saudi Arabia

CONCETTA ZITO, MD, PhD
Department of Clinical and Experimental Medicine – Cardiology Unit, AOU Policlinico G. Martino, University of Messina, Messina, Italy

Contents

Preface: Heart Failure: One, None, and a Hundred Thousand xiii

Francesco Antonini-Canterin and Eduardo Bossone

Stage A Heart Failure: Modern Strategies for an Effective Prevention 167

Pompilio Faggiano, Nicola Bernardi, Emiliano Calvi, Andrea Bonelli, Andrea Faggiano, Francesca Bursi, and Marco Bosisio

Stage A heart failure (HF) patients do not show HF symptoms or any structural heart disease but are at risk of HF development. Cardiovascular risk factors (hypertension, diabetes, metabolic syndrome, sedentary lifestyle, poor diet, and exposure to cardiotoxic agents) characterize subjects affected by stage A HF. It is essential to identify these subjects early and ensure that, despite being asymptomatic, they grasp the importance of undertaking correct lifestyle and therapeutic interventions. A careful stratification of asymptomatic subject's risk profile is needed to adopt proper preventive strategies and to set individualized therapeutic targets that avoid progression to advanced stages of HF.

Asymptomatic Left Ventricular Dysfunction: Is There a Role for Screening in General Population? 179

Salvatore La Carrubba, Roberta Manganaro, Concetta Zito, Gianluca Di Bella, Maria Ludovica Carerj, Luca Longobardo, Maurizio Cusmà Piccione, Antonio Micari, and Scipione Carerj

Stage A and B heart failure (HF) include asymptomatic patients without and with structural cardiac disorder, respectively. Asymptomatic left ventricular (LV) dysfunction represents an early stage of HF that should be recognized to prevent overt HF development. Echocardiography plays a pivotal role in assessment of cardiac structure and function and represents the ideal imaging technique for screening in the general population, thanks to its availability, feasibility, and low cost. Traditional echocardiography, with LV systolic and diastolic function and cardiac remodeling assessment, is usually performed. Development of new technologies may offer additional information and insights in detection of early LV dysfunction.

Prevention of Coronary Artery Disease–Related Heart Failure: The Role of Computed Tomography Scan 187

Michele Fusaro and Giovanni Tessarin

During the past decade, coronary computed tomography angiography has emerged as the primary modality to noninvasively detect and rule out coronary artery disease. Therefore, this technique could play an important role in identifying patients at high risk of heart failure, considering the high prevalence of coronary artery disease in these patients. The latest technologies have also increased diagnostic accuracy, helping to close the gap with the other functional imaging modalities.

Anemia and Management of Heart Failure Patients 195

Carmen C. Beladan and Simona B. Botezatu

Anemia is common in heart failure with preserved and reduced ejection fraction. It is independently associated with poor functional status, hospitalization, and reduced

in patients with abnormal QRS duration and morphology results in a dyssynchronous ventricular activation and contraction leading to cardiac remodeling, worsening systolic and diastolic function, and progressive HF. In this article, the authors aim to explore the current CRT literature, focusing their attentions on the promising innovation in this field.

Combined Effect of Mediterranean Diet and Aerobic Exercise on Weight Loss and Clinical Status in Obese Symptomatic Patients with Hypertrophic Cardiomyopathy **303**

Giuseppe Limongelli, Emanuele Monda, Antonello D'Aponte, Martina Caiazza, Marta Rubino, Augusto Esposito, Giuseppe Palmiero, Elisabetta Moscarella, Giovanni Messina, Paolo Calabro', Olga Scudiero, Giuseppe Pacileo, Marcellino Monda, Eduardo Bossone, Sharlene M. Day, and Iacopo Olivotto

We evaluated the impact of weight loss (WL) using a Mediterranean diet and mild-to-moderate–intensity aerobic exercise program, on clinical status of obese, symptomatic patients with hypertrophic cardiomyopathy (HCM). Compared with nonresponders, responders showed a significant reduction of left atrial diameter, left atrial volume index (LAVI), E/E2b9average, pulmonary artery systolic pressure (PASP), and a significant increase in Vo2max (%) and peak workload. Body mass index changes correlated with reduction in left atrial diameter, LAVI, E/E2b9average, PASP, and increase of Vo2max (mL/Kg/min), Vo2max (%), peak workload. Mediterranean diet and aerobic exercise is associated with clinical-hemodynamic improvement in obese symptomatic HCM patients.

HEART FAILURE CLINICS

FORTHCOMING ISSUES

July 2021
Heart Failure with Preserved Ejection Fraction
Geu-Ru Hong, *Editor*

October 2021
Advanced Heart Failure: From Pathophysiology to Clinical Management
Giuseppe Pacileo, Francesco Grigioni, Daniele Masarone, and Luciano Potena, *Editors*

RECENT ISSUES

January 2021
Cardiovascular Magnetic Resonance
Subha V. Raman, *Editor*

October 2020
Process Improvement in Heart Failure
Clyde W. Yancy and R. Kannan Mutharasan, *Editors*

July 2020
Cardiovascular Emergencies, Part II
Michinari Hieda and Giovanni Esposito, *Editors*

SERIES OF RELATED INTEREST

Cardiology Clinics
http://www.cardiology.theclinics.com/
Cardiac Electrophysiology Clinics
https://www.cardiacep.theclinics.com/
Interventional Cardiology Clinics
https://www.interventional.theclinics.com/

THE CLINICS ARE AVAILABLE ONLINE!
Access your subscription at:
www.theclinics.com

Preface

Heart Failure: One, None, and a Hundred Thousand

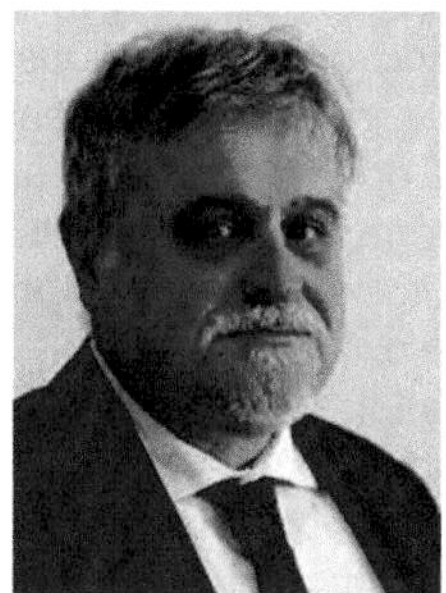

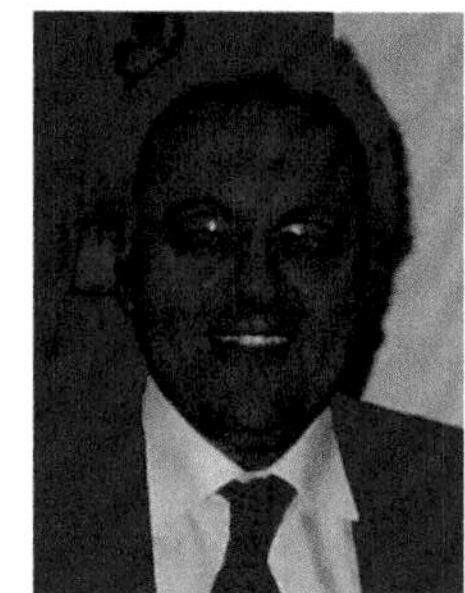

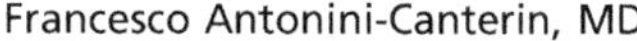

Francesco Antonini-Canterin, MD Eduardo Bossone, MD, PhD, FCCP, FESC, FACC

Editors

Heart failure represents an important public health problem worldwide, with a broad spectrum of clinical scenarios, starting from primary prevention in an asymptomatic phase to acute and chronic congestive heart failure, with use of modern drugs and devices, rehabilitation, and telemedicine strategies.[1–3] So, we can appropriately paraphrase the renowned Italian writer and Nobel Prize recipient, Luigi Pirandello, and his famous novel, written in 1926, as: "Heart Failure: One, None and a Hundred Thousand." Diagnosis and treatment of heart failure are particularly difficult and challenging, especially in these dramatic days, as most medical effort everywhere is devoted to COVID-19 care.[4,5]

The objective of this issue of *Heart Failure Clinics* is to analyze different and peculiar scenarios related to the "heart failure syndrome," ranging from topics such as epidemiology, prevention, sports medicine, integrated diagnostic methods, pharmacologic and nonpharmacologic therapies, to modern and effective health management models.

Specifically, Faggiano discusses in detail the most modern approaches for the early preventive management of stage A patients, in which symptoms have not yet manifested, but insidious risk factors are present.[6,7] Carerj and colleagues provide a complete review on the importance of early detection of asymptomatic left ventricular dysfunction.[8,9] This article describes in-depth the experience of the DAVES (Disfunzione Asintomatica VEntricolare Sinistra) multicenter prospective study conducted by the Italian Society of Echocardiography for a period of more than 10 years.[10]

Fusaro and colleagues describe in a very clear and punctual way, from the radiologist point of view, the actual role of computed tomographic calcium detection and coronary angiography for the prevention of coronary artery disease–related heart failure.[11] Contaldi and colleagues show how cardiac magnetic resonance give us noninvasive morphologic and functional assessment, tissue characterization, blood flow, and perfusion evaluation, providing useful information for early etiologic diagnosis, prognostic stratification, and treatment management in heart failure patients.[12]

Beladan and colleagues treat the complex theme of anemia, which is a highly prevalent comorbidity in patients with heart failure, representing a strong marker of poor outcome in patients with both chronic and acute heart failure, irrespective of the left ventricular ejection fraction. The good news is that treatment of iron deficiency, even in the absence of clear anemia, has proven significant benefit in heart failure patients with systolic dysfunction.[13]

Salzano and colleagues describe in this issue the important clinical role of old and new biomarkers, offering a very practical clinical approach. Therefore, biomarkers are categorized into 5 groups according to their function and suitability: community-based screening, diagnosis, risk stratification, phenotyping, and management/tailoring treatment.[14,15]

Ventricular arterial coupling parameters must be considered when evaluating patients with heart failure. These parameters indicate both the condition and the interaction between the arterial

Heart Failure Clin 17 (2021) xiii–xv
https://doi.org/10.1016/j.hfc.2021.01.011

system and the left ventricle and can be used as prognostic indexes. Ventricular arterial coupling can be used for heart failure patient stratification and tailoring medical therapy. Vriz and colleagues describe in this issue several methods that are suitable for ventricular arterial coupling assessment and how each of them can be applied in different clinical scenarios, such as chronic or acute heart failure.[16,17]

Doimo provides a comprehensive review on the novelties in pharmacologic therapy in chronic heart failure. The cornerstone of the current therapy for heart failure is the inhibition of the sympathetic nervous system and the renin-angiotensin-aldosterone system. Sacubitril/valsartan reduces cardiovascular mortality and hospitalization for heart failure.[18] The research for new treatments for comorbidities has recently led to the discovery of new therapeutic approaches in the treatment of heart failure. Sodium-glucose cotransporters 2 inhibition has nowadays an emerging role in the treatment of heart failure and on cardiovascular outcome.[19]

With regards to exercise-based cardiac rehabilitation programs in heart failure patients, Patti and colleagues clarify some crucial points. Exercise training significantly improves exercise capacity and quality of life and reduces symptoms of depression and anxiety in heart failure patients. Moreover, it can improve survival and reduce the risk for hospitalizations. Exercise-based cardiac rehabilitation can be offered effectively with different modalities, such as continuous interval or aerobic training, resistance, and inspiratory muscle training, and each intervention must be tailored taking into account the general conditions and functional capacity. Unfortunately, to date, adherence to exercise-based programs is still limited, due to socioeconomic factors, patients' characteristics, and lack of referral.[20,21]

The ventricular assist device (VAD) has rapidly emerged as a durable and safe therapy for end-stage heart failure patients.[22] Di Nora and colleagues show in this issue how cardiac rehabilitation should be recognized as a fundamental component to improve outcomes in patients who not only are candidates for VAD therapy but also are carrying the VAD system. The exercise training must be individualized in VAD patients, considering the patient's condition, the previous functional capacity, left VAD parameters, comorbidities, and possible complications after surgery.[23]

Telemonitoring applied to cardiovascular diseases or teleCardiology is a new frontier in the management of cardiac patients, especially in the present post-COVID-19 era. TeleCardiology is defined as the recording, remote transmission, storage, and interpretation of cardiovascular parameters (such as electrocardiographic [ECG] signals, heart rate, blood pressure, oxygen saturation), and, more recently, of diagnostic images (echocardiography, computed tomography, cardiac magnetic resonance, and so forth). Pagliani and colleagues describe the increasing role, emphasized by recent guidelines, of daily monitoring of body weight and other vital signs. The home telemonitoring, integrated with educational interventions, allows an optimized and real-time home clinical management of patients with heart failure by reducing hospitalizations and improving outcome and quality of life.[24]

Cardiac resynchronization therapy (CRT) is an important tool in heart failure patients. However, the last European guidelines for CRT implantation gave very stringent indication, as they require low left ventricular ejection fraction symptoms and the presence of significant electrical dyssynchrony on ECG (left bundle branch block and wide QRS). This has been driven prevalently by MADIT-CRT results, which identified these parameters as powerful predictors to CRT response. Palmiero and colleagues analyze the recent evidence in this field and the promising further applications in the clinical practice.[25]

In addition, Limongelli and colleagues demonstrate that in obese, symptomatic patients with symptoms of heart failure due to hypertrophic cardiomyopathy, weight loss obtained by a combined protocol of Mediterranean diet and aerobic exercise gave markedly favorable effects on left atrium remodeling, diastolic function, exercise capacity, and clinical status.[26]

In conclusion, the present issue of *Heart Failure Clinics* can provide many insights into various themes that not always receive due attention, giving useful information to clinicians and investigators for improving the clinical management of patients with heart failure.

Francesco Antonini-Canterin, MD
Division of Cardiology
High Specialization Rehabilitative Hospital
Via Padre Leonardo Bello, 3/c
31045 Motta di Livenza, Italy

Eduardo Bossone, MD, PhD, FCCP, FESC, FACC
Division of Cardiology
Cardarelli Hospital
Via A. Cardarelli, 9
Naples 80131, Italy

E-mail addresses:
antonini.canterin@gmail.com (F. Antonini-Canterin)
ebossone@hotmail.com (E. Bossone)

REFERENCES

1. Ponikowski P, Voors AA, Anker SD, et al. 2016 ESC guidelines for the diagnosis and treatment of acute and chronic heart failure. The Task Force for the diagnosis and treatment of acute and chronic heart failure of the European Society of Cardiology (ESC). Eur Heart J 2016;37:2129–200.
2. Yancy W, Jessup M, Bozkurt B, et al. 2017 ACC/AHA/HFSA Focused Update of the 2013 ACCF/AHA Guideline for the management of heart failure: a report of the American College of Cardiology/American Heart Association Task Force on Clinical Practice Guidelines and the Heart Failure Society of America. Clinical Practice Guideline: focused update. J Am Coll Cardiol 2017;70:776–803.
3. Paulus WJ. Unfolding discoveries in heart failure. N Engl J Med 2020;382:679–82.
4. Freaney PM, Shah SJ, Khan SS. COVID-19 and heart failure with preserved ejection fraction. JAMA 2020;324:1499–500.
5. Miller JC, Skoll D, Saxon LA. Home monitoring of cardiac devices in the era of COVID-19. Curr Cardiol Rep 2020;23:1.
6. Tanaka H. Future perspectives for management of stage A heart failure. J Atheroscler Thromb 2018; 25:557–65.
7. Carerj S, La Carrubba S, Antonini-Canterin F, et al, Research Group of the Italian Society of Cardiovascular Echography. The incremental prognostic value of echocardiography in asymptomatic stage a heart failure. J Am Soc Echocardiogr 2010;23:1025–34.
8. Pugliese NR, Fabiani I, La Carrubba S, et al, Italian Society of Cardiovascular Echography (SIEC). Classification and prognostic evaluation of left ventricular remodeling in patients with asymptomatic heart failure. Am J Cardiol 2017;119:71–7.
9. Di Bello V, La Carrubba S, Antonini-Canterin F, et al, Research Group of the Italian Society of Cardiovascular Echography (SIEC). Role of electrocardiography and echocardiography in prevention and predicting outcome of subjects at increased risk of heart failure. Eur J Prev Cardiol 2015;22:249–62.
10. Carerj S, Penco M, La Carrubba S, et al. The DAVES (Disfunzione Asintomatica VEntricolare Sinistra) study by the Italian Society of Cardiovascular Echography: rationale and design. J Cardiovasc Med 2006;7:457–63.
11. Waqar Aziz W, Claridge S, Ntalas I. Emerging role of cardiac computed tomography in heart failure. ESC Heart Fail 2019;6:909–20.
12. Aljizeeri A, Sulaiman A, Alhulaimi N, et al. Cardiac magnetic resonance imaging in heart failure: where the alphabet begins! Heart Fail Rev 2017;22:385–99.
13. Anand IS, Gupta P. Anemia and iron deficiency in heart failure: current concepts and emerging therapies. Circulation 2018;138:80–98.
14. Suzuki T. Cardiovascular diagnostic biomarkers: the past, present and future. Circ J 2009;73:806–9.
15. Januzzi JL Jr. Will biomarkers succeed as a surrogate endpoint in heart failure trials? JACC Heart Fail 2018;6:570–2.
16. Antonini-Canterin F, Enache R, Popescu BA, et al. Prognostic value of ventricular-arterial coupling and B-type natriuretic peptide in patients after myocardial infarction: a five-year follow-up study. J Am Soc Echocardiogr 2009;22:1239–45.
17. Antonini-Canterin F, Poli S, Vriz O, et al. The ventricular-arterial coupling: from basic pathophysiology to clinical application in the echocardiography laboratory. J Cardiovasc Echogr 2013;23:91–5.
18. McMurray JJV, Packer M, Desai AS, et al. Angiotensin-neprilysin inhibition versus enalapril in heart failure. N Engl J Med 2014;371:993–1004.
19. Zinman B, Wanner C, Lachin JM, et al. Empagliflozin, cardiovascular outcomes, and mortality in type 2 diabetes. N Engl J Med 2015;373:2117–28.
20. Piepoli MF, Conraads V, Corrà U, et al. Exercise training in heart failure: from theory to practice. A consensus document of the Heart Failure Association and the European Association for Cardiovascular Prevention and Rehabilitation. Eur J Heart Fail 2011;13:347–57.
21. Bjarnason-Wehrens B, Nebel R, Jensen K, et al. Exercise-based cardiac rehabilitation in patients with reduced left ventricular ejection fraction: the Cardiac Rehabilitation Outcome Study in Heart Failure (CROS-HF): a systematic review and meta-analysis. Eur J Prev Cardiol 2020;27:929–52.
22. Kerrigan DJ, Williams CT, Ehrman JK, et al. Cardiac rehabilitation improves functional capacity and patient-reported health status in patients with continuous-flow left ventricular assist devices: the Rehab-VAD randomized controlled trial. JACC Heart Fail 2014;6:653–65.
23. Adamopoulos S, Corrà U, Laoutaris ID, et al. Exercise training in patients with ventricular assist devices: a review of the evidence and practical advice. A position paper from the Committee on Exercise Physiology and Training and the Committee of Advanced Heart Failure of the Heart Failure Association of the European Society of Cardiology. Eur J Heart Fail 2019;21:3–13.
24. Pandor A, Gomersall T, Stevens JW, et al. Remote monitoring after recent hospital discharge in patients with heart failure: a systematic review and network metaanalysis. Heart 2013;99:1717–26.
25. Daubert C, Behar N, Martins RP, et al. Avoiding non-responders to cardiac resynchronization therapy: a practical guide. Eur Heart J 2017;38:1463–72.
26. Limongelli G, Monda E, Tramonte S, et al. Prevalence and clinical significance of red flags in patients with hypertrophic cardiomyopathy. Int J Cardiol 2020;299:186–91.

Stage A Heart Failure
Modern Strategies for an Effective Prevention

Pompilio Faggiano, MD[a,*], Nicola Bernardi, MD[b], Emiliano Calvi, MD[b], Andrea Bonelli, MD[b], Andrea Faggiano, MD[c], Francesca Bursi, MD, PhD, MSc[d], Marco Bosisio, MD[b]

KEYWORDS

- Heart failure • Cardiovascular risk factors • Preventive cardiology • Stage A heart failure
- Early intervention

KEY POINTS

- Patients with stage A heart failure (HF) show no HF symptoms but have related comorbid diseases with a high risk of progressing to HF.
- Early identification of underlying cardiovascular risk factors allows adoption of preventive measures aimed at stopping progression to clinical HF.
- Blood pressure, body weight, and glycemic control with renal function monitoring, smoking cessation, and correct lifestyle adoption are the main measures to be undertaken.
- Stratifying the cardiovascular risk profile and setting individualized targets are the cornerstones of a modern strategy for effective prevention.

INTRODUCTION

Heart failure (HF) is a clinical syndrome characterized by signs and symptoms caused by either a structural or a functional cardiac abnormality, with the result of impaired ventricular filling or reduced cardiac output.[1]

The actual prevalence of HF among the population in developed countries is 2%, with an increase to 10% after 70 years of age.[2] Despite improvement in therapies and medical care, this syndrome is still marked by a poor outcome. Indeed, the calculated 12-month mortality is 17% for hospitalized patients and 7% for stable patients.[3]

The natural history of HF is characterized by a progressive increase in hospital admissions over time, mostly because of fluid overload. For this reason, it confers a substantial burden on health care systems worldwide.[4]

The above-mentioned definition collects those patients with overt clinical features, but this may be, in some ways, restrictive. In fact, even asymptomatic patients can have a structural or functional dysfunction, which is a precursor of future HF.[2] In this context, early detection of subclinical abnormalities can prevent the progression of the disease and reduce mortality.[5]

Left ventricular ejection fraction is the most widely used parameter to categorize patients affected by HF, primarily because of a different response to therapies and a different prognosis.[1]

To describe the severity of symptoms, the New York Heart Association classifies the patients on the basis of dyspnea perception and exercise

Declaration of conflicting interests: The authors declare that there is no conflict of interest.
[a] Cardiology University of Brescia and Fondazione Poliambulanza, Via 4 Novembre, 7, Brescia 25122, Italy; [b] Cardiology Division, Spedali Civili, University of Brescia, Piazzale Spedali Civili, 1, Brescia 25123, Italy; [c] Fondazione IRCCS Ca' Granda Ospedale Maggiore Policlinico, University of Milan, Via Francesco Sforza, 28, Milano 20122, Italy; [d] Division of Cardiology, Heart and Lung Department, San Paolo Hospital, ASST Santi Paolo and Carlo, University of Milan, Via Antonio di Rudini', 8, Milano 20142, Italy
* Corresponding author.
E-mail address: cardiologia@pompiliofaggiano.it

Heart Failure Clin 17 (2021) 167–177
https://doi.org/10.1016/j.hfc.2021.01.004

intolerance (**Table 1**). In addition, the American College of Cardiology (ACC) and the American Heart Association (AHA) have conceived a 4-stage classification (see **Table 1**) based on both structural changes and symptoms.[1] This scale underlines the progressive history of the disease, from absence of structural abnormalities and symptoms (stage A) to refractory HF (stage D).[6] Of interest, a population cohort study evaluated the 5-year survival rates for stages A, B, C, and D, which were 97%, 96%, 75%, and 20%, respectively.[7]

Given the high prevalence, the economic impact, and the natural history of this syndrome, physicians and clinical investigators should focus on the underlying disease process in order to slow and prevent HF progression, rather than on the treatment of worsening episodes that require hospitalization. In this review, the authors focused on "presymptomatic" HF and its management in terms of preventive strategies. They expose the clinical and prognostic features of ACC/AHA stage A HF patients and highlight modern and future approaches to HF prevention.

STAGE A PATIENT'S CHARACTERISTICS

According to the ACC and the AHA, stage A patients do not show HF symptoms or any structural heart disease, but they are at risk of development of HF.[1] In fact, these are patients with comorbidities that can lead to HF, such as hypertension, diabetes mellitus (DM), obesity, metabolic syndrome, atherosclerotic disease, as well as a history of familial cardiomyopathy or of exposure to cardiotoxic agents.

Hypertension is the most common risk factor for the development of HF.[8] The Framingham Heart Study showed a 2- and a 3-fold higher hazard ratio, respectively, for men and women, for hypertensive than for normotensive patients.[9]

Hypertension is also a main risk factor for coronary artery disease, another important condition responsible for HF development; therefore, they are often simultaneously present.

In hypertensive patients, the increased left ventricular overload can result in left ventricular hypertrophy with impaired relaxation and diastolic dysfunction, which consequently lead to HF with preserved or reduced ejection fraction (HFpEF, HFrEF).[10] Among other abnormalities, hypertension-related fibrosis and abnormalities of large and small vessels contribute to increase the risk of HF.

Many trials have proved that an early and intensive treatment of hypertension can prevent new onset HF.[11,12]

DM and HF often coexist and influence each other; in fact, HF increases the risk of diabetes.

Table 1
American College of Cardiology Foundation/American Heart Association stages of heart failure compared with the New York Heart Association functional classification

ACC/AHA Stages		NYHA Functional Classification	
A	At high risk for HF but without structural heart disease or HF symptoms	None	
B	Structural heart disease but without signs or symptoms of HF	I	No limitation of physical activity. Ordinary physical activity does not cause symptoms of HF
C	Structural heart disease with prior or current symptoms of HF	I	No limitation of physical activity. Ordinary physical activity does not cause symptoms of HF
		II	Slight limitation of physical activity. Comfortable at rest, but ordinary physical activity results in HF symptoms
		III	Marked limitation of physical activity. Comfortable at rest, but less than ordinary activity causes symptoms of HF
D	Refractory HF requiring specialized interventions	IV	Unable to carry on any physical activity without symptoms of HF, or symptoms of HF at rest

Data from YANCY, Clyde W., et al. 2013 ACCF/AHA guideline for the management of heart failure: executive summary: a report of the American College of Cardiology Foundation/American Heart Association Task Force on practice guidelines. Circulation, 2013, 128.16: 1810-1852.

On the other hand, patients with diabetes are 2- to 5-fold more likely to develop HF.[13] Their risk is further enhanced by older age, coronary artery disease, peripheral arterial disease, nephropathy, retinopathy, longer duration of DM and poor glycemic control, obesity, hypertension, as well as higher NT-proBNP (N-terminal pro-B-type natriuretic peptide).[13] The pathophysiological mechanisms that subtend this association are multifactorial, both dependent and independent from diabetes itself. Diabetes is often related to many other conditions (hypertension, coronary artery disease, and obesity), which contribute to the incidence and progression of HF. In addition, even in the absence of risk factors, hyperglycemia can cause diabetic cardiomyopathy.[9]

When simultaneously present, HF and diabetes are associated with worse outcomes in terms of increased mortality and morbidity.[14]

Recently, a strong relationship has been established between obesity, measured as body mass index (BMI), and HF. The Framingham Heart Study observed a 5% to 7% (for men and women, respectively) increased risk of HF for every 1-unit BMI increase above normality range.[15] Among other indexes, BMI is the best predictor of HF in obese patients.[16] In this case, the supposed underlying mechanisms are related to obesity-dependent metabolic, inflammatory, and hormonal changes.[9] In contrast, obesity is not a predictor of adverse outcomes in patients with established HF; this condition is known as "obesity paradox."[17]

A similar counterintuitive result has been observed for hypercholesterolemia. In fact, in the case of overt HF, several studies have shown an inverse relationship between cholesterol levels and outcome, with an increased mortality if the cholesterol level is low.[18] Moreover, beneficial effects of statins in patients with established HF were not confirmed by large randomized clinical trials (RCTs).

Conversely, in the general population and in the case of atherosclerotic disease, the presence of hypercholesterolemia is related to worse outcomes, including mortality, cardiovascular (CV) events, and the development of HF.[19]

The metabolic syndrome is an established risk factor for the development of HF. As a matter of fact, every component of this syndrome is a proven CV risk factor, such as elevated blood glucose, hypertension, central obesity, hypertriglyceridemia, and low levels of high-density lipoprotein cholesterol. One study observed a greater than 3-fold increase in HF incidence for patients with metabolic syndrome, and this result remained significant even after adjustment for other HF risk factors. Interestingly, the divergence of incident HF in patients with metabolic syndrome compared with those without was only observed after 10 years of follow-up.[20]

Lastly, patients treated with known cardiotoxic agents belong to ACC/AHA stage A HF find a place those patients treated with known cardiotoxic agents.[21] Cardiotoxicity includes a wide spectrum of drug-related abnormalities that did not involve only the heart. However, left ventricular dysfunction is common among patients who were administered cancer therapies. The risk of developing HF is variably increased after chemotherapy, mainly depending on the drug used. In particular, anthracyclines have a dose-related risk of incident HF, as well as trastuzumab, an inhibitor of human epidermal growth factor receptor 2, and tyrosine kinase inhibitors. Age and preexisting CV risk factors increase the occurrence of left ventricular dysfunction in this population.[21]

STAGE A PATIENT'S DETECTION

ACC/AHA stage A subjects are at risk of developing HF in the absence of structural heart disease. The authors formerly presented several risk factors related to the incidence of HF. Given their high prevalence in the general population, the early detection of individuals with risk factors for HF is useful for the implementation of preventive strategies. The importance of addressing this group of patients is related to the established reduced risk of HF when risk factors are well controlled.

Despite the absence of unique recommendations on how to detect stage A patients, there is a large amount of literature about HF prediction models that have demonstrated a high discrimination.[22] Actually, very few models have been externally validated.[23,24] The benefit is that most of the risk factors in these models can be easily obtained in community care or outpatient settings.

Moreover, biomarkers may be helpful to identify subjects at high risk of CV events and subsequently HF development. In particular, brain-type natriuretic peptide (BNP), a protein produced in response to increased ventricular filling pressures and established CV damage, is one of the molecules proposed as screening. The STOP-HF (St Vincent's Screening to Prevent Heart Failure) randomized 1374 patients with at least 1 CV risk factor to receive routine primary care physician management (control group) or screening with BNP-guided care (intervention group). Intervention-group participants, with high BNP levels, underwent echocardiography and collaborative care between their primary care physician and specialist CV service. The primary end point of left ventricular dysfunction and HF was met in 8.7% of control-group patients and 5.3% of intervention-group patients. Thus, the study demonstrated a reduction in new-onset HF, asymptomatic left ventricular dysfunction, and emergency CV hospitalizations by using BNP-guided care compared with standard care.[25]

The assessment of global longitudinal strain (GLS) by speckle-tracking echocardiography is a relatively new method helpful in detecting subtle left ventricular dysfunction (**Fig. 1**). Although it does not play a major role in clinical practice, it has been proved to be a sensitive marker of myocardial abnormalities and, in some settings, superior to conventional echocardiographic parameters.

Some studies have observed that altered GLS may predict CV outcome in the general population. Similarly, GLS can be reduced in ACC/AHA stage A patients, being an early marker of left ventricular dysfunction. Therefore, it may potentially help in the detection of a group of asymptomatic people that need a strong strategy of preventive intervention.[6]

Therefore, in order to stop the progression of HF, it is essential to identify the risk factors early and thus intervene with coordinated preventive measures, both behavioral and pharmacologic (**Fig. 2**). The guideline-based strategies for prevention are discussed later.

NUTRITION

Nutrition plays a crucial role in the prevention of HF, according to the numerous evidence on the causal association between diet and cardiovascular diseases (CVDs).[26]

The influence of dietary factors on the development of HF, and in general of CVDs, is related to their impact on the traditional CV risk factors. Hence, any preventive strategy should consider the preservation, through proper nutrition, of normal plasma lipids, blood pressure (BP), or glucose levels.[27]

The most extensively evaluated dietary patterns are the DASH (Dietary Approaches to Stop Hypertension) diet and the Mediterranean diet, both effective in preventing CVDs. The major difference between these 2 validated diets consists of the emphasis of the Mediterranean diet on extravirgin olive oil consumption. In this regard, the PREDIMED trial showed a 30% incidence reduction of major CV events for the Mediterranean diet, compared with a traditional low-fat diet.[28] As a consequence, the risk of developing HF from coronary heart disease is mitigated.

In this context, the dietary recommendations with greater impact on CVD development are the limitation of salt intake, the avoidance of saturated fats and trans fats, and the reduction of monosaccharides/disaccharides intake, along with an increased intake of dietary fiber. In general, the consumption of fruit, vegetables, nuts, and fish should be preferred against red meats, processed meats, and foods high in sugar.[29]

However, it should be considered that foods are a complex blend of different macronutrients and micronutrients; thus, attributing the beneficial effect of a food (or a category of foods) to only one of its components may be simplistic.[27]

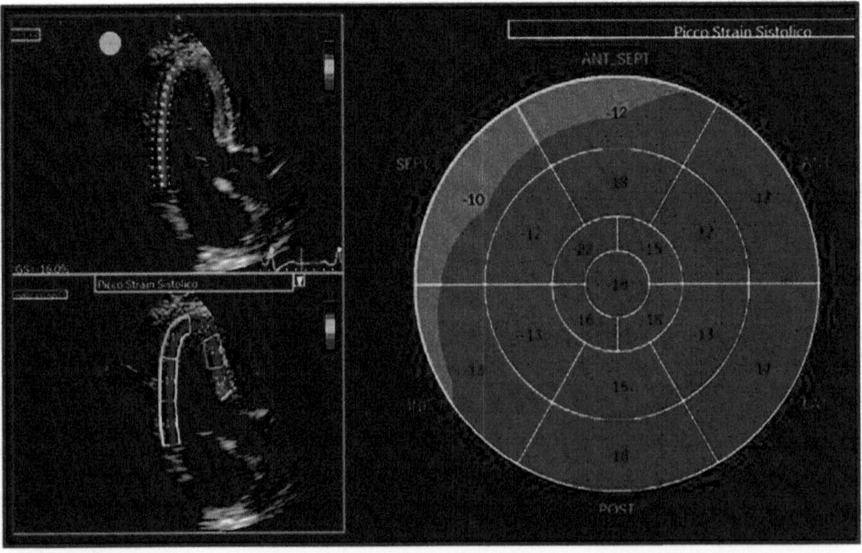

Fig. 1. GLS obtained by speckle-tracking echocardiography reveals a septal basal dysfunction in an asymptomatic hypertensive patient with normal ejection fraction.

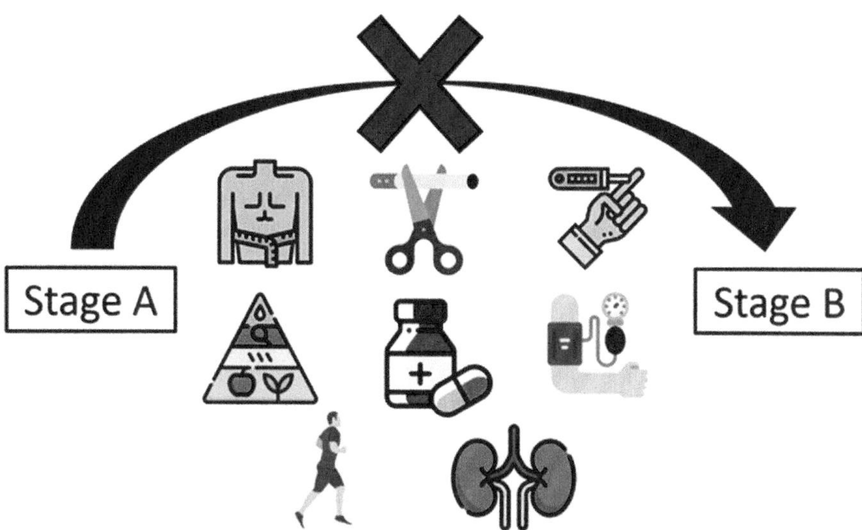

Fig. 2. Eight preventive measures needed to prevent HF progression: BMI, BP and glycemic control, quit smoking, healthy diet, physical activity, renal function monitoring, and guideline pharmacologic interventions.

LIFESTYLE MODIFICATIONS

Body weight reduction and physical activity should be primary targets for the reduction of DM, dyslipidemia, and hypertension, and, as a result, atherosclerotic cardiovascular disease (ASCVD) and HF incidence.[30]

A 5% to 10% body weight reduction can result in significant improvements in lipid and glycemic profile, favorably affecting the total CV risk. Weight loss is generally induced by a sustained caloric deficit of at least 300 to 500 kcal/d as long as a proper and balanced nutrition is maintained.[27]

The new 2020 European Society of Cardiology (ESC) Guidelines on sports cardiology and exercise in patients with CVDs recommend physical activity, both aerobic and endurance exercise, for at least 150 minutes per week, or at least 75 minutes per week for vigorous strength exercise (with additional benefit by doubling the time to 300 minutes and 150 minutes, respectively).[30]

Smoking cessation is mandatory, and it has undoubtable benefits in ASCVD risk reduction. The beneficial effects of this single intervention on mortalities are seen even among elderly persons, supporting the idea that it is never too late to quit smoking for decreasing CV-associated risks.[31] The importance of quitting smoking completely rather than just cutting back is proved by a recent meta-analysis showing that even 1 cigarette daily is associated with a significant increase in the risk for stroke, coronary heart disease, and HF. In fact, researchers found that smoking 1 cigarette a day equaled half the risk of smoking 20 cigarettes, thus demonstrating that there is not a linear dose-response curve associating CVD with the amount of tobacco exposure.[31] In regard to moderate alcohol consumption, it is acceptable only if the intake does not exceed 10 to 15 g/d (ie, 1 alcohol unit).[27]

DYSLIPIDEMIAS

As aforementioned, dyslipidemias, and in particular, elevated low-density lipoprotein cholesterol (LDL-C) levels, represent a major CV risk factor, strongly contributing to the total CVD risk.

There is strong evidence that high LDL-C levels, meeting the Bradford Hill criteria, are causally associated with an increased risk of ASCVD, and thus, lowering LDL-C proportionally reduces the risk. LDL-C has both a causal and a time-cumulative effect, because the ASCVD risk is determined by the LDL-C concentration but also by the duration of exposure.[32] A large-scale meta-analysis showed a 22% risk reduction in major vascular events for each 1.0 mmol/L reduction in LDL-C levels. Therefore, the goal is the reduction of LDL-C levels to as low as possible, with either lifestyle or pharmacologic interventions.

In addition to coronary artery disease, dyslipidemia is also a risk factor for HF.[27] Results from clinical trials proved that lipid-lowering treatments decrease the incidence of HF, mainly by preventing myocardial infarction (and consequent cardiac damage) but also as an independent factor.[33]

However, in patients with established HF, a paradoxically inverse association between lower cholesterol levels and increased mortalities can be observed.[34] In this regard, 2 prospective trials (CORONA and GISSI-HF) showed that, in patients with overt HF, treatment with rosuvastatin does not reduce CV death. For these reasons, routine lipid-lowering therapies in overt HF patients (stages C–D) are not recommended outside of primary and secondary prevention strategies of ASCVD.[35]

These considerations do not concern stage A HF, in which a lipid-lowering treatment is strongly recommended as part of a primary prevention strategy. The 2019 ESC Guidelines for the management of dyslipidemias identify LDL-C reduction as the primary treatment goal, with target levels inversely proportional to the patient's CV risk profile (**Table 2**).

The ESC Guidelines also set the secondary treatment goals. HDL-C levels should be at least 30 mg/dL (0.8 mmol/L); in addition, the target for non–HDL-C levels is less than 85 mg/dL (<2.2 mmol/L) in very-high-risk patients, less than 100 mg/dL (<2.6 mmol/L) in high-risk patients, and less than 130 mg/dL (<3.4 mmol/L) in moderate-risk patients. ApoB levels should be maintained at less than 65 mg/dL, less than 80 mg/dL, and less than 100 mg/dL in very-high-, high-, and moderate-risk patients, respectively.[27]

As a final note, it has to be considered that the CV risk profile is a continuum, but establishing these thresholds allows a more precise identification of stage A HF patients, and setting treatment goals helps provide the optimal prevention strategy.

Table 2
2019 European Society of Cardiology guidelines low-density lipoprotein cholesterol targets according to patient's cardiovascular risk profile

	Risk	LDL-C Target
Extremely high	History of a second vascular event within 2 y while in maximally tolerated statin therapy	<40 mg/dL (<1.0 mmol/L)
Very high	Documented ASCVD, including previous acute coronary syndrome or stroke/transient ischemic attack or peripheral arterial disease or significant plaque on coronary angiography/computed tomographic scan Diabetes mellitus with organ damage Severe CKD with eGFR <30 mL/min/1.73 m^2 Familial hypercholesterolemia Calculated SCORE ≥10% for 10-y risk	≤55 mg/dL (≤1.4 mmol/L)
High	Diabetes mellitus without organ damage Moderate CKD with eGFR 30–59 mL/min/1.73 m^2 Familial hypercholesterolemia Calculated SCORE 5%–10% for 10-y risk	≤70 mg/dL (≤1.8 mmol/L)
Moderate	Young patients (type 1 DM <35 y, type 2 DM <30 y) with diabetes mellitus duration <10 y Calculated SCORE 1%–5%	≤100 mg/dL (≤2.6 mmol/L)
Low	Calculated SCORE <1%	≤116 mg/dL (≤3.0 mmol/L)

Data from MACH, François, et al. 2019 ESC/EAS Guidelines for the management of dyslipidaemias: lipid modification to reduce cardiovascular risk. European heart journal, 2020, 41.1: 111-188.

Statins

Statin therapy seems to have a beneficial effect in reducing the incidence of HF (about 20%) in patients with stable coronary artery disease or previous acute coronary syndrome, as proven by several RCTs.[36]

Furthermore, a meta-analysis comparing many primary- and secondary-prevention RCTs demonstrated that statin therapy provides a slight reduction in the risk of HF death (10%) and of nonfatal HF hospitalization regardless of a previous history of coronary artery disease or myocardial infarction. The beneficial effect of statin therapy on the *development* of HF was also observed in the CORONA trial, which demonstrated how rosuvastatin reduces the risk of HF hospitalization.[35] These findings are consistent with the WOSCOPS study results, showing that a 5-year statin therapy reduces by 35% the 20-year risk of hospitalization for HF.[37]

In conclusion, statin therapy reduces HF risk through mechanisms that are partly independent of the prevention of acute myocardial infarction.

Other Lipid-Lowering Agents

Reduction of LDL-C levels can be achieved through the use of other drugs, alone or in association with statins, with a resulting additional decrease in those CV events potentially responsible for the development of HF.

Ezetimibe lowers LDL-C levels by inhibiting the intestinal uptake of cholesterol, stimulating an upregulation of LDL-receptor (LDLR) expression in the liver and thus an increased clearance of LDL particles. Many RCTs (SEAS, SHARP, IMPROVE-IT) confirmed the beneficial role of Ezetimibe in CV events reduction when associated with a statin.[38–40]

PCSK9 inhibitors are a new class of lipid-lowering drugs that targets a protein (PCSK9) involved in the downregulation of LDLR. As demonstrated by the FOURIER and the ODYSSEY-OUTCOMES trials, the average LDL-C reduction is approximately 50% with both evolocumab and alirocumab, resulting in a 15% to 20% reduction in CV events in the context of primary prevention.[41,42]

DIABETES MELLITUS

Patients with diabetes are known to be at high risk for CV events, such as coronary artery disease, stroke, and CV death, and, particularly, they have a 2-fold increased risk for men and 4-fold risk for women of developing HF.[43] There is also evidence that impaired fasting glucose levels and insulin resistance are linked to increased risk of HF.[44] As stated, the better strategy to reduce HF progression (from stage A to worse stages) is to strongly treat risk factors, including diabetes.

Risk stratification of diabetic patients is strongly recommended by ESC guidelines.[45] Every patient should be screened for organ damage because those with cardiac organ damage should be reclassified in stage B HF.

Patients with diabetes with target organ damage or more than 2 CV risk factors are considered at very high risk for CV events; those with long-standing (>10 years) diabetes without organ damage are at high risk, whereas young patients (type 2 DM <50 years) are at moderate risk.[46] As a consequence, in diabetic patients, clinicians must adopt more intensive preventive interventions to reach a stricter target of LDL-C and BP. In diabetic patients, BP has been broadly investigated. A recent meta-analysis showed that reaching a systolic blood pressure (SBP) of 130 to 140 mm Hg reduces CV death, all-cause mortality, and incidence of HF (−13%); a stronger reduction less than SBP 130 mm Hg resulted in a little reduction only for stroke.[47] These observations have been implemented in the most updated ESC guidelines on hypertension, which recommend 130 to 140 mm Hg as a first target in diabetics and to decrease to less than 130 mm Hg only if tolerated.[10]

The drugs of choice in these patients are renin-angiotensin-aldosterone system inhibitors because of their beneficial renal effects. In fact, compared with beta-blockers, angiotensin-converting-enzyme inhibitor (ACE-I) and angiotensin receptor blocker (ARB) reduced not only albuminuria and CV mortality but also HF.[48] Recent glucose-lowering drugs, such as sodium-glucose transport protein 2 (SGLT2) -inhibitors and glucagon-like peptide-1 receptor agonists (GLP1-Ras), have shown a slight, but significant, BP decrease; this should be considered.

A good marker to evaluate glycemic control is certainly hemoglobin A1c (HbA1c), but its relationship with CV outcomes is still controversial. In a meta-analysis of 3 major controlled randomized trials, lowering HbA1c by 1% results only in a small reduction of nonfatal myocardial infarction, and no positive effects were recorded regarding HF. Again, clinical trials testing more intensive glucose control have not demonstrated a benefit in HF reduction.[49] On the other hand, reducing HbA1c levels is linked to a decrease in microvascular complication. Guidelines recommend HbA1c less than 7% as a good target but stress that this goal must be individualized for each patient with much attention to hypoglycemia episodes.

In diabetic patients at high/very-high risk, guidelines suggest considering the use of low-dose aspirin to reduce CV events, but effects on HF were not recorded. It is important to underline that in patients with and without diabetes, chronic kidney disease (CKD) is considered an additional important risk factor for HF and CV death. A moderate level of CKD (estimated glomerular filtration rate [eGFR] <60 mL/min), even in the absence of diabetes and hypertension at baseline, is associated with a higher risk of developing HF and CVD death in men.[50]

As mentioned above, the only classes of medication that have been shown to slow the decline in kidney function are ACE-I and ARB.

In recent studies (DECLARE-TIMI and EMPA-REG), SGLT-2 inhibitors showed a lower progression of CKD compared with placebo. Furthermore, in DECLARE-TIMI patients with type 2 DM and established CVD (secondary prevention) but also patients considered at high risk of CVD (primary prevention, stage A HF) were admitted.[51] In a recent study (DAPA-CKD), dapagliflozin was demonstrated to slow progression of renal disease only in patients with established HF.[52] Considering these results, SGLT-2 inhibitors are now new standard-of-care drugs in HFrEF, but their role in patients with CKD (and high risk of HF) should be a new research field.

HYPERTENSION

Elevated levels of diastolic BP and especially SBP are major risk factors for the development of HF.[8] Recent meta-analysis suggests that lowering SBP by 10 mm Hg and diastolic BP by 5 mm Hg results in a reduction of main adverse cardiovascular events (MACE) of 20%, death from any cause by 10% to 15%, ictus by 35%, and HF by 40%.[53] The HF risk associated with hypertension may be accentuated by its confounding effect on ischemic heart disease, but hypertension seems to independently contribute to cardiac dysfunction through increased afterload, proatherogenic effect on vessels, and endothelial disfunction.

Most recent ESC guidelines on arterial hypertension recommend starting pharmacologic treatment in patients with grade 2 to 3 hypertension. A more challenging choice is in patient with grade 1 hypertension; guidelines suggest introducing pharmacologic treatment only if patient is at high CV risk, whereas if the patient is at low to moderate CV risk, guidelines suggest starting with lifestyle intervention alone. Patients with high-normal BP are in a particular class; in this situation, guidelines suggests beginning drug treatment only in the presence of CVDs (stage B HF), and no pharmacologic intervention should be done in stage A HF.[10]

Regarding BP targets in patients with stage A HF, guidelines suggest reaching SBP less than 140 mm Hg; SBP less than 130 mm Hg is an option in younger patients who tolerate treatment, but this reduces only the rate of stroke. It is important to consider that in primary prevention a goal of less than 120/70 mm Hg is associated with a major incidence of CV events and CV death.[54]

ACE-I and ARB are first-line drugs for hypertension; these 2 classes of drugs have demonstrated their efficacy and safety in reducing HF development and in determining regression of hypertension-induced organ damage (HMOD), particularly left ventricle hypertrophy (thus preventing the progression to HF stage B) and left ventricle remodeling. As a consequence of inverse remodeling, ACE-I and ARB lead also to a decrease in the incidence of new-onset atrial fibrillation.[53]

Calcium-channel blocking agents have demonstrated a consistent effect on BP levels, on HMOD, and on MACE, but unlike ACE-I/ARB, they show no reduction in HF incidence.[55] Last, beta-blockers, first-line drugs in the treatment of HFrEF, have demonstrated a favorable effect on BP levels but ARE less effective than ACE-I, ARB in reducing incidence of HMOD and left ventricle remodeling; this class of drugs has no demonstrated role in patients with stage A HF.[10]

SUMMARY

In conclusion, the preventive strategies to be adopted in stage A HF patients are comparable to those for primary prevention of CVDs in subjects with CV risk factors. Therefore, the real challenge is to identify these subjects early and ensure that, despite being asymptomatic, they grasp the importance of undertaking correct lifestyles and therapeutic interventions. In this context, the clinician must pay a great amount of attention to the stratification of the asymptomatic subject's risk profile in order to set individualized therapeutic targets that prevent progression to advanced stages of HF.

CLINICS CARE POINTS

- Profile carefully your patient's global cardiovascular risk and identify if they have stage A heart failure.
- Stress the importance of a healthy lifestyle, a balanced diet, and physical activity according to the guidelines.
- Set individualized targets based on risk profile and ensure that they are achieved through behavioural interventions and also through an ad-hoc pharmacological therapy.

REFERENCES

1. Yancy CW, Jessup M, Bozkurt B, et al. 2017 ACC/AHA/HFSA focused update of the 2013 ACCF/AHA Guideline for the management of heart failure. J Am Coll Cardiol 2017. https://doi.org/10.1016/j.jacc.2017.04.025.
2. Ponikowski P, Voors AA, Anker SD, et al. 2016 ESC Guidelines for the diagnosis and treatment of acute and chronic heart failure: the Task Force for the diagnosis and treatment of acute and chronic heart failure of the European Society of Cardiology (ESC). Developed with the special contribution. Eur J Heart Fail 2016. https://doi.org/10.1002/ejhf.592.
3. Maggioni AP, Dahlström U, Filippatos G, et al. EURObservational Research Programme: Regional differences and 1-year follow-up results of the Heart Failure Pilot Survey (ESC-HF Pilot). Eur J Heart Fail 2013. https://doi.org/10.1093/eurjhf/hft050.
4. Ziaeian B, Fonarow GC. Epidemiology and aetiology of heart failure. Nat Rev Cardiol 2016. https://doi.org/10.1038/nrcardio.2016.25.
5. Wang TJ, Evans JC, Benjamin EJ, et al. Natural history of asymptomatic left ventricular systolic dysfunction in the community. Circulation 2003. https://doi.org/10.1161/01.CIR.0000085166.44904.79.
6. Tanaka H. Future perspectives for management of stage a heart failure. J Atheroscler Thromb 2018. https://doi.org/10.5551/jat.RV17021.
7. Ammar KA, Jacobsen SJ, Mahoney DW, et al. Prevalence and prognostic significance of heart failure stages: application of the American College of Cardiology/American Heart Association Heart Failure Staging Criteria in the community. Circulation 2007. https://doi.org/10.1161/CIRCULATIONAHA.106.666818.
8. Sorrentino MJ. The evolution from hypertension to heart failure. Heart Fail Clin 2019. https://doi.org/10.1016/j.hfc.2019.06.005.
9. Bozkurt B, Aguilar D, Deswal A, et al. Contributory risk and management of comorbidities of hypertension, obesity, diabetes mellitus, hyperlipidemia, and metabolic syndrome in chronic heart failure: a scientific statement from the American Heart Association. Circulation 2016. https://doi.org/10.1161/CIR.0000000000000450.
10. Williams B, Mancia G, Spiering W, et al. 2018 ESC/ESH Guidelines for the management of arterial hypertension. Eur Heart J 2018. https://doi.org/10.1093/eurheartj/ehy339.
11. Kostis JB, Davis BR, Cutler J, et al. Prevention of heart failure by antihypertensive drug treatment in older persons with isolated systolic hypertension. J Am Med Assoc 1997. https://doi.org/10.1001/jama.278.3.212.
12. Staessen JA, Fagard R, Thijs L, et al. Randomised double-blind comparison of placebo and active treatment for older patients with isolated systolic hypertension. Lancet 1997. https://doi.org/10.1016/S0140-6736(97)05381-6.
13. Dunlay SM, Givertz MM, Aguilar D, et al. Type 2 diabetes mellitus and heart failure: a scientific statement from the American Heart Association and the Heart Failure Society of America. Circulation 2019. https://doi.org/10.1161/CIR.0000000000000691.
14. Aguilar D, Solomon SD, Koøber L, et al. Newly diagnosed and previously known diabetes mellitus and 1-year outcomes of acute myocardial infarction: the Valsartan in Acute Myocardial infarction (VALIANT) trial. Circulation 2004. https://doi.org/10.1161/01.CIR.0000142047.28024.F2.
15. Kenchaiah S, Evans JC, Levy D, et al. Obesity and the risk of heart failure. N Engl J Med 2002;347(5):305–13.
16. Hu G, Jousilahti P, Antikainen R, et al. Joint effects of physical activity, body mass index, waist circumference, and waist-to-hip ratio on the risk of heart failure. Circulation 2010. https://doi.org/10.1161/CIRCULATIONAHA.109.887893.
17. Oreopoulos A, Padwal R, Kalantar-Zadeh K, et al. Body mass index and mortality in heart failure: a meta-analysis. Am Heart J 2008. https://doi.org/10.1016/j.ahj.2008.02.014.
18. Horwich TB, Hamilton MA, MacLellan WR, et al. Low serum total cholesterol is associated with marked increase in mortality in advanced heart failure. J Card Fail 2002. https://doi.org/10.1054/jcaf.2002.0804216.
19. Pekkanen J, Linn S, Heiss G, et al. Ten-year mortality from cardiovascular disease in relation to cholesterol level among men with and without preexisting cardiovascular disease. N Engl J Med 1990. https://doi.org/10.1056/nejm199006143222403.
20. Ingelsson E, Ärnlöv J, Lind L, et al. Metabolic syndrome and risk for heart failure in middle-aged men. Heart 2006. https://doi.org/10.1136/hrt.2006.089011.
21. Zamorano JL, Lancellotti P, Rodriguez Muñoz D, et al. 2016 ESC Position Paper on cancer treatments and cardiovascular toxicity developed under the auspices of the ESC Committee for Practice Guidelines. Eur Heart J 2016;37(36):2768–801.
22. Sahle BW, Owen AJ, Chin KL, et al. Risk prediction models for incident heart failure: a systematic review of methodology and model performance. J Card Fail 2017. https://doi.org/10.1016/j.cardfail.2017.03.005.
23. Nambi V, Liu X, Chambless LE, et al. Troponin T and N-terminal pro-B-type natriuretic peptide: a biomarker approach to predict heart failure risk-the atherosclerosis risk in communities study. Clin Chem 2013. https://doi.org/10.1373/clinchem.2013.203638.
24. Schnabel RB, Rienstra M, Sullivan LM, et al. Risk assessment for incident heart failure in individuals with atrial fibrillation. Eur J Heart Fail 2013. https://doi.org/10.1093/eurjhf/hft041.

25. Ledwidge M, Gallagher J, Conlon C, et al. Natriuretic peptide-based screening and collaborative care for heart failure: the STOP-HF randomized trial. JAMA 2013. https://doi.org/10.1001/jama.2013.7588.
26. Eckel RH, Jakicic JM, Ard JD, et al. 2013 AHA/ACC Guideline on lifestyle management to reduce cardiovascular risk. Circulation 2014. https://doi.org/10.1161/01.cir.0000437740.48606.d1.
27. Mach F, Baigent C, Catapano AL, et al. 2019 ESC/EAS guidelines for the management of dyslipidaemias: lipid modification to reduce cardiovascular risk. Atherosclerosis 2019. https://doi.org/10.1016/j.atherosclerosis.2019.08.014.
28. Estruch R, Ros E, Salas-Salvadó J, et al. Primary prevention of cardiovascular disease with a Mediterranean diet supplemented with extra-virgin olive oil or nuts. N Engl J Med 2018. https://doi.org/10.1056/nejmoa1800389.
29. Mozaffarian D. Natural trans fat, dairy fat, partially hydrogenated oils, and cardiometabolic health: the Ludwigshafen Risk and Cardiovascular Health Study. Eur Heart J 2016. https://doi.org/10.1093/eurheartj/ehv595.
30. Pelliccia A, Sharma S, Gati S, et al. 2020 ESC Guidelines on sports cardiology and exercise in patients with cardiovascular disease. Eur Heart J 2020. https://doi.org/10.1093/eurheartj/ehaa605.
31. Hackshaw A, Morris JK, Boniface S, et al. Low cigarette consumption and risk of coronary heart disease and stroke: meta-analysis of 141 cohort studies in 55 study reports. BMJ 2018. https://doi.org/10.1136/bmj.j5855.
32. Ference BA, Ginsberg HN, Graham I, et al. Low-density lipoproteins cause atherosclerotic cardiovascular disease. 1. Evidence from genetic, epidemiologic, and clinical studies. A consensus statement from the European Atherosclerosis Society Consensus Panel. Eur Heart J 2017. https://doi.org/10.1093/eurheartj/ehx144.
33. Martin JH, Krum H. Statins and clinical outcomes in heart failure. Clin Sci 2007. https://doi.org/10.1042/CS20070031.
34. Horwich TB, Fonarow GC, Hamilton MA, et al. The relationship between obesity and mortality in patients with heart failure. J Am Coll Cardiol 2001. https://doi.org/10.1016/S0735-1097(01)01448-6.
35. Rogers JK, Jhund PS, Perez AC, et al. Effect of rosuvastatin on repeat heart failure hospitalizations: The CORONA trial (controlled rosuvastatin multinational trial in heart failure). JACC Heart Fail 2014. https://doi.org/10.1016/j.jchf.2013.12.007.
36. Khush KK, Waters DD, Bittner V, et al. Effect of high-dose atorvastatin on hospitalizations for heart failure: subgroup analysis of the Treating to New Targets (TNT) study. Circulation 2007. https://doi.org/10.1161/CIRCULATIONAHA.106.625574.
37. Isles C. West of Scotland Coronary Prevention Study: identification of high-risk groups and comparison with other cardiovascular intervention trials. Lancet 1996. https://doi.org/10.1016/S0140-6736(96)04292-4.
38. Farmer JA. Intensive lipid lowering with simvastatin and ezetimibe in aortic stenosis (the SEAS trial). Curr Atheroscler Rep 2009;11(2):82–3.
39. Baigent C, Landray MJ, Reith C, et al. The effects of lowering LDL cholesterol with simvastatin plus ezetimibe in patients with chronic kidney disease (Study of Heart and Renal Protection): a randomised placebo-controlled trial. Lancet 2011. https://doi.org/10.1016/S0140-6736(11)60739-3.
40. Cannon CP, Blazing MA, Giugliano RP, et al. Ezetimibe added to statin therapy after acute coronary syndromes. N Engl J Med 2015. https://doi.org/10.1056/nejmoa1410489.
41. Sabatine MS, Giugliano RP, Keech AC, et al. Evolocumab and clinical outcomes in patients with cardiovascular disease. N Engl J Med 2017. https://doi.org/10.1056/nejmoa1615664.
42. Schwartz GG, Steg PG, Szarek M, et al. Alirocumab and cardiovascular outcomes after acute coronary syndrome. N Engl J Med 2018. https://doi.org/10.1056/nejmoa1801174.
43. Kannel WB, McGee DL. Diabetes and cardiovascular disease: the Framingham Study. JAMA 1979. https://doi.org/10.1001/jama.1979.03290450033020.
44. Matsushita K, Blecker S, Pazin-Filho A, et al. The association of hemoglobin A1c with incident heart failure among people without diabetes: the atherosclerosis risk in communities study. Diabetes 2010. https://doi.org/10.2337/db10-0165.
45. Cosentino F, Grant PJ, Aboyans V, et al. 2019 ESC Guidelines on diabetes, pre-diabetes, and cardiovascular diseases developed in collaboration with the EASD. Eur Heart J 2020. https://doi.org/10.1093/eurheartj/ehz486.
46. Piepoli MF, Hoes AW, Agewall S, et al. 2016 European Guidelines on cardiovascular disease prevention in clinical practice. Eur Heart J 2016;37(29):2315–81.
47. Emdin CA, Rahimi K, Neal B, et al. Blood pressure lowering in type 2 diabetes: a systematic review and meta-analysis. JAMA 2015. https://doi.org/10.1001/jama.2014.18574.
48. Lindholm LH, Ibsen H, Dahlöf B, et al. Cardiovascular morbidity and mortality in patients with diabetes in the Losartan Intervention For Endpoint reduction in hypertension study (LIFE): a randomised trial against atenolol. Lancet 2002. https://doi.org/10.1016/S0140-6736(02)08090-X.
49. Turnbull FM, Abraira C, Anderson RJ, et al. Intensive glucose control and macrovascular outcomes in type 2 diabetes. Diabetologia 2009. https://doi.org/10.1007/s00125-009-1470-0.

50. Dhingra R, Gaziano JM, Djoussé L. Chronic kidney disease and the risk of heart failure in men. Circ Hear Fail 2011. https://doi.org/10.1161/CIRCHEARTFAILURE.109.899070.
51. Wiviott SD, Raz I, Bonaca MP, et al. Dapagliflozin and cardiovascular outcomes in type 2 diabetes. N Engl J Med 2019. https://doi.org/10.1056/nejmoa1812389.
52. Wheeler DC, Stefansson BV, Batiushin M, et al. The dapagliflozin and prevention of adverse outcomes in chronic kidney disease (DAPA-CKD) trial: baseline characteristics. Nephrol Dial Transplant 2020. https://doi.org/10.1093/ndt/gfaa234.
53. Thomopoulos C, Parati G, Zanchetti A. Effects of blood-pressure-lowering treatment in hypertension: 9. Discontinuations for adverse events attributed to different classes of antihypertensive drugs: meta-analyses of randomized trials. J Hypertens 2016. https://doi.org/10.1097/HJH.0000000000001052.
54. Böhm M, Schumacher H, Teo KK, et al. Achieved blood pressure and cardiovascular outcomes in high-risk patients: results from ONTARGET and TRANSCEND trials. Lancet 2017. https://doi.org/10.1016/S0140-6736(17)30754-7.
55. Turnbull F, Neal B, Algert C, et al. Effects of different blood-pressure-lowering regimens on major cardiovascular events: results of prospectively-designed overviews of randomised trials. Lancet 2003. https://doi.org/10.1016/S0140-6736(03)14739-3.

Asymptomatic Left Ventricular Dysfunction

Is There a Role for Screening in General Population?

Salvatore La Carrubba, MD, PhD[a], Roberta Manganaro, MD, PhD[b], Concetta Zito, MD, PhD[b], Gianluca Di Bella, MD, PhD[b], Maria Ludovica Carerj, MD[c], Luca Longobardo, MD[d], Maurizio Cusmà Piccione, MD, PhD[b], Antonio Micari, MD, PhD[c], Scipione Carerj, MD[b,*]

KEYWORDS

• Asymptomatic left ventricular dysfunction • Echocardiography • General population

KEY POINTS

- Asymptomatic left ventricular dysfunction represents an early stage of HF that should be promptly recognized to prevent overt heart failure development.
- Echocardiography is the technique of choice for screening in the general population.
- New technologies, such as myocardial strain and myocardial work, could help in early detecting of subclinical myocardial dysfunction.

INTRODUCTION

Left ventricular (LV) dysfunction is a progressive disorder, characterized by the development of cardiac remodeling, which usually precedes the development of symptoms, continues after their appearance, and contributes to their worsening, leading to overt heart failure (HF).[1]

According to the American College of Cardiology/American Heart Association HF classification, stage A and B include asymptomatic patients at high risk of HF, without and with structural cardiac disease, respectively.[2] It was shown that LV dysfunction is present also in asymptomatic patients. These silent abnormalities may lead over time to symptomatic LV dysfunction, and the progression of the disease is positively affected by early treatment.[3–5]

Therefore, it has been proposed that asymptomatic LV dysfunction should be treated as an early stage of a chronic HF continuum. For this reason, there is a great interest in identifying asymptomatic patients to prevent overt HF development and thus cardiovascular (CV) morbidity and mortality.

Echocardiography plays a pivotal role in the assessment of cardiac structure and function, being a noninvasive, low-cost, available, feasible, and reliable tool, compared with other imaging techniques. Many studies have been performed with the aim to demonstrate the utility of echocardiographic screening in the general population in patients with or without CV risk factors.

[a] Villa Sofia Hospital, Palermo, Italy; [b] Department of Clinical and Experimental Medicine – Cardiology Unit, AOU Policlinico G. Martino, University of Messina, Messina, Italy; [c] Department of Biomedical and Dental Sciences and of Morphological and Functional Images, AOU Polclinico G. Martino, University of Messina, Messina, Italy; [d] Department of Clinical and Experimental Medicine, AOU Policlinico G. Martino, University of Messina, Messina, Italy

* Corresponding author. Department of Clinical and Experimental Medicine, Section of Cardiology, University of Messina, Via Consolare Valeria n.12, Messina 98100, Italy.

E-mail addresses: scipione2@interfree.it; scarerj@unime.it

Heart Failure Clin 17 (2021) 179–186
https://doi.org/10.1016/j.hfc.2020.12.001

CONVENTIONAL ECHOCARDIOGRAPHY IN ASYMPTOMATIC LEFT VENTRICULAR DYSFUNCTION

Redfield and colleagues[6] investigated, in the general population, LV systolic and diastolic function by means of traditional parameters, namely ejection fraction (EF) and Doppler-derived indices of diastolic function. They demonstrated that systolic and diastolic dysfunction were frequently present in individuals without recognized HF.[6] The prevalence of any systolic dysfunction (EF ≤50%) was 6.0% with moderate or severe systolic dysfunction (EF ≤40%) being present in 2.0%; multivariate analysis showed that, after controlling for age, sex, and EF, mild diastolic dysfunction and moderate or severe diastolic dysfunction were predictive of all-cause mortality.[6]

Another cross-sectional study demonstrated that preclinical functional or structural myocardial abnormalities could be detected by echocardiography in asymptomatic subjects with two or more CV risk factors and without electrocardiogram abnormalities (stage A of HF classification). In this study, the presence or absence of LV systolic or diastolic dysfunction had an incremental value to CV risk factors in predicting the evolution toward more severe HF stage C and the occurrence of CV events.[7]

However, patients in stage B are ideal targets for HF prevention. These individuals with prevalent CV diseases but without symptomatic HF include most patients whose hearts are undergoing progressive maladaptive cardiac remodeling, which leads to HF.

In asymptomatic patients, different pathologic conditions can determinate molecular, cellular, and interstitial changes, responsible for structural alterations of the heart, defined as "cardiac remodeling."[8] The diagnosis of cardiac remodeling is based on the detection of morphologic changes, changes in the LV cavity diameter, mass, geometry, areas of scar after myocardial infarction, fibrosis, and inflammatory infiltrate (eg, in myocarditis).[9] Patients with asymptomatic HF (stage B) are characterized by maladaptive LV remodeling.[8,10] Thus, conventional echocardiographic evaluation should not rely only on assessment of systolic and diastolic function, but should focus also on morphologic and structural findings. Classic four-group classification of remodeling considers only LV mass index and relative wall thickness as variables. Complex remodeling classification includes also LV end-diastolic volume index.[10]

In a population of asymptomatic hypertensive patients, cardiac remodeling was found to be an independent predictor of composite end point (total mortality, myocardial infarction, myocardial revascularizations, cerebrovascular events, and acute pulmonary edema), confirming the role of echocardiography in prognostic stratification of patients in stage B.[11]

TISSUE DOPPLER IMAGING

The significant role of echocardiography has been confirmed also by introduction of new techniques. Tissue Doppler imaging (TDI) is a technique using the Doppler principle to measure the velocity of myocardial segments and other cardiac structures. Pulsed TDI is a simple and useful method of assessing LV longitudinal function, which depends on subendocardial fibers. It is known that the subendocardium is more vulnerable to cardiac injury, thus longitudinal function is affected at an early stage of cardiac disease. TDI has been proposed as a useful tool to identify early cardiac functional abnormalities also in the presence of normal EF or diastolic parameters.[12] Moreover, numerous clinical studies reported that TDI mitral annular velocities had a linear positive correlation with the invasively determined LV diastolic pressures in different cardiac diseases.[13–18]

Di Salvo and colleagues[19] evaluated the ability of TDI in detecting early longitudinal LV dysfunction in asymptomatic subjects with LVEF greater than 55%, normal diastolic function, and its relationship with CV risk factors. In this study, TDI allowed to identify early longitudinal LV systolic abnormalities in the presence of apparently normal systolic and diastolic function and it progressively impaired with increasing CV risk factors. These findings could be clinically relevant in identifying asymptomatic subjects who need an early tailored preventive treatment.[19]

Moreover, the same authors demonstrated a significant additional prognostic value of reduced TDI peak systolic velocity compared with the simple presence of coexisting CV risk factors, in asymptomatic subjects.[20]

MYOCARDIAL STRAIN AND MYOCARDIAL WORK

Myocardial strain has emerged in the last decades as a reliable tool for studying myocardial deformation, adding information on cardiac performance when compared with EF.[21–24] Early detection of subclinical LV dysfunction using strain plays a crucial role in the evaluation of many cardiac diseases.[21–28]

Longitudinal, circumferential, and radial strain have been reported to detect LV dysfunction before a decline in LVEF. Myocardial strain is studied using different techniques, including Doppler strain imaging and two-dimensional and three-dimensional speckle-tracking echocardiography.[29,30] Doppler strain imaging was the first method used; however, it has several limitations, including angle dependency, noise interference, and high intraobserver and interobserver variability. Speckle-tracking echocardiography was developed as an alternative technique that analyzes motion by tracking natural acoustic reflections and interference patterns within an ultrasonic window. It seems to be highly reproducible and minimally affected by intraobserver and interobserver variability. Longitudinal LV mechanics, predominantly governed by the subendocardial fibers, are the most vulnerable component of LV mechanics and therefore most sensitive to the presence of myocardial disease. The midmyocardial and epicardial function may remain preserved initially, and therefore circumferential strain and twist may remain normal or show exaggerated compensation for preserving LV systolic performance.[30] Global longitudinal strain (GLS) has been shown to be more reproducible and more useful clinically than circumferential and radial strains.

Beyond its application in identifying LV subclinical dysfunction in known CV disease, GLS seems reduced despite preserved LVEF in several CV risk conditions, such as advancing age,[31] hypertension,[32] diabetes,[33] stable angina,[34] renal dysfunction,[35] and obesity.[36]

LV hypertrophy is a setting in which EF may fail in detection of LV systolic dysfunction, because LV hypertrophy and volume changes allow depressed systolic function to be underestimated if relying only on EF. There has been a growing interest about the role of GLS in the assessment of LV systolic function in hypertensive patients. Several studies have shown a significant reduction of GLS[37,38] and, interestingly, also shown was the presence of regional alterations of longitudinal strain with normal GLS in the first stages of hypertension.[32] Thus, GLS could be a useful tool in predicting CV morbidity and mortality in the general population.[39,40] Recently, impaired LV function as detected by GLS in the general population was shown to be a significant predictor of incident acute myocardial infarction, HF, or CV disease, independent of clinical and other echocardiographic predictors.[41] In addition GLS provided incremental prognostic value in predicting the composite CV outcome and incident HF alone beyond the Framingham Risk score, the SCORE risk chart, and the modified American College of Cardiology/American Heart Association Pooled Cohort Equation. The authors found that GLS was not as predictive of CV morbidity and mortality in women as in men, but it was a stronger predictor of all outcomes in men.

A growing interest in detection of cardiotoxicity secondary to anticancer treatment has emerged in the last years. Even if the definition of cancer-related cardiac dysfunction relies on EF estimation,[26,27] this parameter does not allow to identify subclinical LV dysfunction. Early identification of myocardial damage is of paramount importance in these patients to prevent the development of overt HF and guarantee to patients the best anticancer treatment. Several studies investigated GLS in patients with cancer and confirmed the value of deformation imaging for early detection of LV dysfunction secondary to cancer therapy.[42–44] Other studies showed that GLS reduction in patients treated with anthracyclines anticipates changes in LVEF, providing fundamental information for an early risk stratification of these subjects.[45,46] For these reasons, guidelines incorporate GLS in the algorithm for detection of cardiotoxicity.[26,27] Accordingly, a relative percentage reduction in GLS of greater than 15% from baseline should be considered abnormal and a marker of early LV subclinical dysfunction in patients treated by chemotherapy. However, at this time, a reduction in GLS is not indicated as a key parameter for therapy discontinuation because of the lack of randomized trials demonstrating that the GLS-oriented strategy is superior to an EF-oriented strategy.

Myocardial strain was investigated also in stage B HF, such as asymptomatic patients with heart valve disease. It is known that, in these patients, indication to surgery relies on EF; however, EF usually declines in an advanced stage of the disease. Several studies investigated GLS in heart valve disease and a reduced GLS was found to be associated with aortic regurgitation and mitral regurgitation progression.[47–49] Moreover, low values of GLS predicted HF occurrence[50,51] and impaired outcomes after surgery.[47,51] Accordingly, the use of GLS for a more accurate evaluation of LV function in asymptomatic patients, particularly those with mitral regurgitation, has been suggested,[52] even if longitudinal strain analysis for risk stratification of these patients has not been included in the guidelines for the management of heart valve disease.[53] The most robust findings with regard to the usefulness of GLS have been obtained in patients with aortic stenosis. GLS gradually decreases while aortic stenosis severity increases without any simultaneous change in LVEF[54] and in asymptomatic patients, impaired GLS was associated with an increased risk of cardiac events over traditional risk markers, including EF and aortic stenosis gradient.[55–57]

In the last few years, myocardial work (MW) by pressure-strain loops analysis developed as an interesting tool to study LV performance, allowing to overcome the limits of GLS secondary to its load-dependency (**Fig. 1**).[58] This new tool was investigated in several CV diseases, particularly ischemic cardiomyopathy and patients with cardiac resynchronization therapy,[59–61] and reference normal ranges were recently provided by the NORRE study.[62] Moreover, the NORRE study showed the absence of a strong dependence of MW indices on age, gender, and body mass index, whereas a good correlation with traditional two-dimensional echocardiography parameters of myocardial systolic function and myocardial strain was found.[62,63]

Chan and colleagues[64] investigated MW in hypertensive patients. They found significantly increased global myocardial and constructive work in patients with systolic blood pressure (SBP) greater than 160 mm Hg, but not in those with SBP between 140 and 159 mm Hg. Global wasted work gradually increased from control subjects, throughout patients with SBP between 140 and 159 mm Hg, to those with SBP greater than 160 mm Hg, whereas global myocardial efficiency decreased in the same direction.[64] More recently, it was shown that LV MW and mechanics were significantly deteriorated in hypertensive patients with and without diabetes.[65] Diabetes additionally affected MW in hypertensive patients. The same study revealed that blood pressure and hemoglobin A_{1c} were associated with MW independently of age, sex, body mass index, and LV function and hypertrophy.[65] MW was investigated also in a population of patients with chronic kidney disease and allowed to detect impairment of LV systolic function at an early stage.[66]

Thus, MW could have clinical implications also in patients with early stage of disease when LV is not significantly remodeled (hypertension, diabetes, and chemotherapy-induced cardiotoxicity) and potentially in patients with HF with preserved EF. The main advantage of MW is the implementation of blood pressure in its calculation, allowing to overcome the afterload-dependence of LV longitudinal strain.

NATRIURETIC PEPTIDES

Natriuretic peptides are known biomarkers for diagnosis and guidance of the management of HF. Moreover, they could play a role for the screening of asymptomatic patients, to detect subclinical LV dysfunction. It was demonstrated that natriuretic peptides improve prediction of incident HF and atrial fibrillation in the general population in addition to conventional risk factors.[67] More recently, very low levels of N-terminal pro–B-type natriuretic peptide were shown to be predictive of new-onset HF in middle-aged men from the general population.[68] Therefore, the use of biomarkers in addition to clinical variables could allow the identification of individuals who might benefit

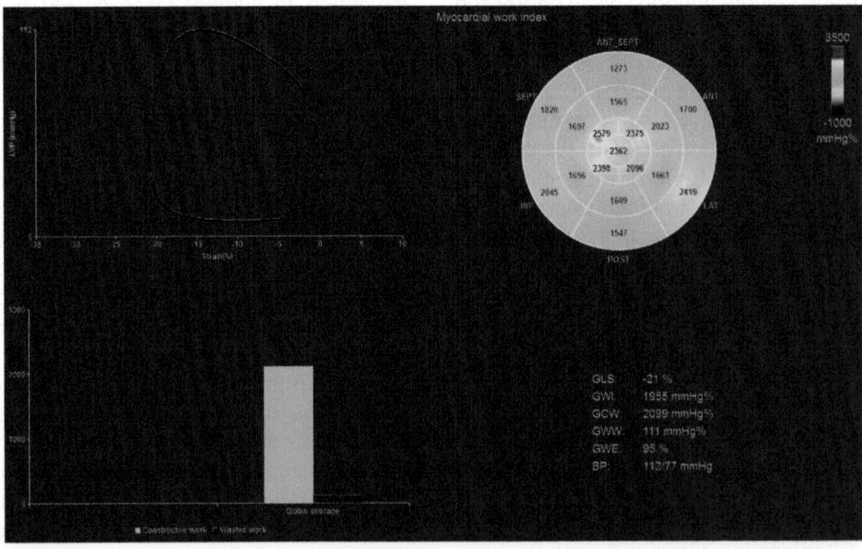

Fig. 1. Myocardial work by pressure-strain loop analysis. LV pressure-strain loop (*top left*), bull's eye of GWI (*top right*), bar graph representing GCW and GWW (*bottom left*), and results from myocardial work analysis (*bottom right*). BP, blood pressure; GCW, global constructive work; GWE, global work efficiency; GWI, global work index; GWW, global work waste; LVP, left ventricular pressure.

from early echocardiography in a broader screening for asymptomatic heart dysfunction.

SUMMARY

Asymptomatic LV dysfunction represents an early stage of HF continuum that should be promptly recognized. For this purpose, echocardiography is the ideal imaging technique to be used for screening of general population. Particularly, the development of new echocardiographic technologies, such as myocardial strain and MW, could allow detection of subclinical LV dysfunction at an early stage. Natriuretic peptides could allow in identifying patients at risk who could benefit from early echocardiography.

CLINICS CARE POINTS

- Asymptomatic left ventricular dysfunction should be considered as an early stage of chronic heart failure.
- Screening of the general population, particularly patients with cardiovascular risk factors, could help in early detection of subclinical left ventricle dysfunction.
- Echocardiography, conventional and advanced, is the technique of choice for screening of the general population.
- Myocardial strain is a recognized tool for assessment of subclinical left ventricle dysfunction. Myocardial work is emerging as a promising technique that allows to overcome the load-dependency of myocardial strain; however, further studies are needed.

DISCLOSURE

The authors have nothing to disclose.

REFERENCES

1. McKee PA, Castelli WP, McNamara PM, et al. The natural history of congestive heart failure: the Framingham study. N Engl J Med 1971;285:1441–6.
2. Hunt SA, Abraham WT, Chin MH, et al. ACC/AHA 2005 guideline update for the diagnosis and management of chronic heart failure in the adult: a report of the American College of Cardiology/American Heart Association task force on practice guidelines (writing committee to update the 2001 guidelines for the evaluation and management of heart failure): developed in collaboration with the American College of Chest Physicians and the International Society for Heart and Lung Transplantation: endorsed by the Heart Rhythm Society. Circulation 2005;112:e154–235.
3. Aronow WS, Ahn C, Kronzon I. Effect of beta blockers alone, of angiotensin-converting enzyme inhibitors alone, and of beta blockers plus angiotensin-converting enzyme inhibitors on new coronary events and on congestive heart failure in older persons with healed myocardial infarcts and asymptomatic left ventricular systolic dysfunction. Am J Cardiol 2001;88(11):1298–300.
4. Investigators SOLVD, Yusuf S, Pitt B, et al. Effect of enalapril on mortality and the development of heart failure in asymptomatic patients with reduced left ventricular ejection fractions. N Engl J Med 1992; 327(10):685–91.
5. Dargie HJ. Effect of carvedilol on outcome after myocardial infarction in patients with left-ventricular dysfunction: the CAPRICORN randomised trial. Lancet 2001;357(9266):1385–90.
6. Redfield MM, Jacobsen SJ, Burnett JC, et al. Burden of systolic and diastolic ventricular dysfunction in the community. JAMA 2003;289:194–202.
7. Carerj S, La Carrubba S, Antonini-Canterin F, et al. Research group of the Italian Society of Cardiovascular Echography (SIEC). The incremental prognostic value of echocardiography in asymptomatic stage a heart failure. J Am Soc Echocardiogr 2010;23(10):1025–34.
8. Cohn JN, Ferrari R, Sharpe N. Cardiac remodeling-concepts and clinical implications: a consensus paper from an international forum on cardiac remodeling. Behalf of an International Forum on Cardiac Remodeling. J Am Coll Cardiol 2000;35(3):569–82.
9. Anand IS, Florea VG, Solomon SD, et al. Noninvasive assessment of left ventricular remodeling: concepts, techniques and implications for clinical trials. J Card Fail 2002;8(6):S452–64.
10. Pugliese NR, Fabiani I, La Carrubba S, et al, Italian Society of Cardiovascular Echography (SIEC). Classification and prognostic evaluation of left ventricular remodeling in patients with asymptomatic heart failure. Am J Cardiol 2017;119(1):71–7.
11. Fabiani I, Pugliese NR, La Carrubba S, et al, Italian Society of Cardiovascular Echography (SIEC). Incremental prognostic value of a complex left ventricular remodeling classification in asymptomatic for heart failure hypertensive patients. J Am Soc Hypertens 2017;11(7):412–9.
12. Yu CM, Sanderson JE, Marwick TH, et al. Tissue Doppler imaging: a new prognosticator for cardiovascular diseases. J Am Coll Cardiol 2007;49: 1903–14.
13. Dokainish H, Zoghbi WA, Lakkis NM, et al. Optimal noninvasive assessment of left ventricular filling pressures: a comparison of tissue Doppler echocardiography and B-type natriuretic peptide in patients

with pulmonary artery catheters. Circulation 2004; 25:2432–9.
14. Nagueh SF, Middleton KJ, Kopelen HA, et al. Doppler tissue imaging: a noninvasive technique for evaluation of left ventricular relaxation and estimation of filling pressures. J Am Coll Cardiol 1997; 30:1527–33.
15. Ommen S, Nishimura RA, Appleton CP, et al. Clinical utility of Doppler echocardiography and tissue Doppler imaging in the estimation of left ventricular filling pressures: a comparative simultaneous Doppler-catheterization study. Circulation 2000; 102:1788–94.
16. Nagueh SF, Lakkis NM, Midleton KJ, et al. Doppler estimation of left ventricular filling pressures in patients with hypertrophic cardiomyopathy. Circulation 1999;99:254–61.
17. Kim YJ, Sohn DW. Mitral annulus velocity in the estimation of left ventricular filling pressure: prospective study in 200 patients. J Am Soc Echocardiogr 2000; 13:980–5.
18. Arques S, Roux E, Sbragia P, et al. Accuracy of tissue Doppler echocardiography in the emergency diagnosis of decompensated heart failure with preserved left ventricular systolic function. Comparison with B-type natriuretic peptide measurement. Echocardiography 2005;22:657–64.
19. Di Salvo G, Di Bello V, Salustri A, et al. Research group of the Italian Society of Cardiovascular Echography (SIEC). Early left ventricular longitudinal systolic dysfunction and cardiovascular risk factors in 1,371 asymptomatic subjects with normal ejection fraction: a tissue Doppler study. Echocardiography 2011;28(3):268–75.
20. Di Salvo G, Di Bello V, Salustri A, et al, Research Group of the Italian Society of Cardiovascular Echography. The prognostic value of early left ventricular longitudinal systolic dysfunction in asymptomatic subjects with cardiovascular risk factors. Clin Cardiol 2011;34(8):500–6.
21. Stanton T, Leano R, Marwick TH. Prediction of all-cause mortality from global longitudinal speckle strain: comparison with ejection fraction and wall motion scoring. Circ Cardiovasc Imaging 2009;2: 356–64.
22. Ersboll M, Valeur N, Mogensen UM, et al. Prediction of all-cause mortality and heart failure admissions from global left ventricular longitudinal strain in patients with acute myocardial infarction and preserved left ventricular ejection fraction. J Am Coll Cardiol 2013;61:2365–73.
23. Haugaa KH, Grenne BL, Eek CH, et al. Strain echocardiography improves risk prediction of ventricular arrhythmias after myocardial infarction. JACC Cardiovasc Imaging 2013;6:841–50.
24. Zito C, Longobardo L, Citro R, et al. Ten years of 2D longitudinal strain for early myocardial dysfunction detection: a clinical overview. Biomed Res Int 2018;2018:8979407.
25. Thavendiranathan P, Poulin F, Lim KD, et al. Use of myocardial strain imaging by echocardiography for the early detection of cardiotoxicity in patients during and after cancer chemotherapy: a systematic review. J Am Coll Cardiol 2014;63:2751–68.
26. Zamorano JL, Lancellotti P, Rodriguez Mu~noz D, et al. 2016 ESC Position Paper on cancer treatments and cardiovascular toxicity developed under the auspices of the ESC Committee for Practice Guidelines: the task force for cancer treatments and cardiovascular toxicity of the European Society of Cardiology (ESC). Eur Heart J 2016;37:2768–801.
27. Plana JC, Galderisi M, Barac A, et al. Expert consensus for multimodality imaging evaluation of adult patients during and after cancer therapy: a report from the American Society of Echocardiography and the European Association of Cardiovascular Imaging. Eur Heart J Cardiovasc Imaging 2014; 15:1063–93.
28. Zito C, Manganaro R, Khandheria B, et al. Usefulness of left atrial reservoir size and left ventricular untwisting rate for predicting outcome in primary mitral regurgitation. Am J Cardiol 2015;116(8): 1237–44.
29. Mor-Avi V, Lang RM, Badano LP, et al. Current and evolving echocardiographic techniques for the quantitative evaluation of cardiac mechanics: ASE/EAE consensus statement on methodology and indications endorsed by the Japanese Society of Echocardiography. J Am Soc Echocardiogr 2011;24(3): 277–313.
30. Geyer H, Caracciolo G, Abe H, et al. Assessment of myocardial mechanics using speckle tracking echocardiography: fundamentals and clinical applications. J Am Soc Echocardiogr 2010;23(4):351–69.
31. Kuznetsova T, Herbots L, Richart T, et al. Left ventricular strain and strain rate in a general population. Eur Heart J 2008;29:2014–23.
32. Narayanan A, Aurigemma GP, Chinali M, et al. Cardiac mechanics in mild hypertensive heart disease: a speckle-strain imaging study. Circ Cardiovasc Imaging 2009;2:382–90.
33. Jensen MT, Sogaard P, Andersen HU, et al. Global longitudinal strain is not impaired in type 1 diabetes patients without albuminuria. JACC Cardiovasc Imaging 2015;8:400–10.
34. Biering-Sørensen T, Hoffmann S, Mogelvang R, et al. Myocardial strain analysis by 2-dimensional speckle tracking echocardiography improves diagnostics of coronary artery stenosis in stable angina pectoris. Circ Cardiovasc Imaging 2014;7:58–65.
35. Nasir K, Rosen BD, Kramer HJ, et al. Regional left ventricular function in individuals with mild to moderate renal insufficiency: the multi-ethnic study of atherosclerosis. Am Heart J 2007;153:545–51.

36. Wong CY, O'Moore-Sullivan T, Leano R, et al. Alterations of left ventricular myocardial characteristics associated with obesity. Circulation 2004;110: 3081–7.
37. Afonso L, Kondur A, Simegn M, et al. Two-dimensional strain profiles in patients with physiological and pathological hypertrophy and preserved left ventricular systolic function: a comparative analyses. BMJ Open 2012;2(4):e001390.
38. Imbalzano E, Zito C, Carerj S, et al. Left ventricular function in hypertension: new insight by speckle tracking echocardiography. Echocardiography 2011;28(6):649–57.
39. Russo C, Jin Z, Elkind MSV, et al. Prevalence and prognostic value of subclinical left ventricular systolic dysfunction by global longitudinal strain in a community-based cohort. Eur J Heart Fail 2014;16: 1301–9.
40. Cheng S, McCabe EL, Larson MG, et al. Distinct aspects of left ventricular mechanical function are differentially associated with cardiovascular outcomes and all-cause mortality in the community. J Am Heart Assoc 2015;4:e002071.
41. Biering-Sørensen T, Biering-Sørensen SR, Olsen FJ, et al. Global longitudinal strain by echocardiography predicts long-term risk of cardiovascular morbidity and mortality in a low-risk general population: the Copenhagen City Heart Study. Circ Cardiovasc Imaging 2017;10(3):e005521.
42. Jurcut R, Wildiers H, Ganame J, et al. Strain rate imaging detects early cardiac effects of pegylated liposomal doxorubicin as adjuvant therapy in elderly patients with breast cancer. J Am Soc Echocardiogr 2008;21(12):1283–9.
43. Sawaya H, Sebag IA, Plana JC, et al. Assessment of echocardiography and biomarkers for the extended prediction of cardiotoxicity in patients treated with anthracyclines, taxanes, and trastuzumab. Circ Cardiovasc Imaging 2012;5(5):596–603.
44. Voigt J-U, Pedrizzetti G, Lysyansky P, et al. Definitions for a common standard for 2D speckle tracking echocardiography: consensus document of the EACVI/ASE/industry task force to standardize deformation imaging. J Am Soc Echocardiogr 2015;28(2): 183–93.
45. Poterucha JT, Kutty S, Lindquist RK, et al. Changes in left ventricular longitudinal strain with anthracycline chemotherapy in adolescents precede subsequent decreased left ventricular ejection fraction. J Am Soc Echocardiogr 2012;25(7):733–40.
46. Charbonnel C, Convers-Domart R, Rigaudeau S, et al. Assessment of global longitudinal strain at low-dose anthracycline-based chemotherapy, for the prediction of subsequent cardiotoxicity. Eur Heart J Cardiovasc Imaging 2017;18(4):392–401.
47. Olsen NT, Sogaard P, Larsson HBW, et al. Speckle-tracking echocardiography for predicting outcome in chronic aortic regurgitation during conservative management and after surgery. JACC Cardiovasc Imaging 2011;4(3):223–30.
48. Lancellotti P, Cosyns B, Zacharakis D, et al. Importance of left ventricular longitudinal function and functional reserve in patients with degenerative mitral regurgitation: assessment by two-dimensional speckle tracking. J Am Soc Echocardiogr 2008;21(12):1331–6.
49. Di Salvo G, Rea A, Mormile A, et al. Usefulness of bidimensional strain imaging for predicting outcome in asymptomatic patients aged ≤ 16 years with isolated moderate to severe aortic regurgitation. Am J Cardiol 2012;110(7):1051–5.
50. Smedsrud MK, Pettersen E, Gjesdal O, et al. Detection of left ventricular dysfunction by global longitudinal systolic strain in patients with chronic aortic regurgitation. J Am Soc Echocardiogr 2011;24(11): 1253–9.
51. Zito C, Carerj S, Todaro MC, et al. Myocardial deformation and rotational profiles in mitral valve prolapse. Am J Cardiol 2013;112(7):984–90.
52. Witkowski TG, Thomas JD, Debonnaire PJMR. Global longitudinal strain predicts left ventricular dysfunction after mitral valve repair. Eur Heart J Cardiovasc Imaging 2013;14(1):69–76.
53. Lancellotti P, Moura L, Pierard LA, et al. European Association of Echocardiography recommendations for the assessment of valvular regurgitation. Part 2: mitral and tricuspid regurgitation (native valve disease). Eur Heart J Cardiovasc Imaging 2010;11(4):307–32.
54. Miyazaki S, Daimon M, Miyazaki T, et al. Global longitudinal strain in relation to the severity of aortic stenosis: a two dimensional speckle-tracking study. Echocardiography 2011;28(7):703–8.
55. Kearney LG, Lu K, Ord M, et al. Global longitudinal strain is a strong independent predictor of all-cause mortality in patients with aortic stenosis. Eur Heart J Cardiovasc Imaging 2012;13(10):827–33.
56. Dahl JS, Videbæk L, Poulsen MK, et al. Global strain in severe aortic valve stenosis relation to clinical outcome after aortic valve replacement. Circ Cardiovasc Imaging 2012;5(5):613–20.
57. Zito C, Salvia J, Cusm-Piccione M, et al. Prognostic significance of valvuloarterial impedance and left ventricular longitudinal function in asymptomatic severe aortic stenosis involving three-cuspid valves. Am J Cardiol 2011;108(10):1463–9.
58. Russell K, Eriksen M, Aaberge L, et al. A novel clinical method for quantification of regional left ventricular pressure-strain loop area: a non-invasive index of myocardial work. Eur Heart J 2012;33(6):724–33.
59. Boe E, Russell K, Eek C, et al. Non-invasive myocardial work index identifies acute coronary occlusion in patients with non-ST-segment elevation-acute coronary syndrome. Eur Heart J Cardiovasc Imaging 2015;16(11):1247–55.

60. Galli E, Leclercq C, Hubert A, et al. Role of myocardial constructive work in the identification of responders to CRT. Eur Heart J Cardiovasc Imaging 2018;19(9):1010–8.

61. Galli E, Leclercq C, Fournet M, et al. Value of myocardial work estimation in the prediction of response to cardiac resynchronization therapy. J Am Soc Echocardiogr 2018;31(2):220–30.

62. Manganaro R, Marchetta S, Dulgheru R, et al. Echocardiographic reference ranges for normal non-invasive myocardial work indices: results from the EACVI NORRE study. Eur Heart J Cardiovasc Imaging 2019;20(5):582–90.

63. Manganaro R, Marchetta S, Dulgheru R, et al. Correlation between non-invasive myocardial work indices and main parameters of systolic and diastolic function: results from the EACVI NORRE study. Eur Heart J Cardiovasc Imaging 2020;21(5):533–41.

64. Chan J, Edwards NFA, Khandheria BK, et al. A new approach to assess myocardial work by non-invasive left ventricular pressure-strain relations in hypertension and dilated cardiomyopathy. Eur Heart J Cardiovasc Imaging 2019;20(1):31–9.

65. Tadic M, Cuspidi C, Pencic B, et al. Myocardial work in hypertensive patients with and without diabetes: an echocardiographic study. J Clin Hypertens (Greenwich) 2020. https://doi.org/10.1111/jch.14053.

66. Ke QQ, Xu HB, Bai J, et al. Evaluation of global and regional left ventricular myocardial work by echocardiography in patients with chronic kidney disease. Echocardiography 2020. https://doi.org/10.1111/echo.14864.

67. Smith JG, Newton-Cheh C, Almgren P, et al. Assessment of conventional cardiovascular risk factors and multiple biomarkers for the prediction of incident heart failure and atrial fibrillation. J Am Coll Cardiol 2010;56(21):1712–9.

68. Ergatoudes C, Thunström E, Hansson PO, et al. Natriuretic and inflammatory biomarkers as risk predictors of heart failure in middle-aged men from the general population: a 21-year follow-up. J Card Fail 2018;24(9):594–600.

Prevention of Coronary Artery Disease–Related Heart Failure: The Role of Computed Tomography Scan

Michele Fusaro, MD[a,*], Giovanni Tessarin, MD[b]

KEYWORDS

• Coronary artery disease • Heart failure • Coronary CT angiography

KEY POINTS

- CCTA is a robust technique for non-invasive detection of both coronary artery calcium and coronary artery disease.
- CCTA has the highest diagnostic accuracy compared to other non-invasive techniques for diagnosing coronary heart disease.
- Fractional flow reserve CT (FFR-CT) and CT perfusion (CTP) are two promising techniques that could significantly increase the diagnostic accuracy and specificity of CCTA in clinical practice.

INTRODUCTION

Heart failure (HF) can be defined as a syndrome caused by any functional or physical damage that impairs ventricular filling or ejection of the blood. This syndrome is characterized by a variety of signs and symptoms including breathlessness, fatigue, low tolerance for physical activity, and ankle swelling, peripheral edema, pulmonary crackles, and splanchnic congestion, linked to fluid retention.[1,2]

Even if HF is defined only when symptoms are apparent, patients may experience asymptomatic left ventricle (LV) function reduction that, if promptly detected and managed, can decrease mortality rate.[1]

The estimated prevalence of HF is 1% to 3% in the global adult population, increasing to 5% to 9% for patients aged 65 years and older.[3] Given the increasing burden of HF on the health system, Australian guidelines have suggested the need to redesign the system of care to reduce hospitalization for these patients. This goal could be achieved through the improvement of collaborative care between the general practitioner, HF nurse, and specialist physician.[4]

In 2002, the Framingham Heart Study stated the importance of both hypertension and myocardial infarction (MI) as risk factors for the development of HF.[5] Other investigators further stressed the prevalence role of coronary artery disease (CAD) in the development of HF, present in up to 50% in patients with HF, in Europe and North America and even in patients with HF with a preserved ejection fraction.[6,7] Moreover CAD also leads to higher morbidity and mortality.[8]

Coronary computed tomography angiography (CCTA) is a rapidly evolving technique. Currently, 64-detector computed tomography (CT) is considered the minimal standard to perform a diagnostic cardiac CT angiography. However different CT vendors produce CT scanners with wide detectors up to 320 slices or dual -source CT scanner, both able to significantly increase time resolution.[9] Two major concerns over the wide use of CCTA are the radiation dose and the contrast medium dosage. Recent developments enable CCTA to be performed with a low radiation dose, approximately 2 to 3 mSv. Some investigators have also suggested that the introduction of reduced tube current voltage to 100

The study was approved by our Institutional Review Board and written informed consent was obtained from all patients.

[a] Department of Radiology, Santa Maria di Ca' Foncello Hospital, Treviso, Italy; [b] Department of Medicine-DIMED, Institute of Radiology, University of Padova, Via Giustiniani 1 - 35128 Padua, Italy
* Corresponding author.
E-mail address: fusaro341@gmail.com

Heart Failure Clin 17 (2021) 187–194
https://doi.org/10.1016/j.hfc.2021.01.005

kVp will further reduce both the radiation dose to patients and the contrast medium dosage required.[10,11] Finally new reconstruction algorithms such iterative reconstruction, have proved useful to further lower the radiation dose up to 50%, without affecting diagnostic accuracy.[12,13]

CORONARY EVALUATION

Calcium Score and Coronary Plaque

Calcium score

An important aspect in coronary evaluation is coronary calcium, assessed with a nonenhanced heart CT scan and defined as a coronary lesion with a density value of more than 130 HU.[14] The most used score to quantify coronary calcium is the Agatston score, first proposed by Agatston and colleagues[15] in 1990.

Over the years, coronary artery calcium (CAC) has emerged as robust technique and a strong predictor tool for cardiovascular disease risk assessment.[14,16–18] It is also well known that the risk of cardiovascular events increases linearly with the CAC score.[19]

In 2009, Sarwar and colleagues[20] investigated the prognostic value of the absence of CAC over a cohort of 85,000 patients. The investigators discovered that the absence of CAC was linked to a very low risk of cardiovascular events. Other studies addressed this issue, coming to similar conclusions.[21,22]

Over the years, large-scale trials have addressed the prognostic value of CAC, such as the St. Francis Heart study, the MESA study, the Heinz Nixdorf Recall Study, the Rotterdam study, and the Dallas Heart Study. All these large trials concluded that calcium score, more accurately than risk factors alone,[18,23–26] is a strong predictor of cardiovascular events. The largest was the MESA study of 6722 adults from 4 ethnic or racial groups aged between 45 and 84 years. New eventual cardiovascular events were recorded for a median of 3.9 years. The investigators found out that a doubling in calcium score increased the risk of major events and coronary events by approximately 25% during a median follow-up of 3.8 years.[18]

Another study focused on prognostic values of CAC in young adults aged between 32 and 46 years old; the investigators concluded that the presence of CAC, including an Agatston score of less than 20, in these patients is associated with an increased risk of fatal and nonfatal coronary heart disease during 12.5 years of follow-up.[27]

The Rotterdam study also investigated the association between CAC and the development of HF. The investigators found that patients with an Agatston score above 400 were more than 4 times more likely to develop HF.[28] Similar results from the Heinz Nixdorf Recall Study showed significantly increased levels of CAC in patients with chronic HF compared with patients without chronic HF, independent from other cardiovascular risk factors.[29] Moreover, Sakuragi and colleagues[30] evaluated the association between CAC and HF, concluding that severe CAC is a predictor of HF in a population with no history of CAD. Finally CAC progression has proved to be an independent predictor of incident HF.[31]

CAC measurement also can be used to exclude CAD as a cause of HF in symptomatic patients, in order to distinguish ischemic from nonischemic cause of HF.[32,33]

Coronary plaque

CCTA has proved to be a solid technique that allows a noninvasive study of coronary arteries, to rapidly and safely assess or rule out CAD in patients with low to intermediate cardiovascular risk.[34,35]

With the use of CCTA, the quantification of coronary arterial stenosis may be performed in different ways. The most used is the estimation of the luminal diameter stenosis, followed by area stenosis, minimum lumen diameter, and minimum lumen area.[36] The Society of Cardiovascular Computed Tomography Guidelines for the interpretation of CCTA (2014), suggest a stenosis grading scale to evaluate coronary artery. A coronary is considered normal if any plaque or stenosis is absent, minimally stenotic if the stenosis is less than 25% of the coronary lumen, mildly stenotic (25% to 49%), moderately stenotic (50% to 69%), severely stenotic (70% to 99%), or occluded.[37]

One of the most important aspects of CCTA is the ability to directly visualize the plaque causing stenosis. The ICONIC study, a recent multicentric case-control study, aimed to analyze atherosclerotic plaque features, such as absolute quantity (volume, thickness, area) and relative burden as possible sentries of future acute coronary syndromes (ACSs). The investigators concluded that stenosis grading alone is an unreliable predictor of future ACS, with only 12.8% of patients having a stenosis greater than 70% before ACS. They also found out that a fibrofatty composition and the presence of a necrotic core were both significant predictor of futures ACS. Finally the investigators demonstrated that high-risk plaques (defined as plaque possessing ≥2 among positive remodeling, low attenuating plaque, spotty calcifications) are associated with ACS.[38]

ACCURACY AND PROGNOSTIC VALUE

A recent meta-analysis of 65 studies and a total of 5332 patients, evaluated negative predictive value (NPV), positive predictive value (PPV), sensitivity, and specificity of CCTA. Considering a pretest probability of 7% CCTA had a PPV of 50.9% and an NPV 97.8%, that became respectively 82.7% and 85% with a pretest probability of 67%. When removing to the count the nondiagnostic examinations PPV and NPV were, respectively, of 68% and 98.3% with a pretest probability of 7% and 88.9% and 91.5% with a pretest probability of 67%. Overall sensitivity was found to be 95.2% with a specificity of 79.2%.[39] Furthermore, the EVINCI study, conducted on more than 475 patients, compared the diagnostic accuracy of CCTA, single-photon emission CT (SPECT), PET, echocardiography, and cardiac magnetic resonance in diagnosing CAD, using invasive coronary angiography as reference. The investigators found that CCTA had the highest diagnostic accuracy over the other noninvasive techniques.[40]

Prognostic value of CCTA was evaluated by the SCOT-HEART study, performed on 4146 patients with stable chest pain, randomly assigned to standard of care plus CCTA or standard of care alone. The study showed that, after a 5-year follow-up, the former group had a significantly lower rate of death from CAD or nonfatal MI compared with the standard-of-care group (2.3% vs 3.9%, respectively).[41] Accordingly, a metanalysis on 4 randomized trials compared clinical outcomes after the evaluations of patients with stable chest pain with CCTA versus with usual care. The investigators determined that relative risk in the incidence of MI reduced 31% in patients evaluated with CCTA.[42]

In the PARADIGM study, conducted on 1255 patients, CCTA was able to effectively evaluate statin impact on coronary artery plaque progression. The investigators, with the help of serial CCTA, determined that a statin intake is linked to a reduction in high-risk plaque features and with a slower progression of atherosclerosis volume.[43]

IMAGE HF is an on-going randomized controlled trial to compare an invasive coronary angiography based protocol and a CCTA-based protocol for the management of patients with HF. The investigators hypothesize that CTA protocol will result in cost and resource utilization reductions, with similar composite clinical events, reduced number of unnecessary ICA, and a lower rate of procedure-related complications.[44] When published, this study will help in defining the role of CCTA for patients with HF.

Advanced Techniques

Computed tomography–fractional flow reserve

Fractional flow reserve is the current invasive preferred technique for the evaluation of flow-limiting coronary stenosis that could require revascularization treatment. However, current advances allow the measurement of fractional flow reserve (FFR) via CT. FFR-CT is a noninvasive technique that uses post processing to derive FFR from a standard CCTA, without the need for additional contrast medium nor an increase of the radiation dose.[45] This process could be performed using a traditional approach based in computational fluid dynamics (CFD) and a more recent technique relying on machine learning (ML).[46]

Three multicentric studies proved the increased diagnostic accuracy reached with CT-FFR, compared with CCTA alone, using invasive coronary angiography as reference. The first multicentric prospective study was the DISCOVER-FLOW study, in 2011 in which FFR-CT showed greater accuracy (84.3% vs 58.5%), similar sensitivity (87.9% vs 91.4%), and higher specificity (82.2% vs 39.6%) than CCTA, on a per-vessel analysis. The study also showed a good correlation between FFR-CT values and FFR values.[47] The DE FACTO study, similarly demonstrated higher accuracy, sensitivity, and specificity with FFR-CT than CT alone on a per-patient analysis; however, it failed to reach its primary objective of 70% or greater accuracy.[48] Finally in the NXT trial, greater attention was paid to CTA acquisition and the investigators were able to reach a higher level of accuracy (81%) and of specificity (86%), compared with CCTA alone (53% and 34%, respectively), keeping similar levels of sensitivity (86% for FFR-CT and 94% for CCTA).[49]

The 2 current methods to evaluate CT-FFR, CFD, and ML were compared in a multicentric study by Coenen and colleagues[50] on 352 patients. The investigators found excellent correlation between CFD and ML CT-FFR, with a Pearson coefficient of 0.997, and a moderate correlation between ML CT-FFR and invasive FFR. Both ML and CFD reached a higher area under the curve (AUC) than visual classification of stenosis on CTA.[50]

A recent systematic review and metanalysis on 16 studies evaluated the diagnostic performances of FFR-CT to identify hemodynamically significant stenosis, using invasive FFR as reference. The pooled sensitivity and specificity on a per-patient level were found to be respectively of 89% and 71%. Although sensitivity value was similar to CCTA (93%), specificity value was significantly higher for the FFR-CT, both on per-patient (71% vs 32%, $P < .001$) and per-vessel levels (82% vs 46%, $P < .001$).[51]

A comparison between the performance of FFR-CT, CCTA, SPECT, and PET for the diagnosis of cardiac ischemia, was performed by a PACIFC trial substudy. The study was designed on 208 patients who all underwent noninvasive study and ICA with FFR within 2 weeks. The AUC was found to be higher for CCTA + FFR-CT combined than CCTA alone, SPECT, and PET, on a per-vessel analysis. Only PET was found to outperform CCTA + FFR-CT on a per-patient analysis.[52]

In the ADVANCE registry, the investigators evaluated the real-world clinical impact of adding FFR-CT to CCTA alone. In their multicentric prospective study on 5083 patients, enrolled at 38 sites all over the world, the investigators found that FFR-CT induce a modification of the clinical management in up to two-third of patients, when compared with a management based on CCTA alone.[53] After a 1-year follow-up, patients with FFR-CT values >0.80 also showed significantly lower rates of cardiovascular deaths and MI than patients with FFR-CT values ≤0.80.[54]

Recently an NXT substudy was published after approximately 5 years of follow-up. The purpose of this study was to evaluate the prognostic value of noninvasive FFR-CT derived from CCTA. The investigators found that patients with an FFR-CT value of greater than 0.80 had a lower incidence of primary composite endpoint of death from any cause, nonfatal MI, and any revascularization. Moreover, patients with FFR-CT of 0.80 or lower had an increased incidence of major adverse cardiac events; no cardiac deaths or MI occurred in patients with FFR-CT greater than 0.80.[55]

The PLATFORM study evaluated the impact of an FFR-CT guided strategy compared with the standard of care for the management of patients with suspected CAD. It emerged that patients of the FFR-CT arm had a lower rate of ICA with nonobstructive CAD than the standard of care; results also showed a decrease in 90-day medical costs for the patients in the FFR-CT strategy.[56,57] A 1-year follow-up also showed that costs of care for remain lower the FFR-CT arm compared with standard of care.[58]

Computed tomography perfusion imaging

One of the new frontiers of cardiac CT imaging is the potential to combine the anatomic information provided by CCTA with functional evaluation of the myocardial perfusion, to evaluate ischemia or infarction. The 2 main techniques to assess myocardial perfusion via CT are static and dynamic, both at rest and at pharmacologic-induced stress.[59] Static acquisition provides qualitative or semi-quantitative information about myocardial perfusion, at single time point. Dynamic CT perfusion, instead, is the only way to directly quantify myocardial perfusion, acquiring multiple scans over time, assessing the changes in contrast medium concentration.[60]

CORE320 was a large study of 381 patients, aimed to evaluate the performance of a CCTA/CTP strategy to evaluate or rule out hemodynamically significant coronary artery stenosis, using ICA and SPECT as reference. The investigators found out that a combined approach of CCTA and static CTP can identify more than 50% of coronary artery stenosis defined by ICA and SPECT, with an accuracy of 0.93.[61]

Multiple meta analyses evaluated diagnostic performances of CTP with sensitivity and specificity values ranging from 75% to 89% and 78% to 95%, respectively.[62–64] CTP also showed that when added to CCTA, diagnostic specificity significantly improved, maintaining high levels of sensitivity.[64]

Computed tomography myocardial perfusion and computed tomography–fractional flow reserve

The integration of both these advanced functional techniques was investigated by Coenen and colleagues[65] in 2017 in a 2-center study on 74 patients. The investigators were able to demonstrate that the combination of CTP and CT-FFR significantly increased the AUC to 0.85 when compared with the CTP (P = .01) and CT-FFR (P = .03). More recently, Pontone and colleagues[66] in a study on 85 patients similarly demonstrated that a strategy based on CCTA + FFR-CT + CTP has the highest AUC (0.919) and diagnostic accuracy (87%) when compared with strategies based on CCTA or CCTA + FFR-CT or CCTA + CTP. These studies seem to answer to the need for clarification of the role of these 2 techniques, that increasingly appear as allies rather than rivals, suggesting also the importance of tailored diagnostic protocols for different patients.[67]

Left ventricular function and volume assessment

The evaluation and assessment of LV volume and function is one of the main aspects of evaluating patients with HF. Both echocardiography and MRI are widely used techniques for this evaluation, with the latter being considered the gold standard for LV function and volume assessment.[68]

Several studies compared CCTA performances in the assessment of LV function end volumes, to MRI and echocardiography, showing good correlation between these different techniques.[69–72] Recently, some investigators have proved the feasibility of LV strain assessment, with good correlation with transthoracic echocardiography values.[73,74] Dykun and colleagues[75] in 2015 also proved that LV size quantification, performed with nonenhanced cardiac CT, is associated with some cardiovascular risk factors such as body size and hypertension.

However CCTA is often found to overestimate end-diastolic and end-systolic volumes. For this reason, and to avoid unnecessary exposition to ionizing radiation, most investigators suggest the use of CCTA for LV volume and function assessment, only to selected patients, especially those with poor echocardiography compliance and contraindications to MRI.[68–71].

GUIDELINES

European Society of Cardiology (ESC) 2019 guidelines recommend CCTA as a first-line diagnostic examination in symptomatic patients if CAD cannot be confidently ruled out. Moreover, ESC stated that if CCTA showed signs of CAD, functional imaging should be performed (recommendation class I). Coronary CT angiography should be considered as an alternative to invasive coronary angiography if a functional test failed to provide unequivocal information.[76]

The National Institute for Health and Care Excellence published their 2016 guidelines for the management of patients with chest pain of suspected cardiac origin. The major change to the previous 2010 version is the suggestion of the use of 64 slices CCTA (or more), as first-line diagnostic test, in the case of patients suffering of typical or atypical angina or not suffering from anginal chest pain but with electrocardiographic changes suggesting MI.[77] It is also worthwhile noting, as highlighted by Alfakih and colleagues[78] and Carrabba and colleagues[79] in their reviews that coronary calcium score of zero is no longer considered a criterion to rule out CAD.[78,79]

The Society of Cardiovascular Computed Tomography, in their consensus statement of 2017 suggested CAC testing for all asymptomatic patients aged between 40 and 75 years in the 5% to 20% 10-year risk of CAD group and selectively for those in the less than 5% risk group. Moreover, it may be recommended to repeat CAC testing every 5 years for patients with a calcium score of 0 and every 3 to 5 in patients with a calcium score of more than 0.[80]

DISCLOSURE

The authors declare that they have no conflict of interest.

REFERENCE

1. Ponikowski P, Voors AA, Anker SD, et al. 2016 ESC guidelines for the diagnosis and treatment of acute and chronic heart failure. Eur Heart J 2016;37(27): 2129–2200m.
2. Yancy CW, Jessup M, Bozkurt B, et al. 2013 ACCF/AHA guideline for the management of heart failure: executive summary: a report of the American College of Cardiology Foundation/American Heart Association task force on practice guidelines. J Am Coll Cardiol 2013;62(16):1495–539.
3. Van Riet EES, Hoes AW, Wagenaar KP, et al. Epidemiology of heart failure: the prevalence of heart failure and ventricular dysfunction in older adults over time. A systematic review. Eur J Heart Fail 2016; 242–52. https://doi.org/10.1002/ejhf.483.
4. Atherton JJ, Sindone A, De Pasquale CG, et al. National Heart Foundation of Australia and Cardiac Society of Australia and New Zealand: guidelines for the prevention, detection, and management of heart failure in Australia 2018. Heart Lung Circ 2018;1123–208. https://doi.org/10.1016/j.hlc.2018.06.1042.
5. Lloyd-Jones DM, Larson MG, Leip EP, et al. Lifetime risk for developing congestive heart failure: the Framingham heart study. Circulation 2002;106(24): 3068–72.
6. Khatibzadeh S, Farzadfar F, Oliver J, et al. Worldwide risk factors for heart failure: a systematic review and pooled analysis. Int J Cardiol 2013;168(2):1186–94.
7. Hwang S-J, Melenovsky V, Borlaug BA. Implications of coronary artery disease in heart failure with preserved ejection fraction. J Am Coll Cardiol 2014; 63(25):2817–27.
8. Velagaleti RS, Vasan RS. Heart failure in the twenty-first century: is it a coronary artery disease or hypertension problem? Cardiol Clin 2007;25(4):487–95.
9. Maffei E, Seitun S, Guaricci AI, Cademartiri F. Chest pain: coronary CT in the ER. Br J Radiol 2016; 89(1061):20150954.
10. Lee JW, Kim CW, Lee HC, et al. High-definition computed tomography for coronary artery stents: image quality and radiation doses for low voltage (100 kVp) and standard voltage (120 kVp) ECG-triggered scanning. Int J Cardiovasc Imaging 2015;31(1):39–49.
11. Mihl C, Kok M, Wildberger JE, et al. Contrast media injection protocols in CT coronary angiography. Totowa (NJ): Humana; 2019. p. 109–15.
12. Yin WH, Lu B, Li N, et al. Iterative reconstruction to preserve image quality and diagnostic accuracy at reduced radiation dose in coronary CT angiography: an intraindividual comparison. JACC Cardiovasc Imaging 2013;6(12):1239–49.
13. Stocker TJ, Deseive S, Leipsic J, et al. Reduction in radiation exposure in cardiovascular computed tomography imaging: results from the PROspective multicenter registry on radiaTion dose Estimates of cardiac CTanglOgraphy iN daily practice in 2017 (PROTECTION VI). Eur Heart J 2018. https://doi.org/10.1093/eurheartj/ehy552.
14. Hecht HS. Coronary artery calcium scanning: past, present, and future. JACC Cardiovasc Imaging 2015;8(5):579–96.

15. Agatston AS, Janowitz WR, Hildner FJ, et al. Quantification of coronary artery calcium using ultrafast computed tomography. J Am Coll Cardiol 1990; 15(4):827–32.
16. Hecht HS, Cronin P, Blaha MJ, et al. 2016 SCCT/STR guidelines for coronary artery calcium scoring of noncontrast noncardiac chest CT scans: a report of the Society of Cardiovascular Computed Tomography and Society of Thoracic Radiology. J Cardiovasc Comput Tomogr 2017;11(1):74–84.
17. Polonsky TS, McClelland RL, Jorgensen NW, et al. Coronary artery calcium score and risk classification for coronary heart disease prediction. JAMA 2010; 303(16):1610–6.
18. Detrano R, Guerci AD, Carr JJ, et al. Coronary calcium as a predictor of coronary events in four racial or ethnic groups. N Engl J Med 2008;358(13): 1336–45.
19. Goel R, Garg P, Achenbach S, et al. Coronary artery calcification and coronary atherosclerotic disease. Cardiol Clin 2012;30(1):19–47.
20. Sarwar A, Shaw LJ, Shapiro MD, et al. Diagnostic and prognostic value of absence of coronary artery calcification. JACC Cardiovasc Imaging 2009;2(6): 675–88.
21. Wang X, Le EPV, Rajani NK, et al. A zero coronary artery calcium score in patients with stable chest pain is associated with a good prognosis, despite risk of non-calcified plaques. Open Heart 2019; 6(1):1–6.
22. Valenti V, Ó Hartaigh B, Heo R, et al. A 15-year warranty period for asymptomatic individuals without coronary artery calcium: a prospective follow-up of 9,715 individuals. JACC Cardiovasc Imaging 2015; 8(8):900–9.
23. Arad Y, Goodman KJ, Roth M, et al. Coronary calcification, coronary disease risk factors, C-reactive protein, and atherosclerotic cardiovascular disease events: The St. Francis heart study. J Am Coll Cardiol 2005;46(1):158–65.
24. Erbel R, Mhlenkamp S, Moebus S, et al. Coronary risk stratification, discrimination, and reclassification improvement based on quantification of subclinical coronary atherosclerosis: The Heinz Nixdorf Recall study. J Am Coll Cardiol 2010;56(17):1397–406.
25. Elias-Smale SE, Proença RV, Koller MT, et al. Coronary calcium score improves classification of coronary heart disease risk in the elderly: the Rotterdam study. J Am Coll Cardiol 2010;56(17):1407–14.
26. Paixao ARM, Berry JD, Neeland IJ, et al. Coronary artery calcification and family history of myocardial infarction in the dallas heart study. JACC Cardiovasc Imaging 2014;7(7):679–86.
27. Carr JJ, Jacobs DR, Terry JG, et al. Association of coronary artery calcium in adults aged 32 to 46 years with incident coronary heart disease and death. JAMA Cardiol 2017;2(4):391–9.
28. Leening MJG, Elias-Smale SE, Kavousi M, et al. Coronary calcification and the risk of heart failure in the elderly: the Rotterdam study. JACC Cardiovasc Imaging 2012;5(9):874–80.
29. Kälsch H, Lehmann N, Möhlenkamp S, et al. Association of coronary artery calcium and congestive heart failure in the general population: results of the Heinz Nixdorf Recall Study. Clin Res Cardiol 2010;99(3):175–82.
30. Sakuragi S, Ichikawa K, Yamada K, et al. An increase in the coronary calcification score is associated with an increased risk of heart failure in patients without a history of coronary artery disease. J Cardiol 2016;67(4):358–64.
31. Bakhshi H, Ambale-Venkatesh B, Yang X, et al. Progression of coronary artery calcium and incident heart failure: the multi-ethnic study of atherosclerosis. J Am Heart Assoc 2017;6(4). https://doi.org/10.1161/JAHA.116.005253.
32. Sousa PA, Bettencourt N, Dias Ferreira N, et al. Role of cardiac multidetector computed tomography in the exclusion of ischemic etiology in heart failure patients. Rev Port Cardiol 2014;33(10):629–36.
33. Abunassar JG, Yam Y, Chen L, et al. Usefulness of the Agatston score = 0 to exclude ischemic cardiomyopathy in patients with heart failure. Am J Cardiol 2011;107(3):428–32.
34. Goldstein JA, Chinnaiyan KM, Abidov A, et al. The CT-STAT (coronary computed tomographic angiography for systematic triage of acute chest pain patients to treatment) trial. J Am Coll Cardiol 2011; 58(14):1414–22.
35. Hoffmann U, Truong Qa, Schoenfeld Da, et al. Coronary CT angiography versus standard evaluation in acute chest pain. N Engl J Med 2012;367(4):299–308.
36. Arbab-Zadeh A, Hoe J. Quantification of coronary arterial stenoses by multidetector CT angiography in comparison with conventional angiography: methods, caveats, and implications. JACC Cardiovasc Imaging 2011;4(2):191–202.
37. Leipsic J, Co-Chair F, Abbara S, et al. SCCT guidelines for the interpretation and reporting of coronary CT angiography: a report of the society of cardiovascular computed tomography guidelines committee. J Cardiovasc Comput Tomogr 2014;8:342–58.
38. Chang HJ, Lin FY, Lee SE, et al. Coronary atherosclerotic precursors of acute coronary syndromes. J Am Coll Cardiol 2018;71(22):2511–22.
39. Haase R, Schlattmann P, Gueret P, et al. Diagnosis of obstructive coronary artery disease using computed tomography angiography in patients with stable chest pain depending on clinical probability and in clinically important subgroups: meta-analysis of individual patient data. BMJ 2019;365. https://doi.org/10.1136/bmj.l1945.
40. Neglia D, Rovai D, Caselli C, et al. Detection of significant coronary artery disease by noninvasive

anatomical and functional imaging. Circ Cardiovasc Imaging 2015;8(3). https://doi.org/10.1161/CIRCIMAGING.114.002179.

41. Newby DE, Adamson PD, Berry C, et al. Coronary CT angiography and 5-year risk of myocardial infarction. N Engl J Med 2018;379(10):924–33.
42. Bittencourt MS, Hulten EA, Murthy VL, et al. Clinical outcomes after evaluation of stable chest pain by coronary computed tomographic angiography versus usual care: a meta-analysis. Circ Cardiovasc Imaging 2016;9(4):1–9.
43. Lee SE, Chang HJ, Sung JM, et al. Effects of statins on coronary atherosclerotic plaques: the PARADIGM study. JACC Cardiovasc Imaging 2018; 11(10):1475–84.
44. Chow BJW, Green RE, Coyle D, et al. Computed tomographic coronary angiography for patients with heart failure (CTA-HF): a randomized controlled trial (IMAGE HF Project 1-C). Trials 2013;14(1):1–8.
45. Khav N, Ihdayhid AR, Ko B. CT-derived fractional flow reserve (CT-FFR) in the evaluation of coronary artery disease. Heart Lung Circ 2020. https://doi.org/10.1016/j.hlc.2020.05.099.
46. Tesche C, De Cecco CN, Albrecht MH, et al. Coronary CT angiography–derived fractional flow reserve. Radiology 2017;285(1):17–33.
47. Koo BK, Erglis A, Doh JH, et al. Diagnosis of ischemia-causing coronary stenoses by noninvasive fractional flow reserve computed from coronary computed tomographic angiograms: Results from the prospective multicenter DISCOVER-FLOW (Diagnosis of Ischemia-Causing Stenoses Obtained Via Noni). J Am Coll Cardiol 2011;58(19):1989–97.
48. Min JK, Leipsic J, Pencina MJ, et al. Diagnostic accuracy of fractional flow reserve from anatomic CT angiography. JAMA 2012;308(12):1237–45.
49. Nørgaard BL, Leipsic J, Gaur S, et al. Diagnostic performance of noninvasive fractional flow reserve derived from coronary computed tomography angiography in suspected coronary artery disease: The NXT trial (analysis of coronary blood flow using CT angiography: next steps). J Am Coll Cardiol 2014; 63(12):1145–55.
50. Coenen A, Kim YH, Kruk M, et al. Diagnostic accuracy of a machine-learning approach to coronary computed tomographic angiography–Based fractional flow reserve result from the MACHINE Consortium. Circ Cardiovasc Imaging 2018;11(6). https://doi.org/10.1161/CIRCIMAGING.117.007217.
51. Zhuang B, Wang S, Zhao S, et al. Computed tomography angiography-derived fractional flow reserve (CT-FFR) for the detection of myocardial ischemia with invasive fractional flow reserve as reference: systematic review and meta-analysis. Eur Radiol 2020;30(2):712–25.
52. Driessen RS, Danad I, Stuijfzand WJ, et al. Comparison of coronary computed tomography angiography, fractional flow reserve, and perfusion imaging for ischemia diagnosis. J Am Coll Cardiol 2019;73(2):161–73.
53. Fairbairn TA, Nieman K, Akasaka T, et al. Real-world clinical utility and impact on clinical decision-making of coronary computed tomography angiography-derived fractional flow reserve: lessons from the ADVANCE Registry. Eur Heart J 2018;39(41): 3701–11.
54. Patel MR, Nørgaard BL, Fairbairn TA, et al. 1-year impact on medical practice and clinical outcomes of FFRCT: the ADVANCE registry. JACC Cardiovasc Imaging 2020;13(1):97–105.
55. Ihdayhid AR, Norgaard BL, Gaur S, et al. Prognostic value and risk continuum of noninvasive fractional flow reserve derived from coronary CT angiography. Radiology 2019;292(2):343–51.
56. Douglas PS, Pontone G, Hlatky MA, et al. Clinical outcomes of fractional flow reserve by computed tomographic angiography-guided diagnostic strategies vs. usual care in patients with suspected coronary artery disease: the prospective longitudinal trial of FFRCT: outcome and resource impacts stud. Eur Heart J 2015;36(47):3359–67.
57. Hlatky MA, De Bruyne B, Pontone G, et al. Quality-of-life and economic outcomes of assessing fractional flow reserve with computed tomography angiography: PLATFORM. J Am Coll Cardiol 2015; 66(21):2315–23.
58. Douglas PS, De Bruyne B, Pontone G, et al. 1-year outcomes of FFRCT-guided care in patients with suspected coronary disease: the PLATFORM study. J Am Coll Cardiol 2016;68(5):435–45.
59. Assen M van, Vonder M, Pelgrim GJ, et al. Computed tomography for myocardial characterization in ischemic heart disease: a state-of-the-art review. Eur Radiol Exp 2020;4(1). https://doi.org/10.1186/s41747-020-00158-1.
60. Seitun S, De Lorenzi C, Cademartiri F, et al. CT myocardial perfusion imaging: a new frontier in cardiac imaging. Biomed Res Int 2018;2018. https://doi.org/10.1155/2018/7295460.
61. Rochitte CE, George RT, Chen MY, et al. Computed tomography angiography and perfusion to assess coronary artery stenosis causing perfusion defects by single photon emission computed tomography: the CORE320 study. Eur Heart J 2014;35(17): 1120–30.
62. Pelgrim GJ, Dorrius M, Xie X, et al. The dream of a one-stop-shop: meta-analysis on myocardial perfusion CT. Eur J Radiol 2015;84(12):2411–20.
63. Takx RAP, Blomberg BA, El Aidi H, et al. Diagnostic accuracy of stress myocardial perfusion imaging compared to invasive coronary angiography with fractional flow reserve meta-analysis. Circ Cardiovasc Imaging 2015;8(1). https://doi.org/10.1161/CIRCIMAGING.114.002666.

64. Sørgaard MH, Kofoed KF, Linde JJ, et al. Diagnostic accuracy of static CT perfusion for the detection of myocardial ischemia. A systematic review and meta-analysis. J Cardiovasc Comput Tomogr 2016; 10(6):450–7.
65. Coenen A, Rossi A, Lubbers MM, et al. Integrating CT myocardial perfusion and CT-FFR in the work-up of coronary artery disease. JACC Cardiovasc Imaging 2017;10(7):760–70.
66. Pontone G, Baggiano A, Andreini D, et al. Dynamic stress computed tomography perfusion with a whole-heart coverage scanner in addition to coronary computed tomography angiography and fractional flow reserve computed tomography derived. JACC Cardiovasc Imaging 2019. https://doi.org/10.1016/j.jcmg.2019.02.015.
67. Schoepf UJ, van Assen M. FFR-CT and CT myocardial perfusion imaging: friends or foes? JACC Cardiovasc Imaging 2019;12(12):2472–4.
68. Sugeng L, Mor-Avi V, Weinert L, et al. Quantitative assessment of left ventricular size and function: side-by-side comparison of real-time three-dimensional echocardiography and computed tomography with magnetic resonance reference. Circulation 2006;114(7):654–61.
69. Butler J, Shapiro MD, Jassal D, et al. Comparison of multidetector computed tomography and two-dimensional transthoracic echocardiography for left ventricular assessment in patients with heart failure. Am J Cardiol 2007;99(2):247–9.
70. Juergens KU, Grude M, Maintz D, et al. Multi-detector row CT of left ventricular function with dedicated analysis software versus MR imaging: initial experience. Radiology 2004;230(2):403–10.
71. Maffei E, Messalli G, Martini C, et al. Left and right ventricle assessment with Cardiac CT: validation study vs. cardiac MR. Eur Radiol 2012;22(5): 1041–9.
72. Lim SJ, Choo KS, Park YH, et al. Assessment of left ventricular function and volume in patients undergoing 128-slice coronary CT angiography with ECG-based maximum tube current modulation: a comparison with echocardiography. Korean J Radiol 2011;12(2):156–62.
73. Marwan M, Ammon F, Bittner D, et al. CT-derived left ventricular global strain in aortic valve stenosis patients: a comparative analysis pre and post transcatheter aortic valve implantation. J Cardiovasc Comput Tomogr 2018;12(3):240–4.
74. Ammon F, Bittner D, Hell M, et al. CT-derived left ventricular global strain: a head-to-head comparison with speckle tracking echocardiography. Int J Cardiovasc Imaging 2019;35(9):1701–7.
75. Dykun I, Mahabadi AA, Lehmann N, et al. Left ventricle size quantification using non-contrast-enhanced cardiac computed tomography -association with cardiovascular risk factors and coronary artery calcium score in the general population: the Heinz Nixdorf recall study. Acta Radiol 2015;56(8): 933–42.
76. Knuuti J, Wijns W, Achenbach S, et al. 2019 ESC guidelines for the diagnosis and management of chronic coronary syndromes. Eur Heart J 2020; 41(3):407–77.
77. National Institute for Health and Care Excellence (NICE). Recent-onset chest pain of suspected cardiac origin: assessment and diagnosis. Clinical Guideline [CG95] 2016;(November 2016). Available at: https://www.nice.org.uk/guidance/cg95.
78. Alfakih K, Greenwood JP, Plein S. The 2016 update to NICE CG95 guideline for the investigation of new onset stable chest pain: more innovation, but at a cost? Clin Med (Lond) 2017;17(3):209–11.
79. Carrabba N, Migliorini A, Pradella S, et al. Old and new NICE guidelines for the evaluation of new onset stable chest pain: a real world perspective. Biomed Res Int 2018. https://doi.org/10.1155/2018/3762305.
80. Hecht H, Blaha MJ, Berman DS, et al. Clinical indications for coronary artery calcium scoring in asymptomatic patients: expert consensus statement from the Society of Cardiovascular Computed Tomography. J Cardiovasc Comput Tomogr 2017; 11(2):157–68.

Anemia and Management of Heart Failure Patients

Carmen C. Beladan, MD, PhD[a,b,*], Simona B. Botezatu, MD[a]

KEYWORDS

• Anemia • Iron deficiency • Heart failure • Clinical outcomes

KEY POINTS

- Anemia is a highly prevalent comorbidity in patients with heart failure. It has a complex etiology with iron deficiency and chronic inflammation playing the central role.
- Anemia represents a proven marker of poor outcome in patients with both chronic and acute heart failure, irrespective of the left ventricular EF.
- In clinical practice, a careful evaluation for the diagnosis of anemia in heart failure patients is recommended to ensure the best therapeutic strategy.
- The treatment of iron deficiency, even in the absence of anemia, has proven significant benefit in heart failure patients with systolic dysfunction.

INTRODUCTION

Anemia is one of the significant comorbidities in patients with heart failure (HF). It is associated with worse clinical status, increased risk of hospitalization, and decreased survival in this population[1] These observations brought to light new potential pathophysiological links and therapeutic options in patients with HF.

Based on several studies analyzing the clinical impact of anemia, the latest guidelines for the management of HF recognized the importance of anemia and particularly iron deficiency in this setting. Thus, a diagnostic workup to seek a cause for any finding of anemia as a part of the standard management of patients with HF is currently recommended.[1] However, unanswered questions remain, especially regarding the potential benefits of anemia directed therapies in patients with HF, because the data available so far are somewhat conflicting. The present article reviews current information on anemia in patients with HF from epidemiology to management options.

DIAGNOSIS AND EPIDEMIOLOGY

According to the World Health Organization, anemia is defined as low hemoglobin (Hb) concentrations: less than 13 g/dL in men and less than 12 g/dL in nonpregnant women.[2] The prevalence of anemia in the overall HF population varies between studies (from 17% to over 50%) and seems to be higher in patients with a higher EF.[3–7] This wide range of reported prevalences may be explained by different patient demographics, comorbidities, stages of HF severity, and by the definition of anemia applied in respective studies.

Patients with HF and anemia are often older, have a higher prevalence of diabetes, chronic kidney disease (CKD), severe HF with worse functional capacity.[8] Moreover, in patients with HF,

[a] University of Medicine and Pharmacy "Carol Davila", Euroecolab; [b] Emergency Institute for Cardiovascular Diseases "Prof. Dr. C. C. Iliescu", Bucharest, Romania

* Corresponding author. Department of Cardiology, University of Medicine and Pharmacy "Carol Davila", Euroecolab, Emergency Institute for Cardiovascular Diseases "Prof. Dr. C. C. Iliescu", Sos. Fundeni 258, Sector 2, Bucharest 022328, Romania.

E-mail address: carmen.beladan@googlemail.com

Heart Failure Clin 17 (2021) 195–206
https://doi.org/10.1016/j.hfc.2020.12.002

haemodilution is a frequent cause of low Hb levels (also known as pseudoanemia) and should be considered when defining anemia in this setting.[9]

ETIOLOGY AND PATHOPHYSIOLOGY OF ANEMIA IN PATIENTS WITH HEART FAILURE

The etiology of anemia in patients with HF is complex, and multiple coexistent mechanisms have been incriminated. A relationship between the severity of HF syndrome and the complexity of these etiologic ramifications has also been suggested.

Iron Deficiency

One of the most studied mechanisms of anemia in patients with HF is iron deficiency. Furthermore, iron deficiency is a highly prevalent condition in patients with HF, even in the absence of anemia, with an impact on outcomes.[10]

Iron deficiency may be either absolute, defined by severe reduction or depletion of iron stores or functional, defined by normal or increased body iron stores that cannot be mobilized into erythroid precursors.[11] Iron deficiency, defined by serum ferritin of less than 100 μg/L or serum ferritin of 100 to 300 μg/L with a transferrin saturation value of less than 20%, has been reported in more than one-third of all patients with HF.[12,13]

There are several putative mechanisms for iron deficiency in HF, including deficiencies in iron uptake, storage, or iron loss. Decreased intake of iron may be secondary to a recommended diet (ie, a low-protein diet in patients with CKD), to dysgeusia associated with several drugs like angiotensin-converting enzyme (ACE) inhibitors or statins, or to a dysfunction of hypothalamus-regulated appetite.[14,15] Intestinal wall edema specific to right-sided congestion may also contribute to the iron deficiency through malabsorption.[14]

Clinical or subclinical gastrointestinal (GI) bleeding associated with the intake of antiplatelet or anticoagulant drugs, frequently included in the therapeutic regimens of patients with HF, can also lead to iron deficiency. GI malignancies or GI angiodysplasia have been mentioned between the culprit lesions responsible for anemia or iron deficiency in this setting.[14] Moreover, recent data suggested that the presence of HF is associated with increased risk of malignancy and accelerated tumor growth, and several myocardial markers that are chronically elevated in human HF have been associated with effects on tumor growth.[16]

Chronic Inflammation

Chronic HF is associated with a proinflammatory status, responsible for the development of anemia through several mechanisms. Inflammation in HF occurs through multiple pathways. Activation of the cardiac fibroblasts by biomechanical strain in the failing heart, the release of monocytes from the splenic reservoir owing to renin–angiotensin–aldosterone system activation, increased gut permeability with subsequent translocation of bacteria and toxins in the blood or the impairment of the norepinephrine regulation of monocyte inflammatory cytokines balance have been studied in this setting.[17]

The main proinflammatory cytokines increased in HF are tumor necrosis factor-α, IL-1, and IL-6. High levels of IL-6 stimulate the synthesis of a liver-derived peptide hormone, hepcidin, the central regulator of iron absorption and its distribution to tissues. Hepcidin inhibits ferroportin and other iron transport proteins from the GI tract, macrophages, and hepatocytes, leading to low iron levels. Moreover, hepcidin is renally excreted, so its levels are increased in renal failure, which can partially explain the iron deficiency in this setting.[18]

Recent studies have challenged the hypothesis of the inflammation–hepcidin–iron pathway as one of the leading causes of iron deficiency in patients with HF. The argument was the low hepcidin levels reported in patients with advanced HF and iron deficiency, despite the proinflammatory state.[14,19–21] Besides its effects on iron metabolism, inflammation may induce anemia by the direct effects of the cytokines on erythropoiesis. The cytokines IL-1 and tumor necrosis factor-α inhibit erythropoietin synthesis, probably owing to reactive oxygen species which affect the erythropoietin-producing cells and the binding affinities of erythropoietin-inducing transcription factors.[22] Moreover, the activity of tumor necrosis factor-α, IL-1, and IFN-γ may interfere with the proliferation and differentiation of erythroid precursors.[23] Inflammatory anemia may also be a consequence of the macrophage activation by IL-1 and IL-6, especially, leading to increased destruction of the erythrocytes.[23]

Chronic Kidney Disease

In patients with HF, CKD is a frequent association, as a risk factor, as a consequence of HF syndrome, or as a comorbidity in systemic diseases and represents a strong independent predictor of anemia.[24] Several studies suggest that 30% to 50% of the patients with HF may have moderate to severe CKD (defined as a glomerular filtration rate of <60 mL/min) associated with a reduction in erythropoietin production.[25] Erythropoietin resistance owing to the proinflammatory state represents another mechanism of anemia in patients with chronic HF and CKD.[26]

Drugs

The renin–angiotensin–aldosterone system plays an important role in plasma volume regulation and erythropoiesis. Several studies suggested that anemia may be induced or worsened in patients with HF treated with ACE inhibitors. In the Study of Left Ventricular Dysfunction (SOLVD), enalapril was associated with increased odds of developing anemia.[27] The Valsartan Heart Failure (ValHeFT) trial reported the same association for angiotensin II receptors blockers.[28]

With increased renin–angiotensin–aldosterone system activation, angiotensin II level increases with the subsequent activation of hypoxia-inducible factor-1 and erythropoietin gene expression.[24] However, Hb level may not increase despite erythropoietin therapy in patients with HF and anemia concomitantly treated with an ACE inhibitor, possibly owing to other angiotensin II related mechanisms, like the blocking of its direct stimulative effect on erythroid progenitor cell growth.

Moreover, ACE inhibitors have been found to inhibit the recruitment of pluripotent hematopoietic stem cells and normal early progenitors and to reduce the levels of IL-12, a stimulator of erythropoiesis and of insulin-like growth factor-1, which is in direct relationship with the hematocrit level.[29] The decrease in hematocrit in patients on ACE inhibitors reaches a peak during the first 3 months of therapy, maintaining a stable level afterward. The cessation of these drugs tends to normalize the hematocrit level within the next 3 to 4 months.[25]

Concomitant therapy with beta-blockers may also be a cause of anemia in patients with HF. Erythropoietin secreting cells and progenitor red cells have sympathetic innervation with beta-1, beta-2, and alpha surface receptors, with beta-2 having the most important role.[30] Results from the Carvedilol or Metoprolol European Trial (COMET) have shown that carvedilol induced a slight but significant decrease in Hb level (0.2 g/dL) when compared with metoprolol.[31]

PATHOPHYSIOLOGICAL CONSEQUENCES OF ANEMIA

The direct consequence of chronic anemia is tissue hypoxia responsible for the development of hemodynamic and nonhemodynamic compensatory mechanisms. One of the main nonhemodynamic responses is related to the increase in the concentration of 2,3-diphosphoglycerate , leading to a right-shifted Hb–oxygen dissociation curve and a decreased affinity of the Hb for oxygen. An increase in erythropoietin production represents another nonhemodynamic response. Both mechanisms increase tissue oxygen delivery.[32]

A decrease in the systemic vascular resistance represents the initial compensatory hemodynamic response, owing to reduced blood viscosity and to nitric oxide-mediated vasodilatation. The baroreceptor-mediated neurohormonal systems activated by hypotension will eventually lead to an expansion of the extracellular and plasma volume. In the short term, vasodilatation and volume expansion have a beneficial effect by increasing cardiac output and oxygen transport. In the long term, these mechanisms will result in LV remodeling (dilation and hypertrophy) secondary to chronic volume overload and increased wall tension, leading to HF development[32,33] (**Fig. 1**).

Moreover, several disease-specific mechanisms like microinfarctions in sickle-cell disease, coronary vascular occlusions by parasites in malaria, iron overload owing to blood transfusions in thalassemia and reduced myocyte iron stores in iron deficiency anemia may contribute to cardiac alterations in this setting.[34,35]

The reversibility of these structural and functional cardiac changes is still unclear. In a substudy on patients with HF enrolled in the Randomized Etanercept North American Strategy to Study Antagonism of Cytokines (RENAISSANCE) trial, an increase of 1 g/dL in Hb concentrations over 24 weeks was associated with a decrease in LV mass of 4.1 g/m.[2,36]

In subjects with preserved LV function, severe anemia may lead to high-output HF, which can be rapidly and completely reverse by the correction of anemia.[11] There is little information regarding the response of patients with HF with a reduced left ventricular EF to less severe anemia and its progressive correction.

ANEMIA AND CLINICAL OUTCOMES

The presence of anemia has been shown to be independently associated with poor functional status, increased risk of hospitalization, longer hospitalization, rehospitalization, and all-cause mortality in patients with HF.[3,6,36–38] Recent data reported a prognostic role for anemia on mortality in patients with both chronic and acute HF.[39]

The increased risk of anemic patients with HF for all-cause mortality or a combined end point (all-cause mortality or hospitalization for HF) has been manifest irrespective of the left ventricular ejection fraction (EF) (reduced, preserved, or mildly reduced).[40] However, when looking to the clinical outcome of patients with HF with anemia

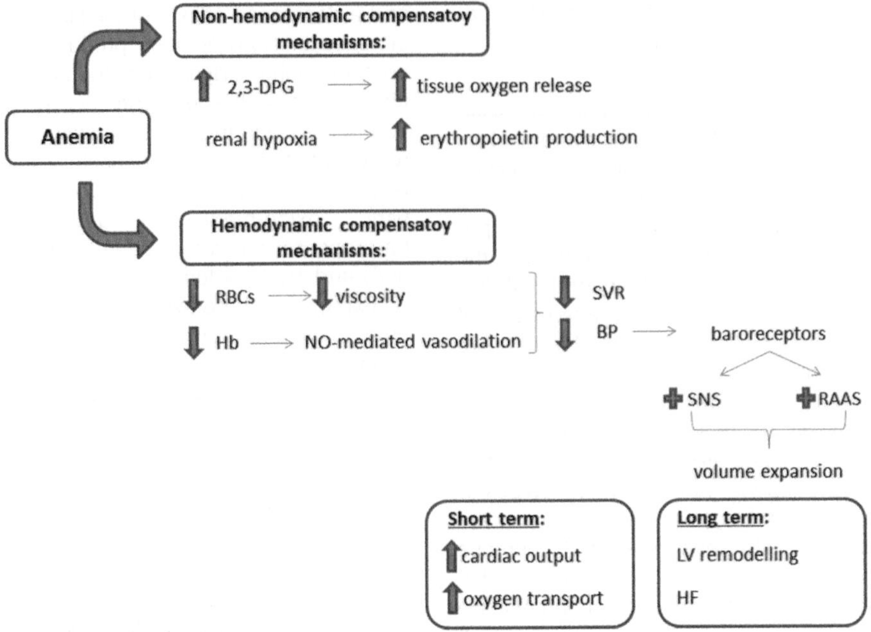

Fig. 1. Pathophysiological consequences of anemia. In chronic anemia, human body responses with several compensatory mechanisms, which in the short term have beneficial effects, but in the long term can lead to the development of HF. 2,3-DPG, 2,3-diphosphoglycerate; BP, blood pressure; RAAS, renin–angiotensin–aldosterone system; RBCs, red blood cells; SNS, sympathetic nervous system; SVR, systemic vascular resistance. (*Data from* Anand IS. Heart failure and anemia: mechanisms and pathophysiology. Heart Fail Rev 2008;13:379-386; and Locatelli F, Pozzoni P, Del Vecchio L, et al. Effect of anemia on left ventricular hypertrophy in end-stage renal disease. The European Journal of Heart Failure Supplements 2003;207-212.)

stratified according to the left ventricular EF, there is no firm consensus of reported data (**Table 1**)

The analysis from the Meta-Analysis Global Group in Chronic Heart Failure (MAGGIC) dataset revealed that patients with HF with reduced EF (HFrEF) and anemia had the worst prognosis, whereas patients with HF with preserved EF (HFpEF) and anemia had a similar prognosis to those with HFrEF without anemia.[38] On the other hand, when analyzing the population with acute decompensated HF from the Atherosclerosis Risk in Communities (ARIC) study, the authors concluded that the incremental risk of death and longer hospitalization associated with anemia was higher in patients with HFpEF (defined by an EF of $\geq$40%) than in those with HFrEF (EF of <40%).[41]

A more recent study, assessing the prognostic role of anemia in patients with HF classified according to the most recent classification proposed by the European Guidelines for the diagnosis and treatment of acute and chronic HF, showed no differences in risk across the left ventricular EF spectrum for all-cause mortality. However, a significantly higher risk for the composite outcome (all-cause death and HF hospitalization) has been reported in HFpEF and HF with mid-range EF versus HFrEF.[7]

An interesting observation emerged from several studies reporting an increased risk for mortality not only in patients with HF with anemia, but also in those with polycythemia. A U-shaped relationship has been suggested between Hb level and mortality. Thus, Evaluation of Losartan In The Elderly (ELITE II) substudy analyzed the all-cause mortality and reported that anemic and polycythemic patients had the worst survival rate. Moreover, the Prospective Randomized Amlodipine Survival Evaluation (PRAISE) study showed that the U-shaped relationship between the Hb level and mortality is related to other causes of death than pump failure.[42,43]

The U-shaped relationship between Hb levels and survival was not confirmed by the analysis of the Study of Effects of Nebivolol Intervention on Outcomes and Rehospitalization in Seniors With Heart Failure (SENIORS) database.[40] Likewise, no evidence to support the U-shaped relationship between Hb levels and survival emerged from the subgroup analysis of the Randomized Etanercept North American Strategy to Study Antagonism of Cytokines (RENAISSANCE) trial.[36]

Table 1
Impact of anemia on clinical outcomes in patients with HF

Author	Study Design	Inclusion Criteria	No. of Patients	Anemic Patients (%)	HF Phenotypes (%)	Results
Mozaffarian et al[42]	Secondary analysis of a multicenter clinical trial (PRAISE)	Left ventricular ejection fraction <30%; New York Heart Association functional class III–IV; Treatment with digoxin, diuretics and an ACE inhibitor	1130			A lower hematocrit was strongly associated with death from progressive HF, rather than sudden death or other deaths.
O'Meara et al[4]	Secondary analysis of a clinical trial (CHARM)	≥18 y of age; New York Heart Association functional class II–IV congestive HF for ≥4 wk	2653	26%	HFrEF: 59.7% HFpEF: 40.3%	Anemia was an independent predictor for both the combined end point (cardiovascular death or HF hospitalization) and all-cause mortality.
Komajda et al[31]	Secondary analysis of a clinical trial (COMET)	Left ventricular ejection fraction <35%; New York Heart Association functional class II–IV	3029	15.9%	–	All-cause mortality (RR 1.47) death or hospitalization (RR 1.28), and HF hospitalization (RR 1.43, all *P*<.0001) were higher in anemic when compared with nonanemic patients.
Anand et al[36]	Secondary analysis of a clinical trial (RENAISSANCE)	Age: 18–55 y; New York Heart Association functional class II–IV Ischemic/nonischemic Left ventricular ejection fraction <30% Stable doses of diuretic, ACE inhibitor and β-blocker (if taking) for ≥3 mo 6-min walk distance of <375 m or <425 m if hospitalized for congestive HF within previous 6 mo)	912	12%	–	An increase in Hb over time was associated with a decrease in LV mass and lower mortality, whereas a decrease in Hb over time was associated with an increase in LV mass and higher mortality.

(*continued on next page*)

Table 1
(continued)

Author	Study Design	Inclusion Criteria	No. of Patients	Anemic Patients (%)	HF Phenotypes (%)	Results
Young et al[37]	Secondary analysis of a clinical trial (OPTIMIZE-HF)	New/worsening HF as the primary cause of admission *or* significant HF symptoms developed during hospitalization for another primary diagnosis and HF was given as the primary discharge diagnosis	48,612	51.2%	HFrEF: 48.8% HFpEF: 51.2%	Lower Hb is associated with higher morbidity and mortality in hospitalized patients with HF.
Von Haehling et al[40]	Secondary analysis of a clinical trial (SENIORS)	$\geq$ 70 y Clinical history of chronic HF with $\geq$1 of: documented hospital admission within the last 12 mo with a discharge diagnosis of congestive HF *or* documentation of an left ventricular ejection fraction $\leq$35% within the previous 6 mo	2069	10%	HFrEF: 64.9% HFpEF: 35.1%	Anemia is an independent predictor of death or hospitalization for cardiovascular reasons among elderly patients with chronic HF and reduced or preserved/mildly reduced left ventricular ejection fraction.
Caughey et al[41]	Secondary analysis of clinical trial (ARIC)	$\geq$55 y of age Hospitalization with acute decompensated HF	15,461	70%	HFrEF: 59% HFpEF: 41%	The incremental risks of death and lengthened hospital stay associated with anemia are more pronounced in acute decompensated patients with HF classified with HFpEF than HFrEF.

Savarese et al[7]	Secondary analysis of Swedish Heart Failure Registry	Age ≥18 and clinician-judged HF, regardless of EF	42,985	34%	HFrEF: 55% HF with mid-range EF: 21% HFpEF: 23%	Over long-term follow-up, anemia was independently associated with increased risk of death or HF hospitalization and of death alone in both HFpEF, HF with mid-range EF and HFrEF, but with higher risk of all-cause death or HF hospitalization in HFpEF and HF with mid-range EF vs HFrEF and no differences in risk across the EF spectrum for all-cause mortality.
Sharma et al[43]	Secondary analysis of a multicenter clinical trial (ELITE-II)	≥60 y of age Left ventricular ejection fraction <40% New York Heart Association functional class II–IV	3044	16.8%	–	Hb is an independent predictor of mortality in patients with congestive HF, with anemic and polycythemic patients having the worst survival.

MANAGEMENT OF ANEMIA IN PATIENTS WITH HEART FAILURE

The comprehensive management of patients with HF aims to improve symptoms and increase patient quality of life and survival. Anemia, among other comorbidities, is one of the therapeutic targets in this setting. It has been demonstrated that in patients with chronic HF, an increase in Hb concentration of 1 g/dL is associated with a 15.8% reduction in mortality risk and a 14.2% decrease in the risk of death or hospitalization for congestive HF.[36]

Erythropoiesis-Stimulating Agents

A possible benefit of using erythropoiesis-stimulating agents to treat anemia in patients with HF emerged from a few small studies and a meta-analysis of 11 randomized control trials, which suggested an improvement in HF symptoms and exercise tolerance in this setting. However, 2 larger trials—STAMINA-HeFT (Study of Anemia in Heart failure Trial) and RED-HF (Reduction of Events by Darbapoetin Alfa in Heart Failure)—concluded there were no significant clinical benefits associated with this treatment.[44–48] The RED-HF trial showed that despite the increase in the median Hb levels in the group treated with darbapoetin, there was no improvement on the primary composite outcome of death of any cause or hospitalization for worsening HF and no significant difference in any secondary outcome. Moreover, there was a higher rate of ischemic stroke and embolic/thrombotic events in patients treated with darbapoetin, similar findings being shown in further studies using erythropoiesis-stimulating agents.[48]

Despite the favorable effects of improving oxygen delivery and the cardioprotective role of erythropoiesis-stimulating agents, the unfavorable effects including higher viscosity, increased vascular resistance and blood pressure as well as hypercoagulability, do not support the use of these agents in patients with HF and anemia to improve the clinical outcome.[8,49]

Iron Therapy

Oral iron therapy seems more convenient than intravenous iron therapy in terms of availability, costs, and administration, but oral iron has some disadvantages. It is not well-absorbed, especially in patients with HF owing to HF effects on the GI tract and hepcidin levels. It also has several side effects like nausea, abdominal bloating, and diarrhea and constipation that can affect patient compliance.[8,50] The largest trial to test oral iron in HF-IRONOUT-HF (Iron Repletion Effects on Oxygen Uptake in Heart Failure) did not show a significant effect on exercise capacity of oral iron compared with placebo in patients with HF with reduced left ventricular EF.[51]

Several studies investigating intravenous iron administration (most of them using ferric carboxymaltose and less frequent iron sucrose) reported beneficial effects on clinical outcomes. Two of the largest trials were FAIR-HF (Ferinject Assessment in Patients with Iron Deficiency and Chronic Heart Failure) and CONFIRM-HF (Ferric Carboxymaltose Evaluation on performance in Patients with Iron Deficiency in Combination with Chronic Heart Failure). Both trials, using ferric carboxymaltose, showed significant improvements on symptoms, functional capacity, and quality of life measurements in patients with HF with systolic dysfunction. The results were independent of the presence of anemia.[52,53] Moreover, CONFIRM-HF reported a significant reduction in the risk of hospitalizations for worsening HF.[53]

The EFFECT-HF (Effect of Ferric Carboxymaltose on Exercise Capacity in Patients with Iron Deficiency and Chronic Heart Failure) trial confirmed the results of the previous studies regarding the improvement of functional status and feeling of well-being. However, no effect has been found on peak oxygen consumption.[54]

Two meta-analyses analyzing the effect of intravenous iron therapy in patients with HF showed a lower incidence of recurrent HF hospitalizations and cardiovascular mortality in the treated groups.[55,56] Based on these findings, the recommendations referring to iron therapy in patients with HF have been recently updated.

The 2016 European Society of Cardiology Guidelines for the diagnosis and treatment of acute and chronic HF states that "IV FCM should be considered in symptomatic patients with HFrEF and iron deficiency (serum ferritin <100 μg/L, or ferritin between 100–299 μg/L and transferrin saturation <20%) to alleviate HF symptoms and improve exercise capacity and quality of life"—class of recommendation IIa, level of evidence A.[1]

The 2017 American College of Cardiology/American Heart Association/Heart Failure Society of America Focused Update of the 2013 American College of Cardiology Foundation/American Heart Association Guideline for the Management of Heart Failure states that "in patients with NYHA [New York Heart Association functional] class II and III HF and iron deficiency (ferritin <100 ng/nL or 100–300 ng/mL if transferrin saturation is <20%), intravenous iron replacement might be reasonable to improve functional status and quality of life"—class of recommendation IIb, level of evidence B.[49] As compared with the European

Table 2
Anemia and iron deficiency in current guidelines

	2016 ESC Guidelines for the Diagnosis and Treatment of Acute and Chronic Heart Failure	2017 ACC/AHA/HFSA Focused Update of the 2013 ACCF/AHA Guideline for the Management of Heart Failure
Recommended tests for initial assessment of patients with HF	Haemoglobin, ferritin, transferrin saturation (I, C)	Evaluation for anemia in addition to other baseline laboratory measurements
Recommended treatment in patients with HF with iron deficiency		
Intravenous ferric carboxymaltose	IIa, A	Intravenous iron (IIb, B)
Other intravenous iron preparations	No	
Oral iron supplementation	No	No
Patients receiving treatment for iron deficiency	Symptomatic with HFrEF	New York Heart Association functional class II–III
Erythropoietin-stimulating agents	Not recommended	No benefit (III)

Data from Ponikowski P, Voors AA, Anker SD, et al. 2016 ESC Guidelines for the diagnosis and treatment of acute and chronic heart failure: The Task Force for the diagnosis and treatment of acute and chronic heart failure of the European Society of Cardiology (ESC). Developed with the special contribution of the Heart Failure Association (HFA) of the ESC. Eur J Heart Fail 2016;18:891–975; and Yancy CW, Jessup M, Bozkurt B, et al. 2017 ACC/AHA/HFSA Focused Update of the 2013 ACCF/AHA Guideline for the Management of Heart Failure: A Report of the American College of Cardiology/American Heart Association Task Force on Clinical Practice Guidelines and the Heart Failure Society of America. Circulation 2017;136:e137-e161.

guidelines, this document does not mention any particular type of intravenous iron preparation that should be used or the HF phenotype (HFrEF, HF with mid-range EF, or HFpEF) but it specifies the stage of the disease prone to derive clinical benefits from iron therapy (New York Heart Association functional classes II and III).

The differences in recommendations between the 2 documents confirm the controversies on this topic and the unanswered questions (**Table 2**).

One of these questions refers to the benefits of intravenous iron therapy in patients with HFpEF, currently evaluated in an ongoing trial—FAIR-HFpEF (NCT03074591).

The use of ferritin levels in the definition of iron deficiency is another debated issues. Some authors consider ferritin levels unreliable to define iron deficiency because it is an acute phase reactant and suggest transferrin saturation less than 20% as the best marker for selecting patients with iron deficiency and identifying patients with HF with the highest mortality risk in this setting.[9,57]

Transfusion Therapy

Blood transfusion in patients with HF is controversial, and there remain a limited number of studies on this subject. Transfusion therapy was associated with volume overload and ischemic events in patients with HF in addition to more classical adverse effects including allergic reactions, acute lung injury, hemolytic reactions, bacterial contamination and endotoxemia. Thus it is supported a more restrictive strategy with a trigger Hb threshold for blood transfusion in patients with HF of 7 to 8 g/dL.[58]

SUMMARY

Anemia is a common comorbidity in patients with HF, with a complex multifactorial etiology and significant consequences on cardiac structure and function. It has a significant impact on the quality of life and prognosis of these patients.

All patients with HF syndrome and anemia should be investigated for the underlying causes and treated according to the current recommendations. Intravenous iron therapy is currently supported as an important therapeutic option in patients with HF with iron deficiency. There are still awaited results regarding the long-term effects of this treatment.

The potential benefits of new therapies targeting anemia in patients with HF are still under evaluation.

CLINICS CARE POINTS

- Within heart failure (HF) patients, anemia and iron deficiency are common comorbidities associated with worse prognosis.

- Laboratory tests to detect the presence of anemia (haemoglobin concentration) and to assess the iron status (serum ferritin and transferrin saturation (TSAT)) should be performed in patients with newly diagnosed HF and in patients with chronic HF during follow-up, particularly in the setting of persistent symptoms despite optimal background HF therapy.
- Additional diagnostic workup is currently recommended in HF patients with anemia (haemoglobin concentration <13.0 g/dL in men and <12.0 g/dL in women) and/or iron deficiency (serum ferritin <100 μg/L or ferritin between 100 and 299 μg/L and TSAT <20%) to seek for any potentially treatable/reversible causes (e.g., gastrointestinal sources of bleeding).
- Intravenous ferric carboxymaltose is currently recommended by the 2016 European Society of Cardiology Guidelines for the Diagnosis and Treatment of Acute and Chronic Heart Failure in symptomatic patients with HF with reduced ejection fraction and iron deficiency in order to alleviate HF symptoms, improve exercise capacity and quality of life. (Class of recommendation IIa, level of evidence A).

DISCLOSURES

The authors have nothing to disclose.

REFERENCES

1. Ponikowski P, Voors AA, Anker SD, et al. 2016 ESC Guidelines for the diagnosis and treatment of acute and chronic heart failure: the Task Force for the diagnosis and treatment of acute and chronic heart failure of the European Society of Cardiology (ESC). Developed with the special contribution of the Heart Failure Association (HFA) of the ESC. Eur J Heart Fail 2016;18:891–975.
2. WHO V. Haemoglobin concentrations for the diagnosis of anaemia and assessment of severity. Geneva (Switzerland): Vitamin and Mineral Nutrition Information System, WHO; 2011.
3. Ezekowitz JA, McAlister FA, Armstrong PW. Anemia is common in heart failure and is associated with poor outcomes: insights from a cohort of 12 065 patients with new-onset heart failure. Circulation 2003; 107:223–5.
4. O'Meara E, Clayton T, McEntegart MB, et al. Clinical correlates and consequences of anemia in a broad spectrum of patients with heart failure: results of the Candesartan in heart failure: assessment of reduction in mortality and morbidity (CHARM) program. Circulation 2006;113:986–94.
5. Wexler D, Silverberg D, Sheps D, et al. Prevalence of anemia in patients admitted to hospital with a primary diagnosis of congestive heart failure. Int J Cardiol 2004;96:79–87.
6. Groenveld HF, Januzzi JL, Damman K, et al. Anemia and mortality in heart failure patients a systematic review and meta-analysis. J Am Coll Cardiol 2008; 52:818–27.
7. Savarese G, Jonsson Å, Hallberg AC, et al. Prevalence of, associations with, and prognostic role of anemia in heart failure across the ejection fraction spectrum [published correction appears in Int J Cardiol 2020 Jan 20]. Int J Cardiol 2020;298:59–65.
8. Anand IS, Gupta P. Anemia and iron deficiency in heart failure: current concepts and emerging therapies. Circulation 2018;138:80–98.
9. Grote Beverborg N, van Veldhuisen DJ, van der Meer P. Anemia in heart failure: still relevant? JACC Heart Fail 2018;6:201–8.
10. Lavoie AJ. Iron deficiency in heart failure: getting to the guidelines. Curr Opin Cardiol 2020;35:133–7.
11. Zusman O, Itzhaki Ben Zadok O, Gafter-Gvili A. Management of iron deficiency in heart failure. Acta Haematol 2019;142:51–6.
12. Jankowska EA, Rozentryt P, Witkowska A, et al. Iron deficiency: an ominous sign in patients with systolic chronic heart failure [published correction appears in Eur Heart J 2011:32:1054]. Eur Heart J 2010;31: 1872–80.
13. von Haehling S, Gremmler U, Krumm M, et al. Prevalence and clinical impact of iron deficiency and anaemia among outpatients with chronic heart failure: the PrEP registry. Clin Res Cardiol 2017;106:436–43.
14. van der Wal HH, Grote Beverborg N, Dickstein K, et al. Iron deficiency in worsening heart failure is associated with reduced estimated protein intake, fluid retention, inflammation, and antiplatelet use. Eur Heart J 2019;40:3616–25.
15. Sîrbu O, Floria M, Dascalita P, et al. Anemia in heart failure - from guidelines to controversies and challenges. Anatol J Cardiol 2018;20:52–9.
16. Meijers WC, Maglione M, Bakker SJL, et al. Heart failure stimulates tumor growth by circulating factors. Circulation 2018;138:678–91.
17. Van Linthout S, Tschöpe C. Inflammation - cause or consequence of heart failure or both? Curr Heart Fail Rep 2017;14:251–65.
18. Silverberg DS, Wexler D, Schwartz D. Is correction of iron deficiency a new addition to the treatment of the heart failure? Int J Mol Sci 2015;16:14056–74.
19. Jankowska EA, Malyszko J, Ardehali H, et al. Iron status in patients with chronic heart failure. Eur Heart J 2013;34:827–34.
20. Weber CS, Beck-da-Silva L, Goldraich LA, et al. Anemia in heart failure: association of hepcidin levels to iron deficiency in stable outpatients. Acta Haematol 2013;129:55–61.

21. Fitzsimons S, Doughty RN. Iron deficiency in patients with heart failure. Eur Heart J Cardiovasc Pharmacother 2015;1:58–64.
22. Weiss G, Goodnough LT. Anemia of chronic disease. N Engl J Med 2005;352:1011–23.
23. Nemeth E, Ganz T. Anemia of inflammation. Hematol Oncol Clin North Am 2014;28:671-vi.
24. Tang YD, Katz SD. Anemia in chronic heart failure: prevalence, etiology, clinical correlates, and treatment options. Circulation 2006;113:2454–61.
25. Caramelo C, Justo S, Gil P. Anemia en la insuficiencia cardiaca: fisiopatología, patogenia, tratamiento e incógnitas [Anemia in heart failure: pathophysiology, pathogenesis, treatment, and incognitae]. Rev Esp Cardiol 2007;60:848–60.
26. van der Putten K, Braam B, Jie KE, et al. Mechanisms of disease: erythropoietin resistance in patients with both heart and kidney failure. Nat Clin Pract Nephrol 2008;4:47–57.
27. Ishani A, Weinhandl E, Zhao Z, et al. Angiotensin-converting enzyme inhibitor as a risk factor for the development of anemia, and the impact of incident anemia on mortality in patients with left ventricular dysfunction. J Am Coll Cardiol 2005;45:391–9.
28. Anand IS, Kuskowski MA, Rector TS, et al. Anemia and change in hemoglobin over time related to mortality and morbidity in patients with chronic heart failure: results from Val-HeFT. Circulation 2005;112:1121–7.
29. Macdougall IC. The role of ACE inhibitors and angiotensin II receptor blockers in the response to epoetin. Nephrol Dial Transplant 1999;14:1836–41.
30. Metra M, Nodari S, Bordonali T, et al. Anemia and heart failure: a cause of progression or only a consequence? Heart Int 2007;3:1.
31. Komajda M, Anker SD, Charlesworth A, et al. The impact of new onset anaemia on morbidity and mortality in chronic heart failure: results from COMET. Eur Heart J 2006;27:1440–6.
32. Anand IS. Heart failure and anemia: mechanisms and pathophysiology. Heart Fail Rev 2008;13:379–86.
33. Locatelli F, Pozzoni P, Del Vecchio L, et al. Effect of anemia on left ventricular hypertrophy in end-stage renal disease. The European Journal of Heart Failure Supplements 2003;Volume 2, Issue S2.p.207–212. Available at: https://onlinelibrary.wiley.com/doi/abs/10.1016/S1567-4215%2803%2980004-8.
34. Hegde N, Rich MW, Gayomali C. The cardiomyopathy of iron deficiency. Tex Heart Inst J 2006;33:340–4.
35. Franzen D, Curtius JM, Heitz W, et al. Cardiac involvement during and after malaria. Clin Investig 1992;70:670–3.
36. Anand I, McMurray JJ, Whitmore J, et al. Anemia and its relationship to clinical outcome in heart failure. Circulation 2004;110:149–54.
37. Young JB, Abraham WT, Albert NM, et al. Relation of low hemoglobin and anemia to morbidity and mortality in patients hospitalized with heart failure (insight from the OPTIMIZE-HF registry). Am J Cardiol 2008;101:223–30.
38. Berry C, Poppe KK, Gamble GD, et al. Prognostic significance of anaemia in patients with heart failure with preserved and reduced ejection fraction: results from the MAGGIC individual patient data meta-analysis. QJM 2016;109:377–82.
39. Ye S, Wang S, Wang G, et al. Association between anemia and outcome in patients hospitalized for acute heart failure syndromes: findings from Beijing acute heart failure registry (Beijing AHF Registry). Intern Emerg Med 2020. https://doi.org/10.1007/s11739-020-02343-x.
40. von Haehling S, van Veldhuisen DJ, Roughton M, et al. Anaemia among patients with heart failure and preserved or reduced ejection fraction: results from the SENIORS study. Eur J Heart Fail 2011;13:656–63.
41. Caughey MC, Avery CL, Ni H, et al. Outcomes of patients with anemia and acute decompensated heart failure with preserved versus reduced ejection fraction (from the ARIC study community surveillance). Am J Cardiol 2014;114:1850–4.
42. Mozaffarian D, Nye R, Levy WC. Anemia predicts mortality in severe heart failure: the prospective randomized amlodipine survival evaluation (PRAISE). J Am Coll Cardiol 2003;41:1933–9.
43. Sharma R, Francis DP, Pitt B, et al. Haemoglobin predicts survival in patients with chronic heart failure: a substudy of the ELITE II trial. Eur Heart J 2004;25:1021–8.
44. Ponikowski P, Anker SD, Szachniewicz J, et al. Effect of darbepoetin alfa on exercise tolerance in anemic patients with symptomatic chronic heart failure: a randomized, double-blind, placebo-controlled trial. J Am Coll Cardiol 2007;49:753–62.
45. Klapholz M, Abraham WT, Ghali JK, et al. The safety and tolerability of darbepoetin alfa in patients with anaemia and symptomatic heart failure. Eur J Heart Fail 2009;11:1071–7.
46. Kotecha D, Ngo K, Walters JA, et al. Erythropoietin as a treatment of anemia in heart failure: systematic review of randomized trials. Am Heart J 2011;161:822–31.e2.
47. Ghali JK, Anand IS, Abraham WT, et al. Randomized double-blind trial of darbepoetin alfa in patients with symptomatic heart failure and anemia. Circulation 2008;117:526–35.
48. Swedberg K, Young JB, Anand IS, et al. Treatment of anemia with darbepoetin alfa in systolic heart failure. N Engl J Med 2013;368:1210–9.
49. Yancy CW, Jessup M, Bozkurt B, et al. 2017 ACC/AHA/HFSA Focused Update of the 2013 ACCF/AHA guideline for the management of heart failure:

a report of the American College of Cardiology/ American Heart Association Task Force on Clinical Practice Guidelines and the Heart Failure Society of America. Circulation 2017;136:e137–61.

50. Chopra VK, Anker SD. Anaemia, iron deficiency and heart failure in 2020. ESC Heart Fail 2020;7: 2007–11.
51. Lewis GD, Malhotra R, Hernandez AF, et al. Effect of oral iron repletion on exercise capacity in patients with heart failure with reduced ejection fraction and iron deficiency: the IRONOUT HF randomized clinical trial [published correction appears in JAMA 2017:317:2453]. JAMA 2017;317: 1958–66.
52. Anker SD, Comin Colet J, Filippatos G, et al. Ferric carboxymaltose in patients with heart failure and iron deficiency. N Engl J Med 2009; 361:2436–48.
53. Ponikowski P, van Veldhuisen DJ, Comin-Colet J, et al. Beneficial effects of long-term intravenous iron therapy with ferric carboxymaltose in patients with symptomatic heart failure and iron deficiency. Eur Heart J 2015;36:657–68.
54. van Veldhuisen DJ, Ponikowski P, van der Meer P, et al. Effect of ferric carboxymaltose on exercise capacity in patients with chronic heart failure and iron deficiency. Circulation 2017;136:1374–83.
55. Jankowska EA, Tkaczyszyn M, Suchocki T, et al. Effects of intravenous iron therapy in iron-deficient patients with systolic heart failure: a meta-analysis of randomized controlled trials. Eur J Heart Fail 2016; 18:786–95.
56. Anker SD, Kirwan BA, van Veldhuisen DJ, et al. Effects of ferric carboxymaltose on hospitalisations and mortality rates in iron-deficient heart failure patients: an individual patient data meta-analysis. Eur J Heart Fail 2018;20:125–33.
57. Grote Beverborg N, Klip IT, Meijers WC, et al. Definition of iron deficiency based on the gold standard of bone marrow iron staining in heart failure patients. Circ Heart Fail 2018;11:e004519.
58. Qaseem A, Humphrey LL, Fitterman N, et al. Clinical guidelines committee of the American College of Physicians. treatment of anemia in patients with heart disease: a clinical practice guideline from the American College of Physicians [published correction appears in Ann Intern Med. 2014:160:144]. Ann Intern Med 2013;159:770–9.

Role of Cardiac Magnetic Resonance Imaging in Heart Failure

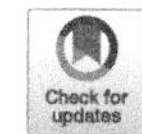

Carla Contaldi, MD, PhD[a,*], Santo Dellegrottaglie, MD, PhD[b,c], Ciro Mauro, MD[d], Francesco Ferrara, MD, PhD[a], Luigia Romano, MD[e], Alberto M. Marra, MD, PhD[f], Brigida Ranieri, PhD[g], Andrea Salzano, MD, MRCP (London)[g], Salvatore Rega[f], Alessandra Scatteia, MD[b], Antonio Cittadini, MD[f], Filippo Cademartiri, MD, PhD, FESC[g], Eduardo Bossone, MD, PhD, FCCP, FESC, FACC[h]

KEYWORDS

• Cardiac magnetic resonance • Heart failure • Etiology • Prognosis • Treatment management

KEY POINTS

- Heart failure (HF) is a growing public health problem affecting heavily on patient survival, quality of life, and health care costs.
- The early and accurate identification of the underlying cause of HF is of great relevance for the diagnostic and prognostic characterization.
- Cardiac magnetic resonance (CMR) allows noninvasive morphologic and functional assessment, tissue characterization, blood flow, and perfusion evaluation.
- In patients with HF with either reduced, midrange or preserved ejection fraction, CMR may provide useful information for early etiologic diagnosis, prognostic stratification, and treatment management.

INTRODUCTION

Heart failure (HF) is a clinical syndrome characterized by typical symptoms that may be accompanied by signs. It may be caused by several structural and/or functional cardiac abnormalities, resulting in a reduced cardiac output and/or elevated intracardiac pressures at rest or during stress.[1] HF is a growing public health problem, with a prevalence of 1% to 2% in the adult population, affecting heavily on patient survival, quality of life, and health care costs.[1,2] In 2016, the European Society of Cardiology proposed a classification of HF based on left ventricular (LV) ejection faction (EF): HF with reduced EF (*HFrEF*; EF <40%); HF with midrange EF (*HFmrEF*; EF between 40% and 49%); and HF with preserved EF (*HFpEF*; EF equal to or greater than 50%).[1] The

[a] Department of Cardiology, University Hospital of Salerno, Via Enrico de Marinis, Cava de' Tirreni, Salerno 84013, Italy; [b] Division of Cardiology, Ospedale Accreditato Villa Dei Fiori, C.so Italia 157, Acerra, Naples I 80011, Italy; [c] Zena and Michael A. Wiener Cardiovascular Institute/Marie-Josee and Henry R. Kravis Center for Cardiovascular Health, Icahn School of Medicine at Mount Sinai, New York, NY, USA; [d] Cardiology Division, A Cardarelli Hospital, Via Cardarelli 9, Naples I 80131, Italy; [e] Department of General and Emergency Radiology, A Cardarelli Hospital, Via Cardarelli 9, Naples I 80131, Italy; [f] Department of Translational Medical Sciences, Federico II University of Naples, Via Pansini 5, Naples I 80131, Italy; [g] IRCCS SDN, Via Gianturco 113, Naples I 80143, Italy; [h] Division of Cardiac Rehabilitation - Echo Lab, A Cardarelli Hospital, Via Cardarelli 9, Naples I 80131, Italy

* Corresponding author. Department of Cardiology, University Hospital of Salerno, Cava de' Tirreni-Amalfi Coast, Via Enrico de Marinis, Cava de' Tirreni, Salerno 84013, Italy.
E-mail address: contaldi.carla@gmail.com

Heart Failure Clin 17 (2021) 207–221
https://doi.org/10.1016/j.hfc.2021.01.001

early and accurate diagnosis of HF paired with proper identification of the underlying cause is of great importance for treatment and ultimately for prognosis and quality of life.[1,3]

Current clinical strategies for the management of patients with HF are heavily based on information provided by cardiac imaging, with echocardiography being the method of choice and additional modalities chosen based on individual characteristics. In many circumstances, cardiac magnetic resonance (CMR) may substantially contribute to early etiologic diagnosis, prognostic stratification, and treatment management of patients with HF.[1,3,4] CMR is a complete and very powerful imaging method that allows noninvasive morphologic and functional assessment, tissue characterization, blood flow, and perfusion evaluation.

This review focuses on describing the current role and potential future applications of CMR for the management of patients with HFrEF, HFmrEF, and HFpEF.

CARDIAC MAGNETIC RESONANCE IMAGING PROTOCOL IN HEART FAILURE

Table 1 summarizes scanning sequences potentially included in a CMR protocol tailored to study patients with HF.[5] Precontrast T1-weighted (T1w) and T2w images can detect areas of increased signal intensity (SI) corresponding to fat and tissue edema, respectively. Cine imaging (generally steady-state free precession sequences that show excellent contrast-to-noise ratio between cardiac different structures) can assess motion of each cardiac structure (eg, assessment of LV and right ventricular [RV] size and function). Phase contrast imaging is useful to assess pulmonary flow-to-systemic flow ratio and valve regurgitation/stenosis severity.[3–5] Late gadolinium enhancement (LGE) imaging (10–15 min after administration of intravenous gadolinium contrast agent [GBCA]) permits visualization/quantification of myocardial damage (eg, myocardial reparative fibrosis/scar).[4–6] Cine and LGE imaging should be considered mandatory, whereas other imaging sequences are variably selected based on the clinical scenario or previous imaging findings.

Although T1w and T2w images are the result of a relative parametrization, mapping techniques allow absolute quantification of changes in myocardial composition directly by measuring the underlying T1 and T2 (and T2*) relaxation times. Native (precontrast) T1 time changes with myocardial extracellular water, focal or diffuse fibrosis, and fat and amyloid content. The myocardial extracellular volume (ECV) (quantified using pre- and postcontrast myocardial and blood T1 values, corrected for the blood hematocrit) is a marker of diffuse interstitial fibrosis when other pathologies increasing the extracellular space can been excluded. T2 mapping is mainly used to detect edematous myocardium. T2* mapping is used for quantification of cardiac iron load and may be used to assess intramyocardial hemorrhage. The mapping techniques are gaining consideration in the evaluation of patients with HF.[7,8]

HEART FAILURE WITH REDUCED EJECTION FRACTION AND HEART FAILURE WITH MIDRANGE EJECTION FRACTION

Etiologic Diagnosis

In the workup of patients with newly diagnosed HF, CMR may provide insights in differentiating between ischemic and nonischemic cause.[8]

Ischemic cardiopathy is generally characterized by LGE (scar) involving the subendocardial ventricular layer with variable extension up to the epicardium (transmural), typically involving myocardial territories in a coronary artery distribution (**Fig. 1**).[8] Thanks to higher spatial resolution, LGE-CMR is more sensitive than single-photon emission computed tomography (SPECT) to detect subendocardial or small-sized myocardial necrosis.[3–5,8] Also, the combination of LGE and T2w imaging enables CMR to differentiate between acute and chronic ischemic injury (**Fig. 2**). In *acute myocardial infarction* (MI), T2w images can detect an area of high SI caused by myocardium edema, which reflects the so-called "area at risk." T1 and T2 mapping may also be applied to quantify the extension of the area at risk.[8] Despite restoration of epicardial flow, in many cases there is lack of restoration of blood flow at myocardial level due to microvascular obstruction (MVO), which can be visualized in early gadolinium enhancement (EGE) and LGE images as hypointense areas within the damaged tissue.[8,9] Intramyocardial hemorrhage potentially associated with reperfusion injury is seen as signal voids on T2w images or as areas with shortened T2, T2*, or T1 on mapping techniques (**Fig. 3**).[8,9]

In *chronic coronary artery disease* (CAD), T2w images normally do not show areas of increased SI (see **Fig. 3**), whereas CMR may be used for the assessment of myocardial ischemia and viability. Sensitivity and specificity of myocardial stress-CMR for the detection of significant stenosis on coronary angiography are 91% and 81%, respectively.[10] Recently, typical patterns of pathologic T1 response to adenosine-CMR have been

Table 1
Cardiac magnetic resonance protocol for heart failure

Technique	Information
CINE (b-SSFP)	• RV and LV dimension, mass, regional, and global function • Atrial dimension
Phase contrast	• QP and QS • Cardiac output and PA flow profile • Valve regurgitation severity • LVOT evaluation
T1w (when indicated)	• Fat infiltration • Pericardial thickness • Anatomic information
T2w STIR	• Myocardial edema • Myocardial hemorrhage • Anatomic information
Perfusion CMR (when indicated)	• Myocardial perfusion defect
EGE (when indicated)	• Ventricular myocardial microvascular obstruction • Thrombus • Myocardial inflammation: hyperemia, capillary leak
LGE	• Ventricular myocardial reparative fibrosis • Ventricular myocardial microvascular obstruction
Coronary angiography (when indicated)	• Course of anomalous coronaries • Coronary aneurysms
T1 mapping (optional)	• Diffuse myocardial fibrosis • Myocardial edema • Amyloidosis and fabry infiltration
T2 mapping (optional)	• Myocardial edema
T2* mapping (optional)	• Myocardial iron overload • Myocardial hemorrhage
Tagging technique/Feature tracking (optional)	• Strain and strain rate analysis • Interventricular asynchrony
Ce-MRA (when indicated)	• Vascular anatomy
3D whole-heart MRA or 3D SSFP (when indicated)	• Vascular anatomy

Abbreviations: b-SSFP, balanced steady-state free precession; Ce-MRA, contrast-enhanced magnetic resonance angiography; EGE, early gadolinium enhancement; LGE, late gadolinium enhancement; LV, left ventricle; LVOT, left ventricular outflow tract; PA, pulmonary artery; QP, pulmonary flow; QS, systemic flow; RV, right ventricle.

demonstrated in patients with significant coronary artery stenosis using native T1 mapping.[11] For the detection/quantification of myocardial viability, the first method is the degree of transmurality of LGE. High degrees of transmural scarring (>75% transmurality) indicate absence of viable myocardium with excellent sensitivity of 95% and low specificity of 51%.[12] The second method is dobutamine stress-CMR. Dysfunctional, but viable, myocardium will improve function during low-dose dobutamine, with a good specificity of 91% and moderate sensibility of 81%. Finally, reduced end-diastolic wall thickness (<5.5 mm) by CMR can be useful in predicting no viability with high sensitivity of 96% but a very poor specificity of 38%.[13]

In patients with new-onset HFrEF or HFmrEF, CMR can also be useful in identifying those with nonischemic cause typically showing either no LGE or LGE with a nonischemic pattern (see **Figs. 1** and **2**). *Dilated cardiomyopathy* (DCM) is characterized by ventricular dilatation and systolic dysfunction in the absence of abnormal loading conditions or significant CAD. Genetic and nongenetic forms of DCM can be observed, as reported in **Table 2**. On CMR, about one-third of patients with DCM show midwall LGE that reflects replacement fibrosis (**Fig. 4**). Also, patchy patterns and

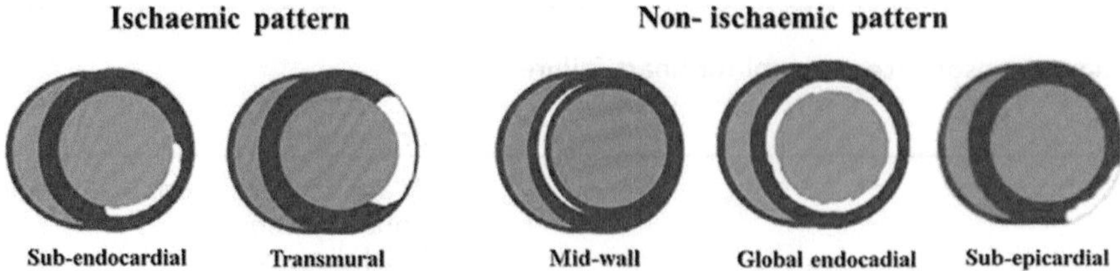

Fig. 1. Ischemic and nonischemic LGE patterns.

subepicardial LGE can be present.[14] Mapping techniques can quantify a diffuse tissue alteration that can be missed by LGE. In DCM, native T1 may be increased also in areas without LGE.[14] ECV, which reflects histology-verified myocardial collagen, is a noninvasive marker of diffuse interstitial fibrosis, and it may be increased also in patients with DCM with positive genotype/negative

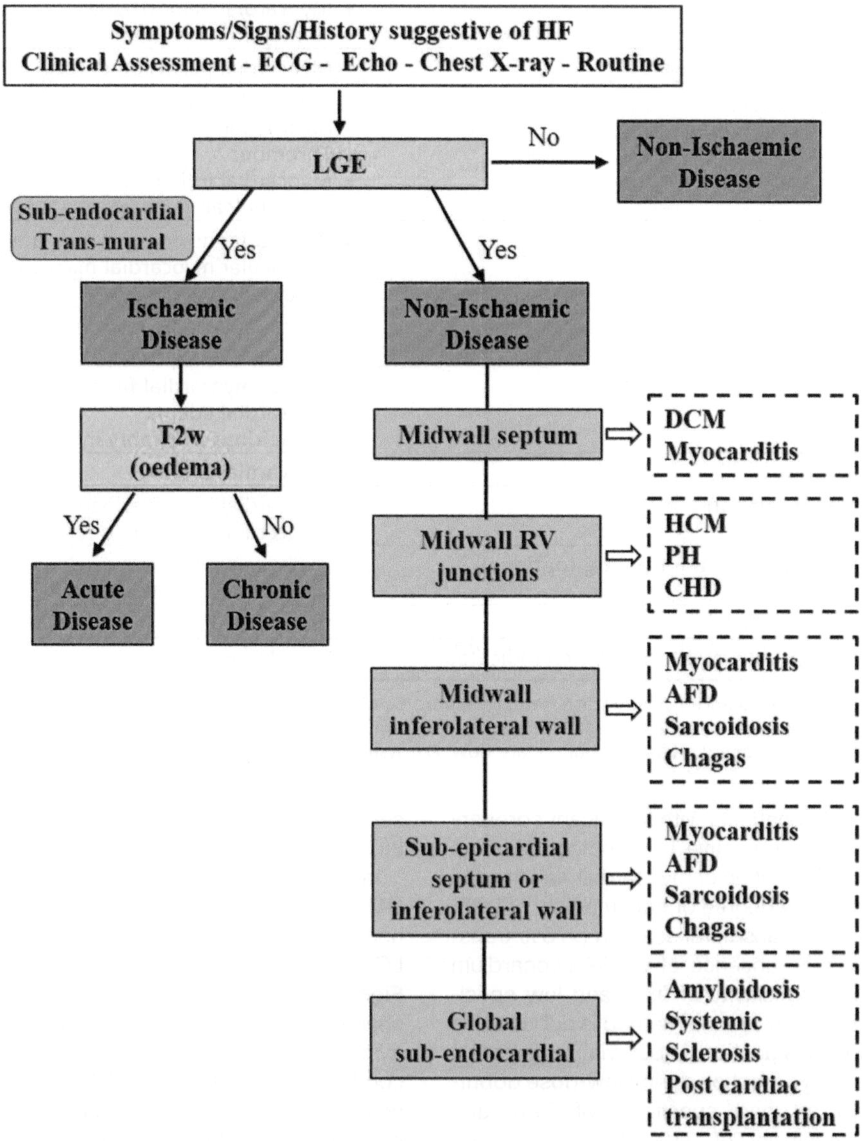

Symptoms/Signs/History suggestive of HF
Clinical Assessment - ECG - Echo - Chest X-ray - Routine

LGE

No → Non-Ischaemic Disease

Sub-endocardial Trans-mural — Yes → Ischaemic Disease

Yes → Non-Ischaemic Disease

Ischaemic Disease → T2w (oedema)

Yes → Acute Disease

No → Chronic Disease

Non-Ischaemic Disease:

Midwall septum ⇨ DCM, Myocarditis

Midwall RV junctions ⇨ HCM, PH, CHD

Midwall inferolateral wall ⇨ Myocarditis, AFD, Sarcoidosis, Chagas

Sub-epicardial septum or inferolateral wall ⇨ Myocarditis, AFD, Sarcoidosis, Chagas

Global sub-endocardial ⇨ Amyloidosis, Systemic Sclerosis, Post cardiac transplantation

Fig. 2. Flowchart depicting the potential value of CMR by LGE and T2w imaging for etiology definition of newly diagnosed HFrEF or HFmrEF.

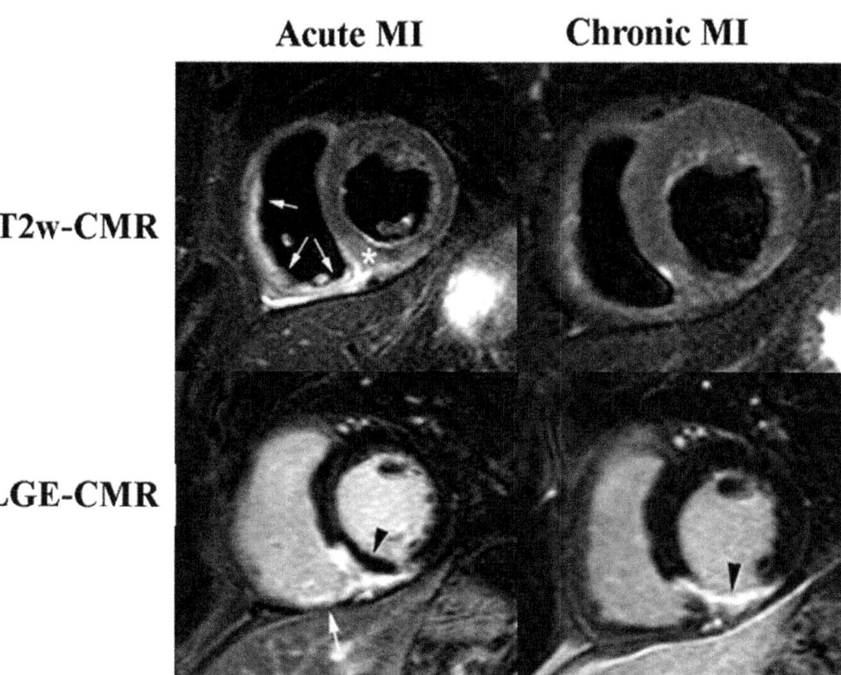

Fig. 3. (*Left panel*) Acute myocardial infarction involving the inferior and inferoseptal LV walls plus the inferior RV wall, with myocardial edema (*white arrows*) and LV hemorrhagic no-reflow (*star*) in T2w images and transmural LGE and LV MVO (*black arrowhead*) in LGE images. (*Right panel*) Chronic myocardial infarction involving the inferior and inferoseptal LV walls, with transmural scar (*black arrowhead*) in LGE images and no myocardial edema in corresponding T2w images.

phenotype.[7,15] *Myocarditis* may clinically present with HF symptoms. CMR, in addition to providing information on ventricular dysfunction and associated pericardial effusion, can also detect myocardial abnormalities related to acute/chronic inflammation. EGE can show increased global myocardial SI relative to skeletal muscle (hyperaemia and capillary leak). T2w imaging can show increased regional (typically with subepicardial or midwall involvement) or global myocardial SI (tissue edema). LGE imaging can show multifocal subepicardium and/or midwall lesions more commonly involving the lateral or inferolateral walls and interventricular septum (myocyte necrosis). Generally, LGE areas become smaller and disappear over time, whereas in some cases they can persist as distinctive linear midwall striae of LGE (similar to that observed in DCM). The Lake Louise Consensus Criteria recommends using a combination of any 2 out of 3 tissue characterization techniques to increase the accuracy in detecting acute myocarditis (**Fig. 5**).[16] Global increase of native T1 and T2 seems to be more accurate for diagnosis than Lake Louise Criteria in acute myocarditis with HF presentation, although for this specific situation standard protocols are still being established. In particular, T2 mapping seems to be more specific to acute inflammation than T1 mapping.[17] In *Takotsubo syndrome,* cine CMR can show specific wall motion abnormalities (about 75% with typical akinesis of the mid- and apical LV segments; 15%–20% with midventricular involvement; 1% with diffuse basal dysfunction), together with possible RV involvement, LV thrombi, and pericardial and/or pleural effusion. T2w images can show diffuse and extended myocardial edema, in particular in akinesis regions. Generally, the absence of significant irreversible tissue injury (LGE) is noted, although subtle fibrosis may be rarely seen (**Fig. 6**). An increase in regional myocardial native T1 and T2 can identify acute myocardial injury with a high diagnostic accuracy.[18]

Prognosis

In *acute MI,* myocardial salvage, infarct size, and MVO are stronger predictors of outcome than LVEF and volumes.[9] Native T1 and T2 mapping may provide prognostic information through the identification of the infarct core and intramyocardial hemorrhage, both associated with adverse prognosis.[7–9] In *chronic CAD*, CMR-LVEF represents a very important prognostic marker, but it

Table 2
Causes of dilated cardiomyopathy

Causes	Aetiology
Genetic	Main pathologic genes: • Titin (sarcomere) • Lamin A/C (nuclear membrane) • Myosin heavy chain (sarcomere) • Troponin T and C (sarcomere) • Myosin-binding protein C (sarcomere) • Actin (sarcomere) • Desmin and dystrophin (cytoskeleton) • SCN5A (ion channel) • Tafazzin (mitochondria) • Desmoplakin (desmosomal junction)
Nongenetic	
Myocarditis (9%)	• Viral and nonviral • Autoimmune
Drug/toxin-related	• Antineoplastic drugs • Psychiatric drugs • Ethanol • Cocaine and amphetamine
Nutritional	• Thiamine deficiency (beri-beri)
Deficiency	• Carnitine deficiency
Endocrinology	• Hypo-/hyperthyroidism • Cushing/Addison disease • Acromegaly • Phaeochromocytoma • Diabetes mellitus
Peripartum cardiomyopathy	• Multifactorial

is very load dependent and limited to patients with EF less than 45%.[1] Stress-CMR has better prognostic value than SPECT for predicting major adverse cardiovascular events (CVEs). High-risk markers on perfusion stress-CMR include large regions of perfusion defects (>5 segments) with 14%/year event rate.[5,19] Infarct size by LGE-CMR and transmurality of LGE are independent predictors of mortality.[20] However, in patients with a large scar (>6 LGE segments), the presence of contractile reserve by low-dose dobutamine is of greater prognostic value after revascularization.[21] The extent of the gray zone by LGE-CMR is related to mortality and is associated with ventricular arrhythmia.[8,9] Among patients without history of MI, the identification of LGE carries a high risk of CVEs.[4,5,8] In *DCM*, CMR-detected RV systolic dysfunction (EF $\leq$45%) is a powerful and independent adverse predictor of HF outcomes.[22] Furthermore midwall septal LGE represents a strong and independent predictor of all-cause mortality, cardiovascular death/transplantation, and sudden cardiac death (SCD), with incremental prognostic value to LVEF.[14] In addition, compared with no-LGE patients, those with midwall LGE with or without cardiac resynchronization therapy (CRT) are less likely to LV reverse remodeling and at higher risk to worse clinical outcome.[5,8] LGE is predictive of ventricular tachycardia even after adjustment for LVEF.[14] High native T1 is associated with an increased risk for CVEs and HF, and ECV increase represents an independent risk factor for major CVEs.[23] In *myocarditis,* LGE showed prognostic relevance in predicting adverse CVEs especially when involving the septum with midwall distribution and persisting at follow-up.[8,16,24]

In *Takotsubo,* T1 values could serve as prognostic marker of clinical outcome.[18]

Treatment Monitoring

In *chronic CAD*, LGE detects treatment effects.[25] In *DCM*, LGE can help to identify the arrhythmogenic substrate and plan an appropriate mapping and ablation strategy.[14] CMR may be useful for accurate estimate of EF when echocardiography documents borderline values in patients candidate for implantable cardioverter defibrillator (ICD) implant.[5] Mechanical dyssynchrony can be assessed using CMR techniques, such as cine wall motion, myocardial tagging, tissue velocity mapping, or displacement imaging.[5,26] A large scar burden, a history of ischemic HF or MI, and fewer viable myocardial segments are associated with no response to CRT. CMR can also be used to assess coronary venous morphology before CRT.[26,27] In summary, CRT guided by CMR demonstrated ability to reduce cardiac mortality along with more LV reverse remodeling and rate of responders.[5,26,27]

HEART FAILURE WITH PRESERVED EJECTION FRACTION

Etiologic Diagnosis

CMR may be useful in differential diagnosis between different types of cardiomyopathy and between restrictive cardiomyopathy and constrictive pericarditis.[28]

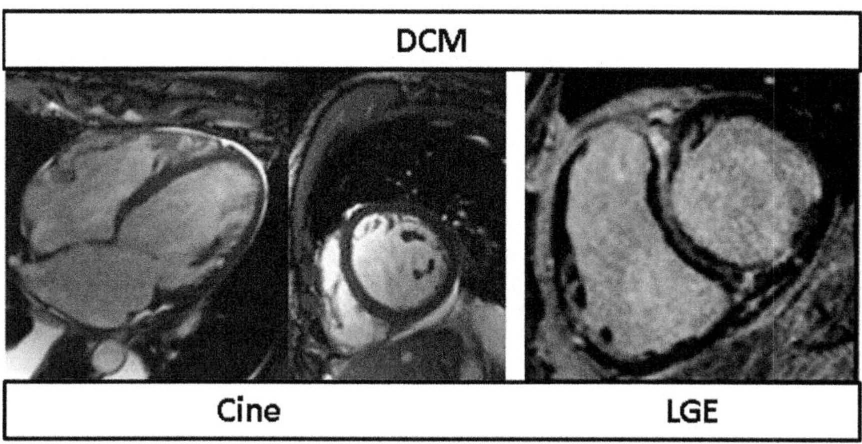

Fig. 4. (*Left panel*) Cine imaging and (*right panel*) midwall LGE of a patient with DCM.

Hypertrophic cardiomyopathy (HCM) is the most common inherited cardiovascular disease caused by mutations in sarcomeric proteins, characterized by replacement and interstitial fibrosis and myocyte disarray.[29] Although echocardiography is typically used for screening, CMR is more sensitive for the identification of more unusual sites of hypertrophy (apex, anterolateral wall, and posterior septum) and is useful in accurate measurements of maximal wall thickness and detection of HCM abnormalities such as apical aneurysms, papillary muscle abnormalities, elongated mitral valve leaflets, and myocardial crypts.[30] These crypts are narrow, deep blood-filled invaginations within the LV myocardium that can be found also in genotype positive-phenotype negative patients with HCM. In HCM, myocardial fibrosis could represent a substrate for ventricular tachyarrhythmias (pathway for SCD) and is responsible for passive diastolic dysfunction (leading cause of dyspnea).[31] Up to 70% of patients with HCM show areas of LGE. The most common LGE pattern is patchy with multiple intramyocardium foci in midmyocardium of both ventricular septum (in particular in the RV insertion areas) and free wall, especially in the regions with the most hypertrophy (**Fig. 7**).[32] ECV gives the most accurate assessment of the diffuse fibrosis as validated by myocardial biopsy.[33] Increased ECV correlates with peak systolic LV outflow tract pressure gradient and energy loss, due to viscous dissipation (evaluated by 4-dimensional [4D] flow CMR), indicating a possible mechanistic link between HCM-related flow abnormalities, increased LV afterload, and LV structural abnormalities (**Fig. 8**).[34] Of interest, ECV is increased in sarcomere mutation carriers even in the absence of LV hypertrophy.[35]

Anderson–Fabry disease (AFD) is an X-linked disease characterized by deficiency of α-galactosidase. The accumulation of sphingolipid in lysosomes in the heart can cause hypertrophy, HF, and SCD. CMR can be useful in detect distribution of hypertrophy, which usually is more symmetric than HCM with substantial RV hypertrophy and sometimes thinning of the inferolateral

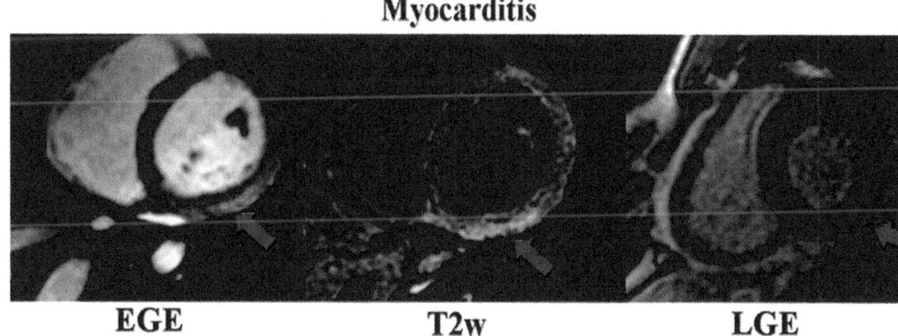

Fig. 5. Acute myocarditis: EGE, T2w, and LGE imaging show increased signal intensity in subepicardial basal inferolateral wall (*red arrows*) consistent with hyperemia, edema, and myocyte necrosis, respectively.

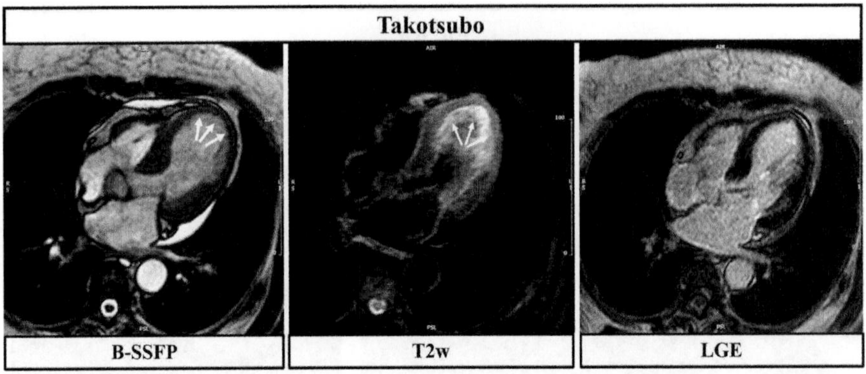

Fig. 6. Typical Takotsubo: akinesis of the mid- and apical LV segments in cine image; extensive myocardial edema in the mid- and apical LV segments without involvement of the basal segments in T2w image; no scar in LGE image.

wall.[36] LGE is typically located in the midwall or subepicardium of the basal inferolateral wall and can become transmural with thinning.[36,37] In around 85% of patients with AFD with hypertrophy, native T1 is characteristically reduced (**Fig. 9**),[7,8,38] which is highly characteristic and diagnostic in the context of LV hypertrophy, despite the rarity of AFD and consequent low pretest probability. A reduction in native T1 occurs early in around half of the patients before the onset of hypertrophy.[7,8,38]

Cardiac amyloidosis (CA) is due to progressive accumulation of amyloid in the myocardial interstitium, associated with increased wall thickness and mass, resulting in diastolic and ultimately systolic dysfunction.[36] CA is often suggested on echocardiography by the presence of severe more concentric LV hypertrophy with preserved systolic function, dilated atria, and restrictive physiology. However, CMR is a valuable tool for the detection of CA. In 80% of patients with CA, there is circumferential mostly subendocardial LGE (most pronounced at the base and midventricle) that is replaced by transmural RV and LV LGE at later stages. Diffuse subendocardial LGE has a specificity of nearly 95% for the diagnosis.[36,39] Typically, blood pool and myocardium tend to have similar signal behavior after GBCA injection. These distinctive alterations can be readily recognized and have a very high sensitivity for the diagnosis

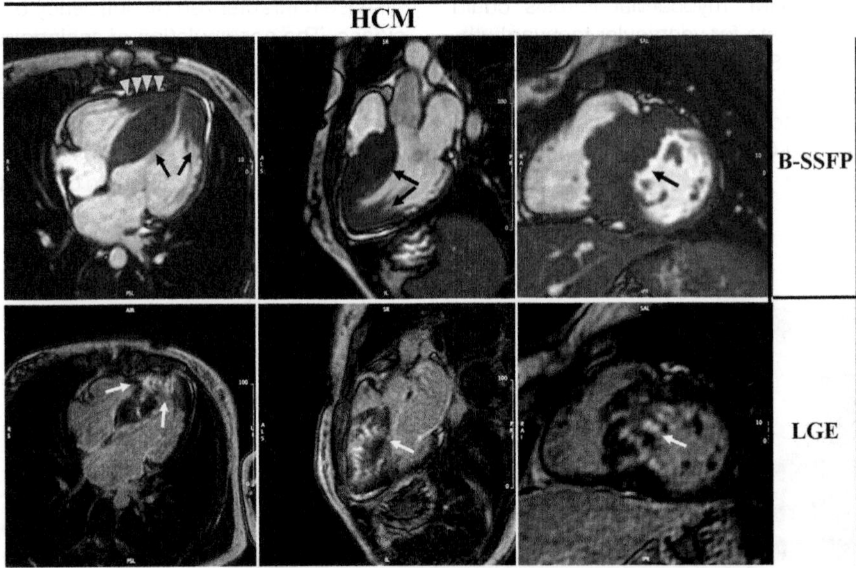

Fig. 7. (*Upper panel*) b-SSFP-images of a patient with HCM showing significant hypertrophy of the interventricular septum and the apex (*black arrows*) with also RV involvement (*arrow heads*). (*Lower panel*) Correspondent LGE images showing diffuse LGE of the hypertrophied segments (*white arrows*).

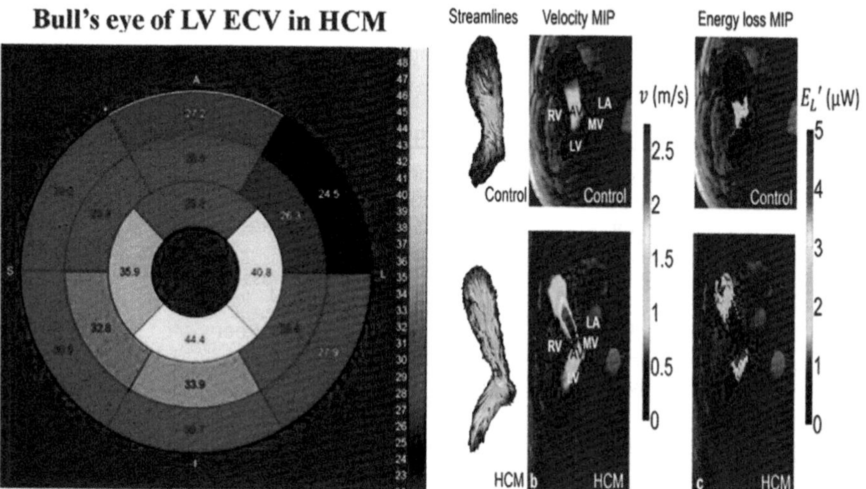

Fig. 8. A patient with HCM (*left panel*) with increased ECV by T1-mapping segmental analysis and (*right panel*) LV outflow tract increased velocity and energy-loss by 4D-flow compared with control.

of CA. In early disease, native T1 and ECV are elevated before LGE appears; these changes are clinically useful when pretest probability is high. ECV can be very high in CA, frequently greater than 50%. The native T1 elevation may be more evident than in any other diffuse disease and, thus, useful in differentiating from HCM.[7,8,28,36,39] *LV noncompaction cardiomyopathy* (LVNC) is characterized by extensive LV trabeculations potentially leading to clinical HF, thromboembolism, and malignant arrhythmias. Dilated, hypertrophic, or restrictive LV can be present. In LVNC, CMR can be useful for the assessment of LV and RV size and function and evaluation of morphology and structure. The trabeculations are preferentially located at LV apex and lateral wall.[28] Proposed CMR criteria for diagnosis of LVNC are listed in **Table 3** and illustrated in **Fig. 10**.[40–42] LGE can be observed in LVNC but is not specific for diagnosis.[7,8,28] *Myocardial iron overload* can occur because of primary disruption of iron regulation or via transfusional iron overload. Without therapy, it is associated with risk of HF, arrhythmias, and SCD.[28,36] CMR T2* mapping is an accurate and reliable method for the quantification of cardiac iron load. A T2* relaxation time less than 20 ms is the cutoff value for diagnosing cardiac siderosis.[43] Low native T1 seems to provide additional information to T2* and seems to be more accurate and reproducible at lower levels of myocardial

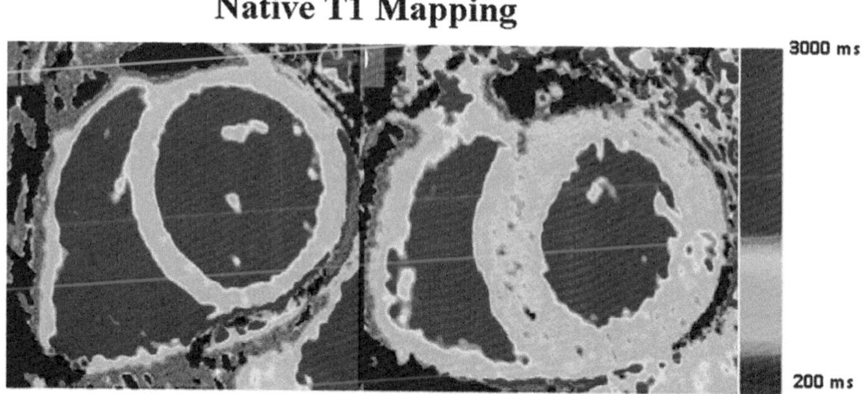

Fig. 9. Native T_1 maps (*basal short-axis*) of a control and a patient with Anderson–Fabry disease that shows low T1 values (*blue areas*) diffusely in the LV myocardium and increasing T1 values (*red areas*) in the inferolateral wall, corresponding to area of LGE.

Table 3
Proposed cardiac magnetic resonance criteria to diagnose left ventricular noncompaction cardiomyopathy

	Petersen[40]	Jacquier[41]	Captur[42]
Method	Long-axis SSFP cine: Thickness of the trabecular myocardial layer Measured at the most pronounced trabeculations, perpendicular to solid myocardium	Short-axis SSFP cine: For obtaining total myocardial mass and solid myocardial mass *Trabecular mass*: difference between total myocardial mass and solid myocardial mass	Short-axis SSFP cine: Fractal dimension (FD) Loss of base-to-apex FD gradient
Cardiac phase	End-diastole	End-diastole	End-diastole
Criteria	Trabecular/Solid layer thickness ratio >2.3	Trabecular mass >20%	Global FD >1.2 Apical FD >1.3
Sensitivity	86%	93.7%	Global FD 83% Apical FD 100%
Specificity	99%	93.7%	Global FD 86% Apical FD 100%

iron loading.[44] ECV may be increased and is associated with cardiac iron overload but not with EF.[7,8,28,36] *Arrhythmogenic cardiomyopathy* (ARVC) is a genetically determined cardiomyopathy, characterized by the replacement of the ventricular myocardium by fibro-fatty tissue, from the epicardium toward the endocardium. The RV can be primarily affected, with RV dilatation and altered regional and/or global function; the LV can also be involved, although LV dimensions or function can be normal. ARVC can be the cause of SCD in young adults, and CMR is the imaging modality of choice for disease early diagnosis.[28,45] Cine CMR is useful for assessment of RV wall motion abnormalities (regional RV akinesia or dyskinesia or dyssynchronous RV contraction) in addition to increased RV volumes and reduced RV EF, which are the CMR diagnostic criteria.[46] LGE images are useful for assessment of RV and, more frequently, LV LGE. The latter has mostly a subepicardial/midwall distribution involving especially posterolateral wall and can be the only sign of LV involvement.[45,46] *Sarcoidosis* is a multiorgan, inflammatory disorder characterized by noncaseating granulomatous infiltration. Cardiac sarcoidosis tends to manifest with a patchy tissue involvement, initially in the absence of evident LV systolic function alterations. Cine CMR can assess the presence of noncaseating granulomas (in few cases).[31,39] An active inflammation can be shown, and increased myocardial T2-values may precede the development of LGE.

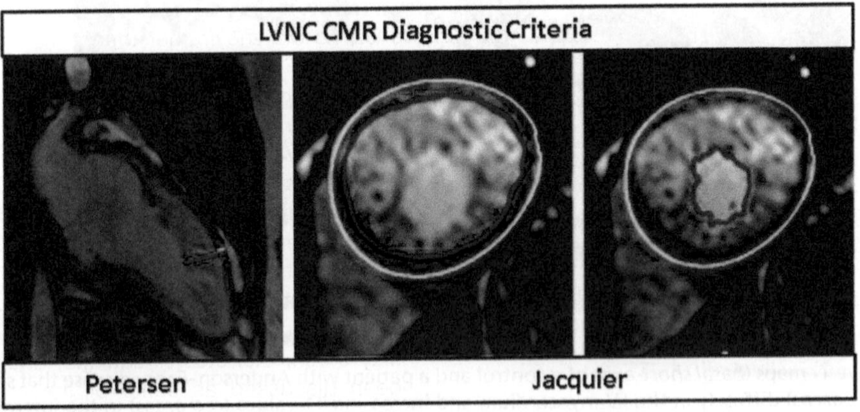

Fig. 10. Examples of CMR criteria for diagnosis of LVNC.

In suspected cases, demonstration of multiple areas of LGE with the coexistence of variable patterns of distribution and involvement of both LV and RV is highly sensitive for diagnosis of cardiac sarcoidosis.[7,28,47] *Constrictive pericarditis* can cause predominant right HF symptoms. CMR can diagnose constrictive pericarditis by providing evidence of a thickened pericardium associated with constrictive physiology.[48] On black-blood anatomical or cine CMR, a pericardial thickness greater than 4 mm suggests possible constriction. Free-breathing real-time cine CMR can depict increased ventricular coupling, with inspiratory interventricular septum inversion and increased right-sided septal motion at onset of expiration on early diastolic ventricular filling. Real-time velocity-encoded CMR typically shows strong respiratory-related variation in cardiac filling. These findings may help differentiate constrictive pericarditis from restrictive cardiomyopathy.[5,48] **Table 4** lists typical changes of myocardial T1, ECV, T2, and T2* observed in some myocardial diseases.

Prognosis

HCM: LGE has prognostic value in predicting adverse CVEs.[32] The LGE extension is an independent predictor of SCD. Patients with LGE mass greater than 15% are at greatest risk.[49] In addition, patients with LGE mass greater than or equal to 20% have increased risk to develop end-stage HCM.[49] Increased global ECV (≥34%), as a marker of diffuse interstitial fibrosis, has shown to be a better predictor of SCD risk compared with LGE.[8,32] ECV is also associated with elevated BNP, which is an independent predictor of morbidity and mortality itself.[8,32]

Table 4
Changes of T1, ECV, T2, and T2* maps in myocardial diseases

	Native T1 Map	ECV	T2 Map	T2* Map
HCM	↑	↑		
AFD	↓↓			
Cardiac Amyloidosis	↑↑	↑↑		
Iron Overload	↓↓		↓↓	↓↓
Myocarditis	↑↑	↑	↑↑	

Abbreviations: AFD, Aderson–Fabry disease; CA, cardiac amyloidosis; HCM, hypertrophic cardiomyopathy; ↑, mild increase; ↑↑, moderate/severe increase; ↓, mild decrease; ↓↓, moderate/severe decrease.

Cardiac amyloidosis: the difference in inversion time between the LV cavity and the myocardium is an important prognostic marker similarly to the transmurality of LGE.[28,36] Both native T1 and ECV are prognostic markers of adverse outcome. Increased ECV (>45%) is associated with a hazard ratio for death of 3.84.[7,8,28,36,50]

LVNC cardiomyopathy: LGE is associated with worse clinical status and LVEF.[8,28]

Myocardial iron overload: myocardial T2* is a biomarker more sensible than LVEF to predict HF events. A T2* relaxation time less than 10 ms is associated with poor prognosis and requires initiation of chelation therapy.[28,36,51]

ARVC: CMR evidence of LV involvement is a strong independent predictor of CVEs in patients with definite, borderline, or possible ARVC diagnosis.[28,45,46]

Sarcoidosis: LGE is associated with an increased risk of death or ventricular arrhythmia even with preserved LVEF. Furthermore, no-LGE is associated with a low risk even with LVEF severely impaired.[28,36,52]

Treatment Monitoring

HCM: LGE could be useful in assessing the grade myocardial tissue involvement and to adjust therapeutic regimens. LGE correlates directly with LV wall thickening and inversely with LVEF. Furthermore, LGE at RV insertion points correlates with increased LV filling pressure (higher E/e' ratio and greater left atrium).[8,32] Patients with large LGE areas should be considered for ICD implant when risk remains ambiguous based on current risk prediction algorithms.[29,32] Detailed description of components contributing to LV outflow tract obstruction may be extremely helpful when surgical myectomy is planned.[29,30]

AFD: CMR has been used to follow regression of LV hypertrophy with enzyme replacement therapy and proposed to define the optimal timing for starting therapy.[53]

Cardiac amyloidosis: ECV might track amyloid regression when a specific treatment can be proposed.[54]

Myocardial iron overload: myocardial T2* measurements represent the current standard for monitoring chelating treatment efficacy.[55]

Sarcoidosis: LGE extension may predict response to steroid treatment.[36,47,52]

Constrictive pericarditis: pericardial LGE may identify inflammatory transient form of constrictive pericarditis that can be reversible with antiinflammatory therapy.[48]

FUTURE PERSPECTIVES

Blood oxygen level–dependent (BOLD)-CMR is a novel technique that permits direct quantification of myocardial tissue oxygenation, based on the changes of paramagnetic properties of hemoglobin due to the effects of oxygenation. An increased myocardial deoxygenation is reelected by increased blood deoxyhemoglobin content that leads to lower signal on $T_2w/T_2{}^*w$ images.[56] In HF, the quantification of myocardial oxygenation by BOLD-CMR correlates with oxygen metabolism during exercise as measured by cardiopulmonary exercise test.[57] Furthermore, BOLD-CMR combined with breathing maneuvers, that exploit the vasodilator effect of the blood CO_2, may be a safe, simple, and fast test for assessment of coronary vascular function, without use of vasodilator drugs. BOLD has shown good correlation with quantitative coronary angiography and perfusion CMR and provides insights into diseases with coronary microvascular impairment.[56] However, for clinical validation, additional studies with large cohorts of patients are needed.

CMR psectroscopy (MRS) allows to study the metabolism of myocardium by exploiting the magnetic properties of chemical nuclei with an odd number of protons.[58] ^{1}H-MRS is mainly used for assessing variations in cardiac triglycerides content, trying to recognize cell damage due to lipid excess. ^{31}P-MRS assesses the adenosine triphosphate to phosphocreatine ratio, a reliable marker of bioenergetics, which is reduced in the failing heart and correlates with cardiac functional status. MRS is a promising tool to study the effects of nutritional and pharmacologic interventions on myocardial metabolism.[58] However, up to now, MRS is technically complex and requires specific expertise; multinuclear MR systems operating at high magnetic field strengths will be needed to allow large-scale trials and clinical application.

Diffusion tensor CMR (DT-CMR) is a novel tool that provides in vivo myocardial microstructure evaluation. DT-CMR assesses the diffusion of water in the heart, thus allowing the fiber and sheet architecture of the myocardium to be resolved.[59] Although technical development is still needed, through the detection of alterations in myocardial microstructure, DT-CMR has the potential to facilitate early diagnosis, identify arrhythmogenic foci, individualize medical therapy, and refine risk stratification in clinically relevant heart diseases, including cardiomyopathies.

4D-flow CMR provides in-vivo qualitative/quantitative assessment of 3-directional blood flow within heart and major vessels throughout the cardiac cycle. 4D-flow CMR offers insights into cardiac and circulatory physiology. Patients with HF exhibit altered intracardiac blood flow, and some 4D-flow–derived hemodynamic parameters have been proposed as new markers of systolic and/or diastolic dysfunction.[60] However, although 4D-flow CMR may provide information with potential clinical impact and prognostic value, additional investigation will be needed before its use in routine clinical management.

Box 1
Role of cardiac magnetic resonance in heart failure

Differentiation of ischemic versus non-ischemic cardiopathy

Differentiation of

- *Acute ischemic injury*:
  - Microvascular obstruction
  - Intramyocardial hemorrhage
  - Complications, such as thrombi, aneurysm

versus

- *Chronic ischemic injury*:
  - Viability detection/quantification
  - Inducible ischemia detection/quantification

Evaluation of Myocarditis

Evaluation of Takotsubo Syndrome

Indication to ICD Implant

Evaluation of Mechanical Dyssynchrony

To Guide Resynchronization Therapy

Evaluation of Anomalous Coronary Origins

Differentiation and Evaluation of Nonischemic Cardiomyopathies:

- Dilated cardiomyopathy
- Hypertrophic cardiomyopathy
- Anderson-Fabry disease
- Cardiac amyloidosis
- Left ventricular noncompaction cardiomyopathy
- Myocardial iron overload
- Arrhythmogenic cardiomyopathy
- Sarcoidosis

Differentiation of Restrictive Cardiomyopathies versus Constrictive Pericarditis

Prognosis and Treatment Monitoring

SUMMARY

CMR overcomes most of the echocardiography limitations (including geometric assumptions, interobserver variability, and poor acoustic window) and provides incremental information in relation to the cause, prognosis, and treatment monitoring of HF.

The role of CMR in HF is summarized in **Box 1**.

Based on current evidence and potential future developments, CMR utilization for initial evaluation and follow-up of patients with HF will grow progressively.

CLINICS CARE POINTS

- The early and accurate diagnosis of heart failure paired with proper identification of the underlying cause is of great importance for treatment, prognosis and quality of life.
- CMR may provide useful information for early etiologic diagnosis, prognostic stratification, and treatment management of heart failure with either reduced, midrange or preserved ejection fraction.
- Limitations of CMR may include low availability, high cost, claustrophobia, safety in patients with ferromagnetic implants and use of gadolinium in patients with severe chronic renal failure.

DISCLOSURE

The authors declare no conflict of interests. This research did not receive any specific grant from funding agencies in the public, commercial, or not-for-profit sectors.

REFERENCES

1. Ponikowski P, Voors AA, Anker SD, et al, ESC Scientific Document Group. 2016 ESC Guidelines for the diagnosis and treatment of acute and chronic heart failure: the task force for the diagnosis and treatment of acute and chronic heart failure of the European society of cardiology (ESC) Developed with the special contribution of the heart failure association (HFA) of the ESC. Eur Heart J 2016;14(37):2129–200.
2. Mosterd A, Hoes AW. Clinical epidemiology of heart failure. Heart 2007;93:1137–46.
3. Contaldi C, Capuano F, Romano L, et al. Cardiovascular magnetic resonance in right heart and pulmonary circulation disorders. Heart Fail Clin 2021;17:57–75.
4. Karamitsos TD, Francis JM, Myerson S, et al. The role of cardiovascular magnetic resonance imaging in heart failure. J Am Coll Cardiol 2009;54:1407–24.
5. Aljizeeri A, Sulaiman A, Alhulaimi N, et al. Cardiac magnetic resonance imaging in heart failure: where the alphabet begins! Heart Fail Rev 2017;22:385–99.
6. Contaldi C, Imbriaco M, Alcidi G, et al. Assessment of the relationships between left ventricular filling pressures and longitudinal dysfunction with myocardial fibrosis in uncomplicated hypertensive patients. Int J Cardiol 2016;202:84–6.
7. Messroghli DR, Moon JC, Ferreira VM, et al. Clinical recommendations for cardiovascular magnetic resonance mapping of T1, T2, T2* and extracellular volume: a consensus statement by the society for cardiovascular magnetic resonance (SCMR) endorsed by the European association for cardiovascular imaging (EACVI). J Cardiovasc Magn Reson 2017;19:75.
8. Karamitsos TD, Arvanitaki A, Karvounis H, et al. Myocardial tissue characterization and fibrosis by imaging. JACC Cardiovasc Imaging 2020;13:1221–34.
9. Bulluck H, Dharmakumar R, Arai AE, et al. Cardiovascular magnetic resonance in acute ST-Segment-elevation myocardial infarction: recent advances, controversies, and future directions. Circulation 2018;137:1949–64.
10. Nandalur KR, Dwamena BA, Choudhri AF, et al. Diagnostic performance of stress cardiac magnetic resonance imaging in the detection of coronary artery disease: a meta-analysis. J Am Coll Cardiol 2007;50:1343–53.
11. Liu A, Wijesurendra RS, Francis JM, et al. Adenosine stress and rest T1 mapping can differentiate between ischemic, infarcted, remote, and normal, myocardium without the need for gadolinium contrast agents. JACC Cardiovasc Imaging 2016;9:27–36.
12. Kim RJ, Wu E, Rafael A, et al. The use of contrast-enhanced magnetic resonance imaging to identify reversible myocardial dysfunction. N Engl J Med 2000;343:1445–53.
13. Dellegrottaglie S, Guarini P, Savarese G, et al. Cardiac magnetic resonance for the assessment of myocardial viability: from pathophysiology to clinical practice. J Cardiovasc Med (Hagerstown) 2013;14:862–9.
14. Assomull RG, Prasad SK, Lyne J, et al. Cardiovascular magnetic resonance, fibrosis, and prognosis in dilated cardiomyopathy. J Am Coll Cardiol 2006;48:1977–85.
15. aus dem Siepen F, Buss SJ, Messroghli D, et al. T1 mapping in dilated cardiomyopathy with cardiac magnetic resonance: quantification of diffuse myocardial fibrosis and comparison with endomyocardial biopsy. Eur Heart J Cardiovasc Imaging 2015;16:210–6.
16. Caforio AL, Pankuweit S, Arbustini E, et al. Current state of knowledge on aetiology, diagnosis,

management, and therapy of myocarditis: a position statement of the European society of cardiology working group on myocardial and pericardial diseases. Eur Heart J 2013;34:2636–48.
17. Bohnen S, Radunski UK, Lund GK, et al. Performance of T1 and T2 mapping cardiovascular magnetic resonance to detect active myocarditis in patients with recent-onset heart failure. Circ Cardiovasc Imaging 2015;8:e003073.
18. Citro R, Okura H, Ghadri JR, et al. EACVI scientific documents committee. Multimodality imaging in takotsubo syndrome: a joint consensus document of the European association of cardiovascular imaging (EACVI) and the Japanese society of echocardiography (JSE). Eur Heart J Cardiovasc Imaging 2020;21:1184–207.
19. Jahnke C, Nagel E, Gebker R, et al. Prognostic value of cardiac magnetic resonance stress tests: adenosine stress perfusion and dobutamine stress wall motion imaging. Circulation 2007;115:1769–76.
20. Kelle S, Roes SD, Klein C, et al. Prognostic value of myocardial infarct size and contractile reserve using magnetic resonance imaging. J Am Coll Cardiol 2009;54:1770–7.
21. Schmidt A, Azevedo CF, Cheng A, et al. Infarct tissue heterogeneity by magnetic resonance imaging identifies enhanced cardiac arrhythmia susceptibility in patients with left ventricular dysfunction. Circulation 2007;115:2006–14.
22. Gulati A, Ismail TF, Jabbour A, et al. The prevalence and prognostic significance of right ventricular systolic dysfunction in nonischemic dilated cardiomyopathy. Circulation 2013;128:1623–33.
23. Vita T, Gräni C, Abbasi SA, et al. Comparing CMR mapping methods and myocardial patterns toward heart failure outcomes in nonischemic dilated cardiomyopathy. JACC Cardiovasc Imaging 2019;12: 1659–69.
24. Aquaro GD, Perfetti M, Camastra G, et al. Cardiac MR with late gadolinium enhancement in acute myocarditis with preserved systolic function: ITAMY Study. J Am Coll Cardiol 2017;70:1977–87.
25. Hare JM, Fishman JE, Gerstenblith G, et al. Comparison of allogeneic vs autologous bone marrow-derived mesenchymal stem cells delivered by transendocardial injection in patients with ischaemic cardiomyopathy: the POSEIDON randomized trial. JAMA 2012;308:2369–79.
26. Helm RH, Lardo AC. Cardiac magnetic resonance assessment of mechanical dyssynchrony. Curr Opin Cardiol 2008;23:440–6.
27. Bilchick KC, Kuruvilla S, Hamirani YS, et al. Impact of mechanical activation, scar, and electrical timing on cardiac resynchronization therapy response and clinical outcomes. J Am Coll Cardiol 2014;63:1657–66.
28. Seferović PM, Polovina M, Bauersachs J, et al. Heart failure in cardiomyopathies: a position paper from the heart failure association of the European society of cardiology. Eur J Heart Fail 2019;21:553–76.
29. Elliott PM, Anastasakis A, Borger MA, et al. 2014 ESC Guidelines on diagnosis and management of hypertrophic cardiomyopathy: the task force for the diagnosis and management of hypertrophic cardiomyopathy of the European society of cardiology (ESC). Eur Heart J 2014;35: 2733–79.
30. Maron MS. Clinical utility of cardiovascular magnetic resonance in hypertrophic cardiomyopathy. J Cardiovasc Magn Reson 2012;14:13.
31. Losi MA, Betocchi S, Chinali M, et al. Myocardial texture in hypertrophic cardiomyopathy. J Am Soc Echocardiogr 2007;20:1253–9.
32. Raiker N, Vullaganti S, Collins JD, et al. Myocardial tissue characterization by gadolinium-enhanced cardiac magnetic resonance imaging for risk stratification of adverse events in hypertrophic cardiomyopathy. Int J Cardiovasc Imaging 2020;36: 1147–56.
33. Flett AS, Hayward MP, Ashworth MT, et al. Equilibrium contrast cardiovascular magnetic resonance for the measurement of diffuse myocardial fibrosis: preliminary validation in humans. Circulation 2010; 122:138–44.
34. van Ooij P, Allen BD, Contaldi C, et al. 4D flow MRI and T1-mapping: assessment of altered cardiac hemodynamics and extracellular volume fraction in hypertrophic cardiomyopathy. J Magn Reson Imaging 2016;43:107–14.
35. Ho CY, Abbasi SA, Neilan TG, et al. T1 measurements identify extracellular volume expansion in hypertrophic cardiomyopathy sarcomere mutation carriers with and without left ventricular hypertrophy. Circ Cardiovasc Imaging 2013;6:415–22.
36. Pereira NL, Grogan M, Dec GW. Spectrum of restrictive and infiltrative cardiomyopathies: Part 1 of a 2-Part series. J Am Coll Cardiol 2018;71:1130–48.
37. Perry R, Shah R, Saiedi M, et al. The role of cardiac imaging in the diagnosis and management of anderson-fabry disease. JACC Cardiovasc Imaging 2019;12:1230–42.
38. Pica S, Sado DM, Maestrini V, et al. Reproducibility of native myocardial T1 mapping in the assessment of Fabry disease and its role in early detection of cardiac involvement by cardiovascular magnetic resonance. J Cardiovasc Magn Reson 2014;16:99.
39. Karamitsos TD, Papanastasiou CA. Cardiac magnetic resonance T1 mapping for cardiac amyloidosis: the best way forward. JACC Cardiovasc Imaging 2020;13:81–2.
40. Petersen SE, Selvanayagam JB, Wiesmann F, et al. Left ventricular non-compaction: insights from cardiovascular magnetic resonance imaging. J Am Coll Cardiol 2005;46:101–5.

41. Jacquier A, Thuny F, Jop B, et al. Measurement of trabeculated left ventricular mass using cardiac magnetic resonance imaging in the diagnosis of left ventricular non-compaction. Eur Heart J 2010; 31:1098–104.
42. Captur G, Muthurangu V, Cook C, et al. Quantification of left ventricular trabeculae using fractal analysis. J Cardiovasc Magn Reson 2013;15:36.
43. Anderson LJ, Holden S, Davis B, et al. Cardiovascular T2-star (T2*) magnetic resonance for the early diagnosis of myocardial iron overload. Eur Heart J 2001;22:2171–9.
44. Sado DM, Maestrini V, Piechnik SK, et al. Noncontrast myocardial T1 mapping using cardiovascular magneticresonance for iron overload. J Magn Reson Imaging 2015;41:1505–11.
45. Haugaa KH, Basso C, Badano LP, et al. Comprehensive multi-modality imaging approach in arrhythmogenic cardiomyopathy-an expert consensus document of the European association of cardiovascular imaging. Eur Heart J Cardiovasc Imaging 2017;18:237–53.
46. Marcus FI, McKenna WJ, Sherrill D, et al. Diagnosis of arrhythmogenic right ventricular cardiomyopathy/dysplasia: proposed modification of the task force criteria. Eur Heart J 2010;31:806–14.
47. Cain MA, Metzl MD, Patel AR, et al. Cardiac sarcoidosis detected by late gadolinium enhancement and prevalence of atrial arrhythmias. Am J Cardiol 2014; 113:1556–60.
48. Bogaert J, Francone M. Cardiovascular magnetic resonance in pericardial diseases. J Cardiovasc Magn Reson 2009;11:14.
49. Chan RH, Maron BJ, Olivotto I, et al. Prognostic value of quantitative contrast enhanced cardiovascular magnetic resonance for the evaluation of sudden death risk in patients with hypertrophic cardiomyopathy. Circulation 2014;130:484–95.
50. Banypersad SM, Fontana M, Maestrini V, et al. T1 mapping and survival in systemic light-chain amyloidosis. Eur Heart J 2015;36:244–51.
51. Kirk P, Roughton M, Porter JB, et al. Cardiac T2* magnetic resonance for prediction of cardiac complications in thalassemia major. Circulation 2009;120:1961–8.
52. Murtagh G, Laffin LJ, Beshai JF, et al. Prognosis of myocardial damage in sarcoidosis patients with preserved left ventricular ejection fraction: risk stratification using cardiovascular magnetic resonance. Circ Cardiovasc Imaging 2016;9:e003738.
53. Hughes DA, Elliott PM, Shah J, et al. Effects of enzyme replacement therapy on the cardiomyopathy of Anderson-Fabry disease: a randomised, double-blind, placebo-controlled clinical trial of agalsidase alfa. Heart 2008;94:153–8.
54. Richards DB, Cookson LM, Berges AC, et al. Therapeutic clearance of amyloid by antibodies to serum amyloid P component. N Engl J Med 2015;373: 1106–14.
55. Pennell DJ, Udelson JE, Arai AE, et al. Cardiovascular function and treatment in β-thalassemia major: a consensus statement from the American Heart Association. Circulation 2013;128:281–308.
56. Sree Raman K, Nucifora G, Selvanayagam JB. Novel cardiovascular magnetic resonance oxygenation approaches in understanding pathophysiology of cardiac diseases. Clin Exp Pharmacol Physiol 2018;45:475–80.
57. Nagao M, Yamasaki Y, Kawanami S, et al. Quantification of myocardial oxygenation in heart failure using blood-oxygen-level-dependent T2* magnetic resonance imaging: Comparison with cardiopulmonary exercise test. Magn Reson Imaging 2017;39: 138–43.
58. Dellegrottaglie S, Scatteia A, Pascale CE, et al. Evaluation of cardiac metabolism by magnetic resonance spectroscopy in heart failure. Heart Fail Clin 2019;15:421–33.
59. Khalique Z, Ferreira PF, Scott AD, et al. Diffusion tensor cardiovascular magnetic resonance imaging: a clinical perspective. JACC Cardiovasc Imaging 2020;13:1235–55.
60. Dyverfeldt P, Bissell M, Barker AJ, et al. 4D flow cardiovascular magnetic resonance consensus statement. J Cardiovasc Magn Reson 2015;17:72.

Biomarkers in Heart Failure

Clinical Insights

Andrea Salzano, MD, PhD, MRCP (London)[a,*,1], Roberta D'Assante, PhD[b,1], Muhammad Zubair Israr, PhD[c], Mohamed Eltayeb, MRCP (UK)[c], Anna D'Agostino, PhD[a], Dennis Bernieh, PhD[c], Mariarosaria De Luca, MD[b], Salvatore Rega[b], Brigida Ranieri, PhD[a], Ciro Mauro, MD[d], Eduardo Bossone, MD, PhD, FCCP, FESC, FACC[d], Iain B. Squire, MD, FRCP[c], Toru Suzuki, MD, PhD, FRCP[c], Alberto M. Marra, MD, PhD[b]

KEYWORDS

• Biomarkers • Heart failure • Prognosis • Risk stratification • Outcomes • Diagnosis

KEY POINTS

- Biomarkers have a preponderant role in Heart Failure general management.
- A novel categorisation of HF biomarkers, grouping them into five groups according to their function and suitability (i.e. community-based screening, diagnosis, risk stratification, phenotyping, and management/tailoring treatment), would allow a more useful clinical approach.
- Natriuretic peptides (i.e. BNP and NT-proBNP) represent, to date, the gold standard biomarkers in HF.
- Emerging biomarkers (e.g. source of tumorigenicity 2, galectin-3, Trimethylamine N-oxide, hormones) showing their importance particularly in risk stratification, phenotyping, and HF management, are currently under investigation with promising results.

Heart failure (HF) is a clinical syndrome caused by structural and/or functional cardiac abnormalities and resulting from impaired cardiac output or an increase of intracardiac pressures at rest and/or during stress. Typical signs and symptoms of HF include ankle swelling, fatigue, dyspnea and peripheral edema, pulmonary crackles, or increased jugular venous pressure. Usually, patients with ejection fraction (EF) greater than or equal to 50% are defined as HF with preserved EF, whereas those with EF less than 40% have HF with reduced EF. Patients with EF between 40% and 49% are now classified as HF with midrange EF.

INTRODUCTION

Heart failure (HF) is a clinical syndrome caused by structural and/or functional cardiac abnormalities and resulting from impaired cardiac output or an increase of intracardiac pressures at rest and/or during stress.[1–3] Typical signs and symptoms of HF include ankle swelling, fatigue, dyspnea and peripheral edema, pulmonary crackles, or increased jugular venous pressure.[1–3] Because of different underlying causes, demographics, comorbidities, and treatment response, the classic classification used to describe HF is based on left ventricle ejection fraction (EF) measurement. Usually, patients with normal EF (accepted as ≥50%) are defined as HF with preserved EF (HFpEF), whereas those with EF less than 40% have HF with reduced EF (HFrEF). In the latest European Society of Cardiology (ESC) guidelines, patients with EF between 40% and 49%, previously considered as a gray area, are now classified as HF with midrange EF (HFmrEF).[1]

[a] IRCCS SDN Nuclear and Diagnostic Research Institute, Naples, Italy; [b] Department of Translational Medical Sciences, Federico II University, Naples, Italy; [c] Department of Cardiovascular Sciences, University of Leicester, Leicester, UK; [d] AORN A Cardarelli, Cardiac Rehabilitation Unit, Naples, Italy
[1] These authors equally contributed.
* Corresponding author. IRCCS SDN Nuclear and Diagnostic Research Institute, Via E Gianturco 113, 80143, Naples, Italy.
E-mail address: andrea.salzano@leicester.ac.uk

Heart Failure Clin 17 (2021) 223–243
https://doi.org/10.1016/j.hfc.2021.01.002

Despite the reduction in total mortality from cardiovascular disease over recent years, HF still maintains high levels of mortality.[4] This high mortality associated with a slow but steady increase in prevalence represents negative HF characteristics[5] and results in a huge economic and social burden.[1,4] Thus, the scientific community is trying to change this tendency, with great efforts in the research and development of biomarkers for the early detection, diagnosis, prognosis, and management of HF to reduce the associated mortality, morbidity, and economic burden. Over the past few years, the level of interest in the discovery of new biomarkers has progressively grown.[6,7] Biomarkers are now routinely used in clinical practice for diagnosis, monitoring, and risk stratification.[8] However, none of the novel biomarkers have shown sufficient prognostic impact when used alone and therefore it has been suggested that, rather than a single biomarker, the integration of multiple biomarkers would represent the best strategy, although further studies are needed to test this hypothesis.[9]

Nowadays, the term biomarker is routinely used, and in some cases misused, to describe several emerging tools, technologies, and strategies intended to progress knowledge about diseases.[10,11] In 2001, the Biomarkers and Surrogate End Point Working Group suggested the following definition: "a characteristic that is objectively measured and evaluated as an indicator of normal biological processes, pathogenic processes, or pharmacologic responses to a therapeutic intervention."[12] Therefore, biomarkers may be derived from the blood, urine, genetic samples, imaging, physiologic tests, and tissue-specimen biopsies.[13]

Biomarkers have been grouped into 3 different categories[14]:

- Type 0: specific disease biomarkers, correlated with clinical indices that can be longitudinally monitored.
- Type I: biomarkers used to evaluate pharmacologic intervention effects together with the mechanism of action of a therapeutic drug.
- Type II: surrogate end points able to predict clinical benefits, representative of the patient's clinical status, disease progression, and outcomes. Surrogate end points are in need of fulfilling at least 4 major criteria.[15,16]:
  - Correlation between the interventional impact on the biomarker and the interventional impact on clinically meaningful end points
  - Ability of therapeutic intervention to modify the outcome of interest
  - Should reflect both benefits and risks related to the intervention
  - Clear knowledge of the sampling strategies, the related relative risk, and the time course between the outcome and the change in the biomarker

Research for the ideal biomarker is focused on the improvement in disease management, and in the reduction of health care costs.[17,18] As a result, a biomarker should be disease specific, easy to detect, cost-effective, and able to provide precise results.[19] New disease biomarkers are identified and reported in several studies; however, many of them do not fulfill the analytical validation process, which requires meeting specific sensitivity and specificity criteria, thus rendering them inapplicable in clinical practice.[20] For this reason, it is necessary to identify appropriate protocols and standards when developing and validating clinical biomarker assays (eg, accurate selection of patients, sample preparation, improvement of laboratory assays, proper statistical/analytical validation).[19]

To expand, Morrow and de Lemos[21] identified 3 criteria a biomarker should fulfill to be useful in the clinic context:

1. The biomarker needs to be accurate, and repeated measurement must be possible with a reasonable cost and time.
2. The biomarker must offer additional information that is not already available from clinical assessment.
3. The biomarker should support clinical decision making.

Outline of the Review

The present article provides clinical insight with straightforward key points and critical commentary on HF biomarkers based on the most recent international recommendations (ie, ESC/Heart Failure Association [HFA] and American College of Cardiology [ACC]/American Heart Association [AHA]/Heart Failure Society of America [HFSA]) and evidence from the literature.

With the aim of offering a more useful clinical approach, biomarkers are categorized here into 5 groups according to their function and suitability: community-based screening, diagnosis, risk stratification, phenotyping, and management/tailoring treatment (**Fig. 1**).

HEART FAILURE SCREENING IN THE COMMUNITY

The use of biomarkers to screen asymptomatic patients with HF in the community (ie, community-based screening) is an emerging

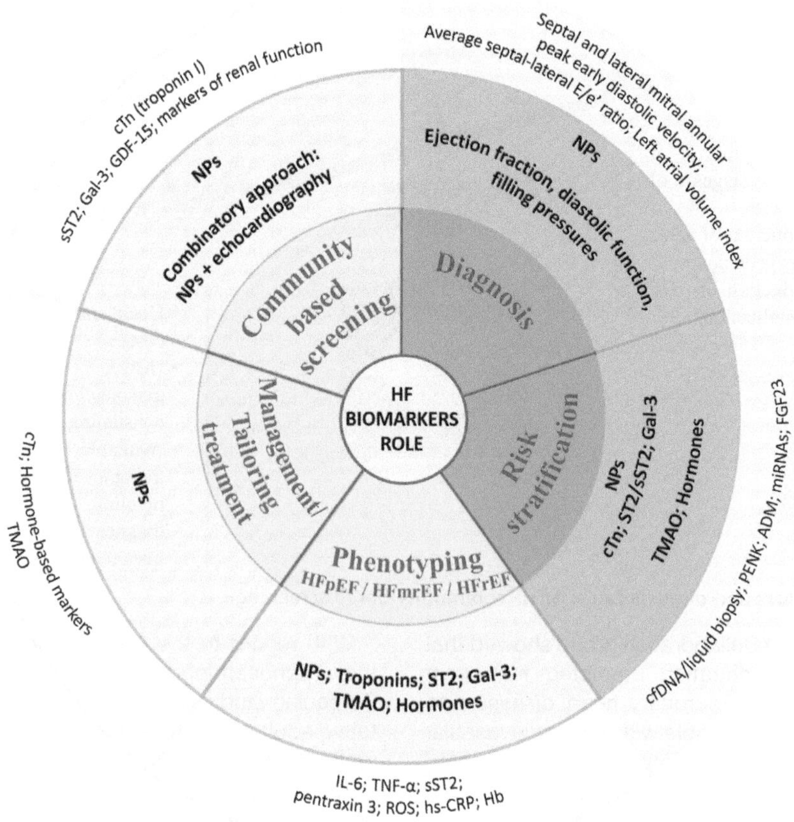

Fig. 1. Biomarkers and Heart Failure: A New Biomarker Classification Proposal. A new biomarker classification proposal based on identified clinical roles for biomarkers in Heart Failure. Green boxes: well-established and supported by data; recommended or suggested by consensus or guidelines. Yellow boxes: promising but not yet recommended in any consensus or guidelines. HF, heart failure; EF, ejection fraction; HFpEF, HF with preserved EF; HFrEF, HF with reduced EF; HFmrEF, HF with mid-range EF; NPs, Natriuretic peptides; cTN, cardia troponins; ST2, source of tumoregenicity 2; Gal-3, Galectin-3; TMAO, Trimethylamine N-oxide; IL-6, Interleukin-6; TNF, Tumor necrosis factor; hs-CRP, High sensitivity C-reactive protein; GDF-15, Growth differentiation factor-15.

issue. This approach is based on the concept that the identification of patients with left ventricular (LV) dysfunction before HF symptoms develop would lead to a delay or a reduction of clinical HF and its related morbidity and mortality. However, apart from the high-risk conditions, currently there are no guideline-based recommended strategies.

Of the different strategies, the most evaluated and promising approach is the evaluation of cardiac-specific biomarkers (mostly natriuretic peptides [NPs] and troponins) in the general population. This approach starts from the concept that B-type natriuretic peptide (BNP) was able to identify patients with AHA/ACC stage A and B HF at higher risk of worse outcome.[3] Furthermore, the St Vincent's Screening to Prevent Heart Failure (STOP-HF) study showed that, between patients at risk of HF, BNP-based screening and collaborative care were able to reduce the rates of systolic dysfunction, diastolic dysfunction, and HF,[22] estimating a good probability of being cost-effective.[23] In the Screening Evaluation of the Evolution of New Heart Failure (SCREEN-HF) study, performed in subjects at high risk of HF (defined as age >60 years plus at least 1 HF risk factor), significant ventricular dysfunction was documented in about 25% of asymptomatic elderly subjects displaying at least 1 HF risk factors and a very high N-terminal proBNP (NT-proBNP) level.[24] Recently, it has been shown that the use of single or serial NT-proBNP measurements for predicting the risk of HF at 5 years has a sensitivity exceeding 75% and specificity in the range of 47% to 69% when specific age cut-offs were applied,[25] confirming previous findings from the literature.[26] An individual-participant-data meta-analysis performed by the Natriuretic

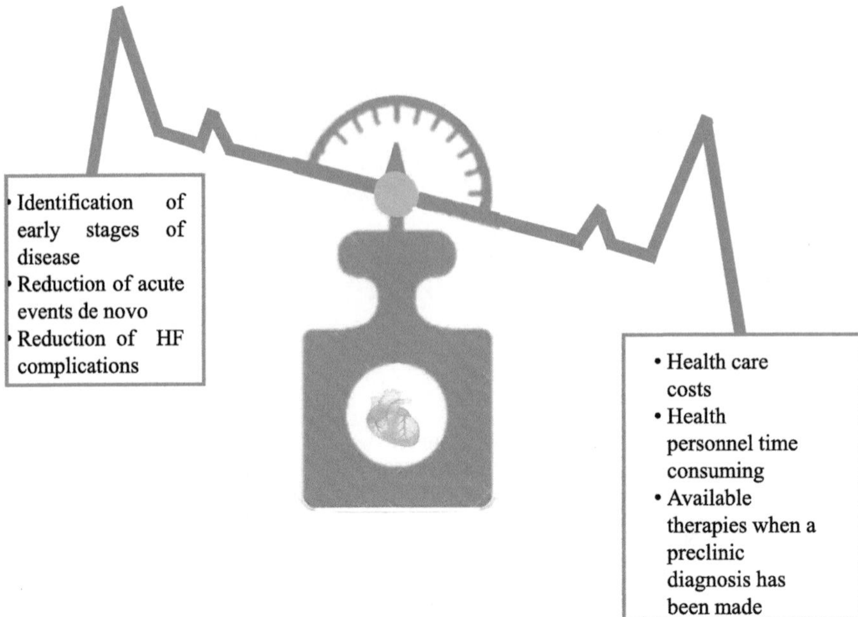
• Identification of early stages of disease
• Reduction of acute events de novo
• Reduction of HF complications
• Health care costs
• Health personnel time consuming
• Available therapies when a preclinic diagnosis has been made

Fig. 2. Advantages and disadvantages of HF community-based screening.

Peptides Studies Collaboration group showed that NT-proBNP concentration predicted first-onset HF and augmented coronary heart disease and stroke prediction in people without cardiovascular disease.[27] As a result, the investigators suggested that NT-proBNP is potentially suitable for general population-level risk assessment.

However, some concerns have been raised around this approach, particularly regarding cost-effectiveness and the possible therapeutic options, particularly for patients with preserved EF, for which treatment options are not yet satisfactory.[28,29]

With regard to cardiac troponins (cTn), recent evidence supports the idea that clinicians would be able to identify individuals at highest risk of developing symptomatic HF, resulting in early diagnosis and improved prognosis.[30,31] The Biomarkers for Cardiovascular Risk assessment in Europe (BiomarCaRE) consortium, a European consortium including 31 institutions, combining data from 4 large populations of healthy people, has shown that high-sensitivity troponin I could independently predict incident HF, with a better predictive value when combined with NT-proBNP.[32]

As for other emerging biomarkers, galectin-3 (Gal-3) and soluble source of tumorigenicity 2 (sST2) have been tested (respectively, in the PREVEND[33] and in the Finnish study[34]), with contrasting results. Multimarker strategy (ie, the addition of multiple biomarkers to clinical variables) could potentially lead to an improvement in discrimination and reclassification abilities of predictive models.[35]

With regard to the use of imaging biomarkers, the Echocardiographic Heart of England Screening study showed that, in a large representative adult population in England, LV dysfunction (defined as LV EF<40%) was detectable in about 1.8% of subjects whereas EF of 40% to 50% was detectable in 3.5% of them.[36] Again, the cost-effectiveness of this approach represents a cause for concern.

Going forward with these concepts, it has been shown that the use of BNP, added to other simple clinical parameters/measurements(eg, electrocardiographic abnormalities) was able to reduce the number of patients needed to perform an echocardiographic study to identify LV systolic dysfunction.[37] Therefore, the combinatory approach seems to be the most effective. Despite the reported effectiveness of this approach in community screening, inadequate access to primary care physicians and its expense have limited the application of echocardiography to screening healthy people (**Fig. 2**).[38,39] Additional strategies to select patients for referral to echocardiography (eg, combine blood and urinary NPs[40] or the addition of other biomarkers such as C-reactive protein and myloperixodases[41]), although fascinating, remain without current clinical application. Results from The Screening of adult Urban Population to Diagnose Heart Failure (SOBOTA-HF) study, currently ongoing (all patients aged >55 years in the large Monska Sobota region are being testing for NT-proBNP and, if increased levels are detected, echocardiographic assessment is performed),[42] will add information about the feasibility of the use of NP screening in the general population.

Community-Based Heart Failure Screening: Should it be Done?

In summary, population screening with NPs followed by echocardiography is a promising approach; however, there is still no evidence of cost-effectiveness to justify its adoption at a large scale[28] (see **Fig. 2**). The AHA, in a recent statement on biomarkers, concluded that the measurement of NPs or cTn alone adds prognostic information to standard risk factors for predicting new-onset HF, with the measurement of emerging biomarkers (ie, sST2, Gal-3, growth differentiation factor 15 [GDF-15], and markers of renal function) alone or in a multimarker strategy, providing additional risk stratification.[11] In contrast, the most recent position paper from European Society of Preventive Cardiology[43] does not recommend HF screening in the community.

DIAGNOSIS

In the latest version of HF guidelines,[1,3] biomarkers (circulating and imaging) have an essential role in HF diagnosis. NPs can be considered the gold standard circulating biomarkers, with increased levels helping to identify patients in need of a further evaluation and lower levels helping to exclude HF diagnosis, regardless of phenotype.[44,45] In parallel, among imaging techniques, echocardiography is considered the most valuable tool owing to its wide availability, easy accessibility, and low cost. EF, ventricle volumes, systolic and diastolic function, valvular diseases, and right ventricle impairment represent fundamental information, changing the clinical management of patients suspected of HF in order to confirm or exclude an HF diagnosis.

Circulating Biomarkers

Among circulating biomarkers, only NPs have shown a clear role in HF diagnosis and have been widely approved with this purpose.[1–3]

Natriuretic peptides

NPs (mainly BNP and NT-proBNP) are strongly linked to the presence and the severity of hemodynamic stress, intracardiac volumes, and filling pressures. Considering this strict correspondence, it is not surprising that other biomarkers

Table 1
Suggested natriuretic peptide cutoffs

	HFrEF		HFpEF	
	Chronic Setting	**Acute Setting**	**Major Criteria**	**Minor Criteria**
BNP	• <35 pg/mL HF unlikely • 35–150 pg/mL gray zone • >150 pg/mL HF likely	• <100 pg/mL HF unlikely • 100–400 pg/mL gray zone • >400 pg/mL HF likely	• >80 pg/mL if sinus rhythm • >240 pg/mL if atrial fibrillation	• 35–80 pg/mL if sinus rhythm • 105–240 pg/mL if atrial fibrillation
NT-proBNP	• <125 pg/mL unlikely • 125–600 pg/mL gray zone • >600 pg/mL HF likely	• <300 pg/mL unlikely • 300–450 pg/mL (<50 y) gray zone • 300–900 pg/mL (50–75 y) gray zone • 300–1800 pg/mL (>75 y) gray zone • >450 pg/mL or >900 or >1800 (>75 y) HF likely	• >220 pg/mL if sinus rhythm • >660 pg/mL if atrial fibrillation	• 125–220 pg/mL if sinus rhythm • 365–660 pg/mL if atrial fibrillation
MR-proANP	—	• 120 pmol/L	—	—

Current guidelines suggested cutoffs for NPs in HF, with regard to phenotype (preserved vs reduced), setting (acute vs chronic), and presence of relevant comorbidities (ie, atrial fibrillation).
Abbreviation: MR-proANP, midregional pro–A-type natriuretic peptide.

have not shown a better performance in HF diagnosis. To date, NPs represent the only circulating biomarkers with an undeniable application, and their use in clinical practice represents the first step for the diagnosis of HF.

What are the cutoffs?

Different cutoffs have been suggested for HFrEF and HFpEF (**Table 1**).

Heart failure with reduced ejection fraction Most recent ESC guidelines[1] and focused NPs practical guidance[46] identified specific cutoffs for chronic and acute setting. These cutoffs, despite being limited by several caveats, should be used in clinical practice in all patients suspected to have HF. Notably, a single-cutoff strategy or a multiple-cut-point strategy can be applied, with higher levels in the acute setting. In the first case, cutoffs have the role of ruling out HF. In the latter case, they also have a good performance in supporting HF diagnosis.

Considering the relationship between age, renal function, and NPs, in the multistep approach, NT-proBNP levels need to be age adjusted, whereas BNP levels do not, because NT-proBNP has a greater degree of correlation with age.

- Chronic setting
  - BNP: less than 35 pg/mL, HF unlikely; 35 to 150 pg/mL, gray zone; greater than 150 pg/mL, HF likely
  - NT-proBNP: less than 125 pg/mL, HF unlikely; 125 to 600 pg/mL, gray zone; greater than 600 pg/mL, HF likely
- Acute setting
  - BNP: less than 100 pg/mL, HF unlikely; 100 to 400 pg/mL, gray zone; greater than 400 pg/mL, HF likely
  - NT-proBNP: less than 300 pg/mL, HF unlikely; 300 to 450 pg/mL if <50 years old, 300 to 900 pg/mL if 50 to 75 years old, and 300 to 1800 pg/mL if >75 years old, gray zone; greater than 450 pg/mL or greater than 900 pg/mL, or greater than 1800 pg/mL if age greater than 75 years, HF likely
  - Midregional pro–A-type natriuretic peptide (MR-proANP): 120 pmol/L

Other cutoffs have been suggested by other experts.[15] However, all the investigators agreed that NPs should be used as continuous variables rather than as singular cutoffs.[1,15,46]

However, there are some categories of patients in whom these cutoffs need to be reconsidered. For instance, patients with altered kidney function (ie, when estimated glomerular filtration [eGFR] is <60 mL/min) are in need of different cutoffs. Therefore, although NT-pro-BNP, when corrected by age, does not need additional changes, for BNP, when eGFR is less than 60 mL/min, it is necessary to increase the rule-out cutoff to 200 pg/mL rather than 100 pg/mL.

Furthermore, there are some groups of patients (eg, obese patients or patients with fatigue as main symptoms) in whom levels are lower than expected. Therefore, in these patients, a lower cutoff (ie, <50 pg/mL BNP in presence of obesity) should be used. With regard to gender differences,[47–50] lower NP levels have been described in men compared with women.[51]

Further, in patients with HF with pre–left ventricle causes (eg, mitral stenosis and acute mitral regurgitation) or pericardial abnormalities, NP levels can be lower than expected or not increased at all, in particular at an early stage, reflecting the lack of the left ventricle overload. In addition, patients of African/African Caribbean origin, and those taking renin angiotensin aldosterone modulators and biotin supplements, also have lower-than-expected NP levels.[46]

Heart failure with preserved ejection fraction For the diagnosis of HFpEF, the ESC suggests the use of a new score (HFA-PEFF score), in which different biomarkers (circulating and imaging) are split into major and minor criteria and combined to strongly suggest or to exclude HFpEF diagnosis.[52] With regard to NPs, different cutoffs are applied depending on the presence or absence of atrial fibrillation (resulting in NP levels about 3 times higher). Notably, normal NP levels do not exclude HFpEF, especially in the presence of obesity.

- BNP:
  - Major criteria: greater than 80 pg/mL if sinus rhythm, greater than 240 pg/mL if atrial fibrillation
  - Minor criteria: 35 to 80 pg/mL if sinus rhythm, 105 to 240 pg/mL if atrial fibrillation
- NT-proBNP:
  - Major criteria: greater than 220 pg/mL if sinus rhythm, greater than 660 pg/mL if atrial fibrillation
  - Minor criteria: 125 to 220 pg/mL if sinus rhythm, 365 to 660 pg/mL if atrial fibrillation

Which is the clinical utility of natriuretic peptides?

Suggested cutoff levels for NPs have very high negative predictive values but very low positive predictive values (in particular in the acute setting). Therefore, they should be used to rule out HF (ie, patients with low levels are unlikely to have an

Box 1
Factors influencing natriuretic peptide levels

Factor that increase NP concentrations

Left ventricular dysfunction

Hypertrophic heart muscle diseases

- Infiltrative myocardiopathies
- Acute cardiomyopathies
- Inflammatory
- Valvular heart disease

Arrhythmias

- Atrial fibrillation
- Atrial flutter

Ischemic heart disease

- Acute coronary syndromes
- Coronary artery ischemia

Cardiotoxic drugs

- Anthracyclines and related compounds

Significant pulmonary or cardiopulmonary diseases

- Acute respiratory distress syndrome
- Pulmonary diseases with right-sided HF
- Obstructive sleep apnea
- Pulmonary hypertension
- Pulmonary embolism

Advanced age

Renal dysfunction

Critical illness

- Burns
- Stroke

High-output states

- Hyperthyroidism
- Cirrhosis
- Sepsis
- Anemia

Myocardial dysfunction

- Systolic dysfunction
- Diastolic dysfunction
- Fibrosis/scar
- Hypertrophy
- Infiltrative disease

Valvular abnormalities

- Mitral stenosis, regurgitation
- Aortic stenosis, regurgitation
- Tricuspid regurgitation
- Pulmonary stenosis

Increased cardiac chamber size

- Ventricular enlargement
- Atrial enlargement

Increased filling pressures

- Atrial
- Ventricular
- Pulmonary

Congenital abnormalities

- Shunts
- Stenotic lesions

Factors that do not show increased NP concentrations as expected

Pericardial constriction

Obesity

Cardiac tamponade

Flash pulmonary edema

HF diagnosis), whereas higher values support but do not make a diagnosis of HF per se (ie, not all patients with high NP levels are have HF). Indeed, several cardiac and noncardiac conditions cause increased NP levels (eg, atrial fibrillation and renal impairment) (**Box 1**).

However, NPs show good diagnostic accuracy in discerning HF from other causes of dyspnea: the higher the NP levels, the higher the likelihood that dyspnea is caused by HF. For example, in patients with preexisting chronic obstructive pulmonary disease, NPs can be valuable in diagnosing masked coexisting HF.

Therefore, in all patients presenting with dyspnea, the American guidelines recommend the measurement of NP levels to support the diagnosis or the exclusion of HF (class I, level of evidence [LOE] A),[2,3,11] with ESC guidelines on the same page.

Are natriuretic peptides interchangeable?

Both NPs (BNP and NT-proBNP) can be used in patient care settings. Overall, they have comparable diagnostic accurateness. However, it is important to consider that their values are not interchangeable. Although some conversion formulas have been suggested, these have no role in clinical practice.[53]

Notably, in patients having angiotensin receptor neprilysin inhibition (ARNI) treatment, BNP assessment is not reliable, and NT-proBNP levels should be considered.[46] In addition, even if both NPs are reported to be predictive of outcome, BNP levels are confusing, particularly in the early phase of switching to and uptitrating ARNI.[54]

Imaging Biomarkers

Among imaging biomarkers, transthoracic echocardiography (TTE) is an indispensable tool in the diagnosis of patients with HF. American guidelines recommend that all patients with suspected, acute, or new-onset HF should have a TTE performed (class I, LOE C).[2,3] European guidelines recommend TTE for the assessment of myocardial structure and function in all patients with suspected HF in order to establish a diagnosis of HFrEF, HFmrEF, or HFpEF (class I, LOE C).[1]

Ejection fraction

EF is the most important parameter to evaluate, and the modified biplane Simpson rule is recommended by international guidelines. LV end-diastolic volume (LVEDV) and LV end-systolic volume (LVESV) should be obtained from apical 4-chamber and 2-chamber views. Based on EF, at least 2 different HF phenotypes can be identified:

- HFrEF: EF less than 40%
- HFpEF: EF greater than 50%

Patients with EF between 40% and 50% are defined as HFpEF borderline in American guidelines, whereas they are defined as a new entity in the latest European guidelines: HF-mrEF.[1]

In this context, the latest British Society of Echocardiography guidelines suggests that an EF of 50% to 54% should be considered as borderline low rather than normal LV EF.[55]

Diastolic function

Evaluation of diastolic function with TTE represents another fundamental imaging biomarker. The evaluation of diastolic function together with evaluation of the filling pressures, through the measurement of parameters such as mitral inflow during early diastole (E) recorded by pulsed Doppler between the tips of the mitral leaflets, the average of septal and lateral mitral annular early diastolic peak velocities (e') recorded by tissue Doppler, and its ratio (E/e'), are now considered mandatory for a basic TTE in patients with HF. Further, the end-systolic maximal volume of the left atrium indexed for body surface area (left atrial volume index) represents a surrogate marker of LV filling pressures.

Full description of these parameters is available[56]; however, for the purpose of the present article, the latest cutoff is reported as suggested by the ESC in the HFA-PEFF diagnostic algorithm for the diagnosis of HFpEF[52]:

- Septal and lateral mitral annular peak early diastolic velocity (e'; the main determinant of e' is LV relaxation)
  - Major criteria:
    - Septal e' less than 7 cm/s; or lateral e' less than 10 cm/s in patients aged less than 75 years
    - Septal e' less than 5 cm/; or lateral e' less than 7 cm/s in patients aged greater than 75 years
- Average septal-lateral E/e' ratio (reflecting the mean pulmonary capillary wedge pressure):
  - Major criterion: average septal-lateral E/e' ratio greater than or equal to 15
  - Minor criterion: average septal-lateral E/e' ratio 9 to 14
- Left atrial volume index
  - Major criteria:
    - Greater than 34 mL/m^2 in sinus rhythm
    - Greater than 40 mL/m^2 in atrial fibrillation
  - Minor criteria:
    - From 29 to 34 mL/m^2 in sinus rhythm
    - From 34 to 40 mL/m^2 in atrial fibrillation

With regard to left atrial volume index, the latest British Society of Echocardiography guidelines introduced a new borderline LA volume range of 34 to 38 mL/m^2.[55]

RISK STRATIFICATION

The most active research topic in biomarkers is the search for biomarkers able to identify patients with HF with worse outcomes. Again, NPs are the most validated, with current guidelines recommending measurement of NPs on admission (class of recommendation (COR) I, LOE A) and predischarge (COR IIa, LOE B) to assess HF prognosis.[3] In addition, it has been suggested that NPs alone have at least the same reclassification capability of HF clinical scores in predicting HF prognosis.[57] Therefore, this article does not discuss these biomarkers here, to avoid redundancy with other publications. However, other biomarkers showed their importance in risk stratification,[58] and, even if they have not yet entered into clinical practice, they warrant further discussion.

Therefore, a quick overview is provided here of the best-validated biomarkers (ie, troponins, ST-2, galectin 3) and the emerging biomarkers with most robust evidence investigated (ie, trimethylamine N-oxide [TMAO] and hormones) are briefly described.

Troponins

cTn are biomarkers of myocyte injury and are the cornerstone of the diagnosis of myocardial infarction.[59] However, in patients with HF, circulating cTn can be detected regardless of the presence of coronary artery disease.[60] For instance, in different cohorts, it has been shown that high-sensitivity assays may detect cTn at greater than the 99th upper reference limit in about 50% (ASCEND-HF trial) or 90% (Relaxin in Acute Heart Failure [RELAX-AHF]) of patients presenting with acute HF.[61–63] cTn was shown to have prognostic value in acute HF. A retrospective analysis from the Acute Decompensated Heart Failure National Registry (ADHERE) suggested that detection of cTn was associated with an increased risk of in-hospital mortality, and the higher the increase, the higher the risk[64]; further, increased cTn level was associated with an increased risk of intensive care admission, mechanical circulatory support, and mechanical ventilation.[64] In the RELAX-AHF study, cTn levels were higher in patients with lower blood pressure, EF, and incidence of atrial fibrillation, and increased baseline cTn levels were associated with adverse cardiovascular events; with regard long-term outcomes (>6 months), inconclusive results were derived from trials. Although in RELAX-AHF they were associated, in the ASCEND-HF, cTn predicted in-hospital outcome but was not an independent predictor of long-term outcomes.[63]

With regard to the chronic setting, it is common to detect circulating cTn in CHF (CHF) and the likelihood increases depending on the sensitivity of the assay used.[65] Increased high-sensitivity cTn level was an independent risk factor for mortality and adverse outcome in patients with CHF in several studies. Troponin level increase may be useful in predicting mortality in patients with CHF and may have a complementary role to NP measurement in this context.[66–68]

In summary, cTn levels are associated with an increased risk of morbidity and mortality in both acute HF and CHF, providing incremental prognostic information. Therefore, it is recommended to assess (COR I, LOE A) baseline levels of cTn on admission to the hospital because of their utility to establish a prognosis in acutely decompensated HF.[3]

Source of Tumorigenicity 2

Source of tumorigenicity 2 (ST2), first described in 1989, is a member of the interleukin (IL)-1 receptor family, secreted in response to mechanical strain, therefore reflecting myocardial stretch.[69,70] The Pro-Brain Natriuretic Peptide Investigation of Dyspnea in the Emergency Department study showed that concentrations of sST2 were higher in patients who were dead at 1 year compared with survivors, with a cutoff of 20 pg/mL predicting mortality.[71] Recently, it has been shown that sST2 has a diurnal rhythm, with lower values in the morning.[72] Notably, sST2 was less influenced by age than NT-proBNP and cTn; the addition of age-specific and outcome-specific cutoffs of sST2 to NT-proBNP and cTn allowed a more accurate risk stratification than NT-proBNP alone or the combination of NT-proBNP and troponins.[73] No ethnicity differences have been shown,[74] whereas men showed higher levels than women.[49] A score based on ST has been proposed as a predictor of sudden cardiac death (ST2-SCD score).[75] Several findings suggest that sST2 granted a strong and independent predictive value for poor outcome in CHF.[76] As a cutoff, a level of 35 pg/mL in the outpatient setting seems to define low-risk patients.[77]

In summary, sST2 seems to be the most promising of the novel biomarkers, with the advantage of not being affected by age, renal function, body mass index, atrial fibrillation, and other comorbidities.[78] On one hand, ESC guidelines concluded that there is no definite evidence to recommend sST2 for clinical practice[1]; however, the American guidelines recommend the use of sST2 in addition to NPs in risk stratification (class IIB, LOE B).[3]

Galectin-3

Gal-3, also known as carbohydrate-binding protein 35, is a protein acting on fibroblasts and macrophages activation[79,80] with profibrotic actions. Women showed higher levels compared with men,[49] possibly related to fat mass.[81] It has been shown among patients with dyspnea referred to emergency departments that Gal-3 concentrations were associated with echocardiographic markers of ventricular dysfunction, with the ability to predict mortality in acute HF.[82]

As a prognostic biomarker, Gal-3 is an independent marker for outcome in HF, and seems to be particularly useful in patients with HFpEF.[83] Further it has been shown that higher Gal-3 levels at discharge after an acute decompensation predict later events[84] and early HF rehospitalization. However, a head-to-head comparison of fibrosis biomarkers ST2 and Gal-3 in CHF revealed superiority of ST2 to Gal-3 in risk stratification.[85]

In summary, similar to sST2, ESC guidelines concluded that there is no definite evidence to recommend Gal-3 for clinical practice, whereas the American guidelines recommend the use of Gal-3 in addition to NPs in risk stratification (class IIB, LOE B).[3]

Trimethylamine N-oxide

A novel pathophysiologic model of interest is the association between HF and the gastrointestinal (GI) system,[86,87] the so-called gut hypothesis.[88]

In recent years, TMAO, a gut microbiota–mediated metabolite originating from the metabolism of choline and carnitine, has been thought to be the missing link between the Western diet and cardiovascular disease risk,[89,90] shown to be a strong prognostic biomarker in both acute[91,92] and stable CHF,[93–98] with some intriguing geographic[99] and ethnicity differences.[100] Further, it seems to be a promising biomarker when combined with NPs in patients with HFpEF.[101]

To date, despite growing evidence, no guideline recommendations have been provided with regard to TMAO's role in HF.

Hormones

A growing body of evidence suggests that, in addition to neurohormonal hyperactivity, the imbalance between catabolic and anabolic hormonal axes depicts HF progression.[102–106] In this context, it has been shown that HF could be considered as a multiple hormone deficiency syndrome (MHDS).[107,108] Each component of MHDS (eg, growth hormone [GH]/insulinlike growth factor [IGF]-1 axes, thyroid hormones, androgens, insulin resistance) is associated with impaired functional capacity and poor clinical outcome.[102,105–113] Furthermore, HF prognosis has been shown to be strictly related to the number of coexistent deficiencies,[105] in line with the important relationship between hormones and the cardiovascular system shown in other clinical settings.[114–117] Notably, the prevalence of hormonal deficiency is increased in HF and consequently is related to poor cardiovascular performance and prognosis[107,108]; further, targeted hormone replacement therapy leads to an improvement in cardiovascular performance and outcomes.[118–122] These data provide strong evidence to suggest that the reversal of MHDS should be considered as an exciting and novel strategy in HF management.[123,124]

In this context, the latest version of the AHA guidelines on dilated cardiomyopathies suggest testing for thyroid disorders (LOE C) and GH/IGF-1 disorders (ie, acromegaly and GH deficiency) (LOE C) in patients with dilated cardiomyopathy and that appropriate therapy should be performed to correct a thyroid disorder (LOE C), acromegaly, or GH deficiency when present (LOE C).[125] Furthermore, thyroid hormone assessment should be considered in the initial HF assessment (LOE C).[2]

With regard to ESC guidelines, thyroid disorders have been confirmed and included as possible causes of dilated cardiomyopathies,[126] with thyroid-stimulating hormone recommended in the initial assessment of patients with HF (class I, LOE C).[1] For GH/IGF-1, acromegaly but not GH deficiency has been indicated as a possible causal factor of dilated cardiomyopathies,[126] whereas GH deficiency has been indicated as a possible cause of HF, both with reduced[1] and preserved EF.[52]

Although the American guidelines do not recommend the use of testosterone,[2] European guidelines cautiously suggest a possible role in the treatment of sarcopenia and cachexia.[1]

Emerging Biomarkers

Cell-free DNA

Circulating cell-free DNA (cfDNA) is genomic DNA released as result of cell death mechanisms.[127] Mostly investigated in oncology, it has been shown to be associated with cardiovascular risk factors,[128–131] cardiovascular diseases (eg, acute myocardial infarction and atrial fibrillation),[130] and with the early diagnosis of heart transplant rejection.[132–134] Recently, in 71 consecutive patients with chronic stable HFrEF and HFmrEF, cfDNA levels showed association with morbidity and mortality in HF; as a result, liquid biopsy may be considered an additional tool in risk stratification.[135]

Proenkephalin

Proenkephalin, a 243-amino-acid precursor for endogenous opioid peptides interacting with delta-receptors for morphine (ie, enkephalins), has been shown to have a role in HF because of its relationship with sympathetic activation.[136] Because of their short-half life, enkephalins are difficult to assess, whereas the product of the proenkephalin cleavage, the proenkephalin molecular form 119-159 (PENK) is stable in plasma and cerebrospinal fluid for at least 48 hours.[136] For this reason, together with the notion that proenkephalin is the predominant source of mature enkephalin, this peptide fragment could serve as a surrogate measurement of systemic enkephalin synthesis. With regard to HF, it has been suggested that higher PENK levels are associated with lower EF and kidney function, and poor outcome in both acute and chronic HFrEF.[137–140] Further, it has been shown that PENK levels are related to body mass index, diastolic dysfunction, and prognosis in HFpEF.[141]

Therefore, PENK represents an interesting emerging biomarker reflecting cardiac, glomerular, and tubular dysfunction, giving remarkable information about the intricate relationship among the opioid systems and HF.

Adrenomedullin

It has been suggested that adrenomedullin (ADM), a vasodilatory peptide originally described in pheochromocytoma tissues and expressed in the heart, vasculature, and the kidneys, has positive inotropic, antiapoptotic, angiogenic, antiinflammatory, and antioxidant effects, acting as a protective factor in HF.[142] Several reports showed that plasma ADM levels are increased in HF, strictly related to HF severity.[143–145] Further, the midregional pro-ADM showed a good role in risk stratification.[146–148] In addition, it has been shown that bioactive ADM in plasma is associated with increased biventricular filling pressures in patients with advanced HF.[149] It has been shown that beneficial vasodilatory, diuretic, natriuretic, and positive inotropic effects are exerted by its acute administration in HF.[142]

MicroRNA

Recent evidence suggests that there are genome portions, previously known as junk DNA, that are transcribed and give rise to a large and heterogeneous family of RNA molecules with a variety of functions. These regulatory molecules seem to be a promising tool in diagnostics, therapeutics, and personalized medicine in HF.[150] For instance, angiogenic early-outgrowth cells from patients with CHF show reduced miR-126 and miR-130a expression levels, with subsequent impaired ability to improve cardiac function,[151] whereas expression levels of miR-126 and miR-508-5p in endothelial progenitor cells have been shown to be prognostic for CHF in patients with cardiomyopathy.[152] Moreover, several studies have shown that circulating microRNAs can react in a dynamic way in response to therapy, indicating potential efficacy of treatment.[153]

Fibroblast growth factor-23

High levels of fibroblast growth factor-23, a phosphaturic hormone regulating phosphate metabolism acting on kidney phosphate absorption and vitamin D production, have been shown to be related to clinical severity and adverse outcomes in HFrEF,[154] with a strict link with volume overload, worse renal function, and an independent association with less successful uptitration of guideline-recommended angiotensin-converting-enzyme inhibitors (ACEi)/angiotensin receptor blocker (ARB) therapy.[155] Notably, it also seems a promising biomarker for patients with HFpEF,[156] showing association with reduced exercise capacity and increased risk of death.[157]

PHENOTYPING

A recent research field of interest, fueled by the unknown HFmrEF group of patients previously considered to be in the gray zone by the ESC,[1] is focused on the possibility of identifying specific biomarkers for specific HF phenotypes.[158] Identifying the pathophysiologic pathways most involved in the different HF phenotypes would allow a better tailoring of management and treatment.

It has been shown that the 3 different HF phenotypes (ie, HFpEF, HFmrEF, and HFrEF), despite sharing some common features, are characterized by different pathophysiologic indices, different clinical comorbidities, different response to treatment, and different prognosis.[159] Therefore, the possibility of distinguishing peculiar biomarker pathways and different pathophysiologic routes involved, with the aim of identifying possible specific therapeutic targets, represents one of the possible uses of biomarkers.

General Features

It has been proved that HFpEF is characterized by myocardial dysfunction driven by a very high proinflammatory systemic state also affecting microvascular endothelium, with increased plasma levels of IL-6, tumor necrosis factor-α, sST2, and pentraxin 3 and resulting in an increase in reactive oxygen species (ROS) production.[160] In contrast, myocardial dysfunction, typical in HFrEF, is characterized by ROS production caused by cardiac ischemia, infections, or toxic agents.[160] As a result, these differences are documented by the different expression of biomarkers, particularly those related to myocardial stress (eg, NPs), myocardial injury (eg, troponins), fibrosis (eg, ST2), inflammation (eg, high-sensitivity C-reactive protein), and hematopoiesis (eg, hemoglobin). In particular, myocardial stress/injury is more pronounced in HFrEF, whereas HFpEF is more characterized by inflammation and fibrosis, after adjustment for several confounders (ie, comorbidities).[161,162]

Recently, a network analysis confirmed that HFrEF showed a peculiar biomarker profile related to cellular proliferation and metabolism, whereas HFpEF biomarker profiles are related to inflammation and extracellular matrix reorganization.[163]

Specific Biomarkers

- NPs: because NPs are released in the blood as a response to LV end-diastolic stress in patients with HFpEF, being wall stress counteracted by the typical hypertrophy of HFpEF, NP levels are less increased or normal in HFpEF.[52]
- Troponins: it has been shown that troponin levels are more increased in HFrEF than in HFpEF.[161,162] To date, no different cutoffs have been suggested in clinic practice.

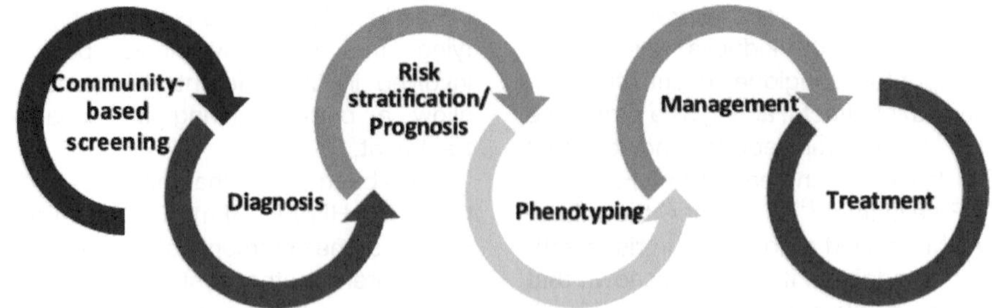

Fig. 3. The 'Biomarkers Continuum' in Heart Failure.

- ST2, galectin: ST2 and Gal-3are more increased in HFpEF.
- TMAO: several studies have shown the role of TMAO in HFrEF.[87,93–98] With regard to HFpEF, results are less consistent[95]; however, it has been shown that the combination of TMAO with NPs is the most valuable tool in this group of patients.[101]
- Hormones: the presence of a catabolic/anabolic imbalance in HF has been clearly shown in HFrEF (discussed next). Patients with HFpEF seem to have a lower prevalence of hormone deficiencies, however, a strong association with outcomes has been showed in HFpEF too.[108]

MANAGEMENT AND TAILORED TREATMENT

An emerging body of evidence suggests that serial measurement of biomarkers could have a positive role in HF management, allowing a tailored management approach. However, despite BNP measurements at discharge/follow-up (ie, serial measurements) showing prognostic association,[164] and BNP reduction in response to guideline-recommended HF treatment being reported to add value to tailoring risk, the proper role of serial NP measurements in clinical practice still remains a matter of debate.[164,165]

It has been clearly shown that HF treatment directly or indirectly affects processes related to increase of NP levels.[164,165] β-Blockers, ACEi/ARBs, magnetic resonance angiography, and cardiac resynchronization therapy lead to a reduction in NP levels.[166–170] Data from several studies showed that NP concentration 2 to 4 weeks after a therapy change gives the best prognostic value, suggesting that this can be considered an appropriate window to reassess NP values after medical titration.[171]

With regard to serial NP measurements, it has been shown that follow-up levels after treatment showed better association with adverse outcomes compared with baseline levels.[172–175] Further, it has been suggested that personalized scheduling of NP measurements performs similarly with respect to the prediction of recurrent events but requires fewer total measurements than fixed scheduling.[176,177]

Given these premises, several trials investigated the role of NP-guided HF management, with conflicting results. Some trials showed a clear benefit (eg, the Use of NT-proBNP Testing to Guide Heart Failure Therapy in the Outpatient Setting [PROTECT] trial,[178] the Systolic Heart Failure Treatment Supported by BNP [STARS-BNP][179] trial, and others[180,181]) or a positive trend (eg, the NT-proBNP-Assisted Treatment to Lessen Serial Cardiac Readmissions and Death [BATTLESCARRED] and the Trial of Intensified vs Standard Medical Therapy in Elderly Patients With Congestive Heart Failure [TIME-CHF] study) when a biomarker-guided HF treatment approach was used. However, other trials have shown neutral results (eg, the Swedish Intervention Study–Guidelines and NT-ProBNP Analysis in Heart Failure [SIGNAL-HF],[171] the Can Pro-brain-natriuretic Peptide Guided Therapy of Chronic Heart Failure Improve Heart Failure Morbidity and Mortality [PRIMA] study,[182] the Use of Peptides in Tailoring Heart Failure Project [UPSTEP],[183] and the Strategies for Tailoring Advanced Heart Failure Regimens in the Outpatient Setting: Brain Natriuretic Peptide Versus the Clinical Congestion Score [STARBITE] study[184]). In this context, although preliminary results of the GUIDE-IT trial showed guideline-directed medical therapy guided by NT-proBNP levels was not superior to guideline-directed medical treatment alone,[185] a following analysis showed that patients whose levels at follow-up decreased (NT-proBNP levels ≤1000 pg/mL) had better outcomes.[186] However, when results from several randomized clinical trials were combined, different metanalyses reported that HF management and treatment titration incorporating serial NPs levels was associated with a significant reduction of outcomes compared with usual care.[187–192]

Recently, an interesting study performed by the BIOSTAT-CHF consortium showed that uptitrating patients with HF based on biomarker values might have resulted in fewer deaths or hospitalizations compared with a hypothetical scenario in which patients were uptitrated without considering biomarkers levels.[193]

With regard to cTn, it has been shown that serial measurements of cTn may have a value in the risk stratification of patients with CHF and perhaps intensification of treatment.[194,195]

Hormone-based markers, testifying to hormone deficiencies, can be directly considered as therapeutic targets, with replacement treatment showing benefit in HF cardiovascular performance and outcome.[118,120,122] Therefore, their serial measurements, after correction of specific hormone deficit, can be specifically used to guide treatment on top of HF guidelines. Second, in the BIOSTAT-CHF consortium, TMAO was not directly affected by medication uptitration, suggesting the need to search for other complimentary treatments to decrease its levels.[97] Neither of these 2 biomarkers has clinical approval; however, given the promising supporting literature, their status as promising emerging biomarkers to clinical translation is well deserved.

SUMMARY

In conclusion, beyond NPs, other well-known or emerging biomarkers are under investigation to provide useful clinical information in HF management, which is becoming ever more personalized and tailored. The most valuable approach seems to be the multiparameter approach, specifically when different types of biomarkers (eg, circulating and imaging) and biomarkers from different pathophysiologic pathways are combined. Further, in the present review, the authors have spotlighted that several biomarkers have different potential roles, identifying the concept of a biomarker continuum in HF (**Fig. 3**). However, further robust randomized trials are needed before novel biomarkers can enter clinical practice.

DISCLOSURE STATEMENT

Dr Salzano receives research grant support from Cardiopath, Department of Advanced Biomedical Sciences, Federico II University of Naples, Naples, Italy, and UniNa and Compagnia di San Paolo, in the frame of the Programme STAR. Dr Marra was supported by an institutional grant from Italian Healthcare Ministry (Ricerca Finalizzata for young researchers) project GR-2016-02364727.

CLINICS CARE POINTS

- Population screening with NPs followed by echocardiography is a promising approach; specifically, the measurement of NPs or cardiac troponins alone adds prognostic information to standard risk factors for predicting new-onset HF, with the measurement of emerging biomarkers (i.e. sST2, Gal-3, GDF-15, and markers of renal function) alone or in a multi-marker strategy, providing additional risk stratification; however there is still no evidence of cost-effectiveness to justify its adoption at a large scale.
- Biomarkers (circulating and imaging) have an essential role in HF diagnosis. Without doubt, NPs can be considered the gold standard circulating biomarkers with elevated levels helping to identify subjects in need of a further evaluation and lower levels helping to exclude HF diagnosis, regardless of phenotype.
- The most active research topic in the biomarker field is the search for biomarkers able to identify HF patients with a worse outcome. Again, NPs are the most validated, with current guidelines recommending measurement of NPs on admission and predischarge to assess HF prognosis. However, other biomarkers showed their importance in risk stratification (e.g. troponins, source of tumorigenicity 2, galectin-3, Trimethylamine N-oxide, hormones) and even if they have not yet entered into clinical practice, they warrant further discussion.
- A recent research field of interest is focused on the possibility of identifying specific biomarkers for specific HF phenotypes. Indeed, the possibility to identify pathophysiological pathways mostly involved in the different HF phenotypes would allow a better tailoring of management and treatment.

REFERENCES

1. Ponikowski P, Voors AA, Anker SD, et al. 2016 ESC Guidelines for the diagnosis and treatment of acute and chronic heart failure: the task force for the diagnosis and treatment of acute and chronic heart failure of the European society of cardiology (ESC). Developed with the special contribution of the heart failure association (HFA) of the ESC. Eur J Heart Fail 2016;18(8):891–975.
2. Yancy CW, Jessup M, Bozkurt B, et al. 2013 ACCF/AHA guideline for the management of heart failure: a report of the American college of cardiology foundation/American heart association task force on practice guidelines. J Am Coll Cardiol 2013;62(16):e147–239 (In eng).
3. Yancy CW, Jessup M, Bozkurt B, et al. 2017 ACC/AHA/HFSA Focused update of the 2013 ACCF/AHA Guideline for the management of heart failure:

a report of the American College of Cardiology/ American heart association task force on clinical practice guidelines and the heart failure society of America. J Am Coll Cardiol 2017;70(6): 776–803 (In eng).
4. Braunwald E. Heart failure. JACC Heart Fail 2013; 1(1):1–20.
5. Benjamin EJ, Virani SS, Callaway CW, et al. Heart disease and stroke statistics-2018 update: a report from the American heart association. Circulation 2018;137(12):e67–492.
6. Suzuki T. Cardiovascular diagnostic biomarkers: the past, present and future. Circ J 2009;73(5): 806–9.
7. Israr MZ, Heaney LM, Suzuki T. Proteomic biomarkers of heart failure. Heart Fail Clin 2018; 14(1):93–107 (In eng).
8. Suzuki T, Bossone E. Biomarkers of heart failure: past, present, and future. Heart Fail Clin 2018; 14(1):ix–x.
9. Nymo SH, Aukrust P, Kjekshus J, et al. Limited added value of circulating inflammatory biomarkers in chronic heart failure. JACC Heart Fail 2017;5(4):256–64.
10. Salzano A, Marra AM, D'Assante R, et al. Biomarkers and imaging: complementary or subtractive? Heart Fail Clin 2019;15(2):321–31 (In eng).
11. Chow SL, Maisel AS, Anand I, et al. Role of biomarkers for the prevention, assessment, and management of heart failure: a scientific statement from the American heart association. Circulation 2017; 135(22):e1054–91 (In eng).
12. Biomarkers Definitions Working G. Biomarkers and surrogate endpoints: preferred definitions and conceptual framework. Clin Pharmacol Ther 2001; 69(3):89–95.
13. Braunwald E. Biomarkers in heart failure. N Engl J Med 2008;358(20):2148–59.
14. Naylor S. Biomarkers: current perspectives and future prospects. Expert Rev Mol Diagn 2003; 3(5):525–9.
15. Ibrahim NE, Gaggin HK, Konstam MA, et al. Established and emerging roles of biomarkers in heart failure clinical trials. Circ Heart Fail 2016;9(9). https://doi.org/10.1161/CIRCHEARTFAILURE.115.002528.
16. Januzzi JL Jr. Will biomarkers succeed as a surrogate endpoint in heart failure trials? JACC Heart Fail 2018;6(7):570–2.
17. Ghashghaei R, Arbit B, Maisel AS. Current and novel biomarkers in heart failure: bench to bedside. Curr Opin Cardiol 2016;31(2):191–5.
18. Suzuki T, Lyon A, Saggar R, et al. Editor's choice-biomarkers of acute cardiovascular and pulmonary diseases. Eur Heart J Acute Cardiovasc Care 2016;5(5):416–33 (In eng).
19. Drucker E, Krapfenbauer K. Pitfalls and limitations in translation from biomarker discovery to clinical utility in predictive and personalised medicine. EPMA J 2013;4(1):7.
20. Mayeux R. Biomarkers: potential uses and limitations. NeuroRx 2004;1(2):182–8.
21. Morrow DA, de Lemos JA. Benchmarks for the assessment of novel cardiovascular biomarkers. Circulation 2007;115(8):949–52.
22. Ledwidge M, Gallagher J, Conlon C, et al. Natriuretic peptide-based screening and collaborative care for heart failure: the STOP-HF randomized trial. JAMA 2013;310(1):66–74 (In eng).
23. Ledwidge MT, O'Connell E, Gallagher J, et al. Cost-effectiveness of natriuretic peptide-based screening and collaborative care: a report from the STOP-HF (St Vincent's Screening TO Prevent Heart Failure) study. Eur J Heart Fail 2015;17(7): 672–9 (In eng).
24. McGrady M, Reid CM, Shiel L, et al. NT-proB natriuretic peptide, risk factors and asymptomatic left ventricular dysfunction: results of the SCReening evaluation of the evolution of new heart failure study (SCREEN-HF). Int J Cardiol 2013;169(2): 133–8 (In eng).
25. Campbell DJ, Gong FF, Jelinek MV, et al. Prediction of incident heart failure by serum amino-terminal pro-B-type natriuretic peptide level in a community-based cohort. Eur J Heart Fail 2019; 21(4):449–59 (In eng).
26. Loke I, Squire IB, Davies JE, et al. Reference ranges for natriuretic peptides for diagnostic use are dependent on age, gender and heart rate. Eur J Heart Fail 2003;5(5):599–606 (In eng).
27. Natriuretic Peptides Studies Collaboration, Willeit P, Kaptoge S, et al. Natriuretic peptides and integrated risk assessment for cardiovascular disease: an individual-participant-data meta-analysis. Lancet Diabetes Endocrinol 2016;4(10):840–9 (In eng).
28. Squire I. Measurement of circulating natriuretic peptides to identify community-based patients at risk of incident heart failure - should we? Eur J Heart Fail 2019;21(4):460–1 (In eng).
29. Gaggin HK, Abboud A. Prediction of incident heart failure: is it time for routine screening? JACC Heart Fail 2020;8(5):412–4 (In eng).
30. Clerico A, Zaninotto M, Passino C, et al. Evidence on clinical relevance of cardiovascular risk evaluation in the general population using cardio-specific biomarkers. Clin Chem Lab Med 2020. https://doi.org/10.1515/cclm-2020-0310 (In eng).
31. deFilippi CR, de Lemos JA, Christenson RH, et al. Association of serial measures of cardiac troponin T using a sensitive assay with incident heart failure and cardiovascular mortality in older adults. JAMA 2010;304(22):2494–502 (In eng).

32. Yan I, Börschel CS, Neumann JT, et al. High-sensitivity cardiac troponin I levels and prediction of heart failure: results from the BiomarCaRE consortium. JACC Heart Fail 2020;8(5):401–11 (In eng).
33. Brouwers FP, van Gilst WH, Damman K, et al. Clinical risk stratification optimizes value of biomarkers to predict new-onset heart failure in a community-based cohort. Circ Heart Fail 2014;7(5):723–31 (In eng).
34. Hughes MF, Appelbaum S, Havulinna AS, et al. ST2 may not be a useful predictor for incident cardiovascular events, heart failure and mortality. Heart 2014;100(21):1715–21 (In eng).
35. Wang TJ, Wollert KC, Larson MG, et al. Prognostic utility of novel biomarkers of cardiovascular stress: the Framingham Heart Study. Circulation 2012; 126(13):1596–604 (In eng).
36. Davies M, Hobbs F, Davis R, et al. Prevalence of left-ventricular systolic dysfunction and heart failure in the echocardiographic heart of England screening study: a population based study. Lancet 2001;358(9280):439–44 (In eng).
37. Ng LL, Loke I, Davies JE, et al. Identification of previously undiagnosed left ventricular systolic dysfunction: community screening using natriuretic peptides and electrocardiography. Eur J Heart Fail 2003;5(6):775–82 (In eng).
38. Heidenreich PA, Gubens MA, Fonarow GC, et al. Cost-effectiveness of screening with B-type natriuretic peptide to identify patients with reduced left ventricular ejection fraction. J Am Coll Cardiol 2004;43(6):1019–26 (In eng).
39. Gori M, Lam CS, D'Elia E, et al. Integrating natriuretic peptides and diastolic dysfunction to predict adverse events in high-risk asymptomatic subjects (In eng). Eur J Prev Cardiol 2020. https://doi.org/10.1177/2047487319899618.
40. Ng LL, Loke IW, Davies JE, et al. Community screening for left ventricular systolic dysfunction using plasma and urinary natriuretic peptides. J Am Coll Cardiol 2005;45(7):1043–50 (In eng).
41. Ng LL, Pathik B, Loke IW, et al. Myeloperoxidase and C-reactive protein augment the specificity of B-type natriuretic peptide in community screening for systolic heart failure. Am Heart J 2006;152(1): 94–101 (In eng).
42. Lainscak M, Omersa D, Sedlar N, et al. Heart failure prevalence in the general population: SOBOTA-HF study rationale and design. ESC Heart Fail 2019;6(5):1077–84 (In eng).
43. Piepoli MF, Abreu A, Albus C, et al. Update on cardiovascular prevention in clinical practice: a position paper of the European association of preventive cardiology of the european society of cardiology. Eur J Prev Cardiol 2020;27(2): 181–205 (In eng).
44. Maisel AS, Duran JM, Wettersten N. Natriuretic peptides in heart failure: atrial and B-type natriuretic peptides. Heart Fail Clin 2018;14(1):13–25 (In eng).
45. Richards AM. N-terminal B-type natriuretic peptide in heart failure. Heart Fail Clin 2018;14(1):27–39 (In eng).
46. Mueller C, McDonald K, de Boer RA, et al. Heart failure association of the European society of cardiology practical guidance on the use of natriuretic peptide concentrations. Eur J Heart Fail 2019; 21(6):715–31 (In eng).
47. Salzano A, Demelo-Rodriguez P, Marra AM, et al. A focused review of gender differences in antithrombotic therapy. Curr Med Chem 2017;24(24): 2576–88 (In eng).
48. Marra AM, Benjamin N, Eichstaedt C, et al. Gender-related differences in pulmonary arterial hypertension targeted drugs administration. Pharmacol Res 2016;114:103–9 (In eng).
49. Suthahar N, Meems LMG, Ho JE, et al. Sex-related differences in contemporary biomarkers for heart failure: a review. Eur J Heart Fail 2020;22(5): 775–88 (In eng).
50. Marra AM, Salzano A, Arcopinto M, et al. The impact of gender in cardiovascular medicine: Lessons from the gender/sex-issue in heart failure. Monaldi Arch Chest Dis 2018;88(3):988 (In eng).
51. Faxén UL, Lund LH, Orsini N, et al. N-terminal pro-B-type natriuretic peptide in chronic heart failure: the impact of sex across the ejection fraction spectrum. Int J Cardiol 2019;287:66–72 (In eng).
52. Pieske B, Tschöpe C, de Boer RA, et al. How to diagnose heart failure with preserved ejection fraction: the HFA-PEFF diagnostic algorithm: a consensus recommendation from the heart failure Association (HFA) of the European society of cardiology (ESC). Eur Heart J 2019;40(40):3297–317 (In eng).
53. Kasahara S, Sakata Y, Nochioka K, et al. Conversion formula from B-type natriuretic peptide to N-terminal proBNP values in patients with cardiovascular diseases. Int J Cardiol 2019;280:184–9 (In eng).
54. Myhre PL, Vaduganathan M, Claggett B, et al. B-Type natriuretic peptide during treatment with Sacubitril/Valsartan: the PARADIGM-HF trial. J Am Coll Cardiol 2019;73(11):1264–72 (In eng).
55. Harkness A, Ring L, Augustine DX, et al. Normal reference intervals for cardiac dimensions and function for use in echocardiographic practice: a guideline from the British Society of Echocardiography. Echo Res Pract 2020;7(1):G1–18 (In eng).
56. Nagueh SF, Smiseth OA, Appleton CP, et al. Recommendations for the evaluation of left ventricular diastolic function by echocardiography: an update from the American society of echocardiography and the European association of cardiovascular

imaging. Eur Heart J Cardiovasc Imaging 2016; 17(12):1321–60 (In eng).
57. Arzilli C, Aimo A, Vergaro G, et al. N-terminal fraction of pro-B-type natriuretic peptide versus clinical risk scores for prognostic stratification in chronic systolic heart failure. Eur J Prev Cardiol 2018; 25(8):889–95 (In eng).
58. Rabkin SW, Tang JKK. The utility of growth differentiation factor-15, galectin-3, and sST2 as biomarkers for the diagnosis of heart failure with preserved ejection fraction and compared to heart failure with reduced ejection fraction: a systematic review. Heart Fail Rev 2020. https://doi.org/10.1007/s10741-020-09913-3 (In eng).
59. Thygesen K, Alpert JS, Jaffe AS, et al. Fourth universal definition of myocardial infarction (2018). J Am Coll Cardiol 2018;72(18):2231–64 (In eng).
60. Kociol RD, Pang PS, Gheorghiade M, et al. Troponin elevation in heart failure prevalence, mechanisms, and clinical implications. J Am Coll Cardiol 2010;56(14):1071–8 (In eng).
61. Pascual-Figal DA, Manzano-Fernández S, Boronat M, et al. Soluble ST2, high-sensitivity troponin T- and N-terminal pro-B-type natriuretic peptide: complementary role for risk stratification in acutely decompensated heart failure. Eur J Heart Fail 2011;13(7):718–25 (In eng).
62. Felker GM, Mentz RJ, Teerlink JR, et al. Serial high sensitivity cardiac troponin T measurement in acute heart failure: insights from the RELAX-AHF study. Eur J Heart Fail 2015;17(12):1262–70 (In eng).
63. Felker GM, Hasselblad V, Tang WH, et al. Troponin I in acute decompensated heart failure: insights from the ASCEND-HF study. Eur J Heart Fail 2012;14(11):1257–64 (In eng).
64. Peacock WF, De Marco T, Fonarow GC, et al. Cardiac troponin and outcome in acute heart failure. N Engl J Med 2008;358(20):2117–26 (In eng).
65. Januzzi JL, Filippatos G, Nieminen M, et al. Troponin elevation in patients with heart failure: on behalf of the third universal definition of myocardial infarction global task force: heart failure section. Eur Heart J 2012;33(18):2265–71 (In eng).
66. Horwich TB, Patel J, MacLellan WR, et al. Cardiac troponin I is associated with impaired hemodynamics, progressive left ventricular dysfunction, and increased mortality rates in advanced heart failure. Circulation 2003;108(7):833–8 (In eng).
67. Tsutamoto T, Kawahara C, Nishiyama K, et al. Prognostic role of highly sensitive cardiac troponin I in patients with systolic heart failure. Am Heart J 2010;159(1):63–7 (In eng).
68. Latini R, Masson S, Anand IS, et al. Prognostic value of very low plasma concentrations of troponin T in patients with stable chronic heart failure. Circulation 2007;116(11):1242–9 (In eng).
69. Aimo A, Januzzi JL, Bayes-Genis A, et al. Clinical and prognostic significance of sST2 in heart failure: JACC review topic of the week. J Am Coll Cardiol 2019;74(17):2193–203 (In eng).
70. McCarthy CP, Januzzi JL. Soluble ST2 in heart failure. Heart Fail Clin 2018;14(1):41–8 (In eng).
71. Januzzi JL, Peacock WF, Maisel AS, et al. Measurement of the interleukin family member ST2 in patients with acute dyspnea: results from the PRIDE (Pro-brain natriuretic peptide investigation of dyspnea in the emergency department) study. J Am Coll Cardiol 2007;50(7):607–13 (In eng).
72. Crnko S, Printezi MI, Jansen TPJ, et al. Prognostic biomarker soluble ST2 exhibits diurnal variation in chronic heart failure patients. ESC Heart Fail 2020;7(3):1224–33 (In eng).
73. Aimo A, Januzzi JL, Vergaro G, et al. Circulating levels and prognostic value of soluble ST2 in heart failure are less influenced by age than N-terminal pro-B-type natriuretic peptide and high-sensitivity troponin T. Eur J Heart Fail 2020. https://doi.org/10.1002/ejhf.1701 (In eng).
74. Savvoulidis P, Snider JV, Rawal S, et al. Serum ST2 and hospitalization rates in Caucasian and African American outpatients with heart failure. Int J Cardiol 2020;304:116–21 (In eng).
75. Lupón J, Cediel G, Moliner P, et al. A bio-clinical approach for prediction of sudden cardiac death in outpatients with heart failure: The ST2-SCD score. Int J Cardiol 2019;293:148–52 (In eng).
76. Emdin M, Aimo A, Vergaro G, et al. sST2 predicts outcome in chronic heart failure beyond NT-proBNP and high-sensitivity troponin T. J Am Coll Cardiol 2018;72(19):2309–20 (In eng).
77. Ky B, French B, McCloskey K, et al. High-sensitivity ST2 for prediction of adverse outcomes in chronic heart failure. Circ Heart Fail 2011;4(2):180–7 (In eng).
78. Rehman SU, Mueller T, Januzzi JL. Characteristics of the novel interleukin family biomarker ST2 in patients with acute heart failure. J Am Coll Cardiol 2008;52(18):1458–65 (In eng).
79. Barondes SH, Castronovo V, Cooper DN, et al. Galectins: a family of animal beta-galactoside-binding lectins. Cell 1994;76(4):597–8 (In eng).
80. Gehlken C, Suthahar N, Meijers WC, et al. Galectin-3 in heart failure: an update of the last 3 years. Heart Fail Clin 2018;14(1):75–92 (In eng).
81. Nayor M, Wang N, Larson MG, et al. Circulating Galectin-3 Is associated with cardiometabolic disease in the community. J Am Heart Assoc 2015; 5(1). https://doi.org/10.1161/JAHA.115.002347 (In eng).
82. Shah RV, Chen-Tournoux AA, Picard MH, et al. Galectin-3, cardiac structure and function, and long-term mortality in patients with acutely decompensated heart failure. Eur J Heart Fail 2010;12(8): 826–32 (In eng).

83. de Boer RA, Lok DJ, Jaarsma T, et al. Predictive value of plasma galectin-3 levels in heart failure with reduced and preserved ejection fraction. Ann Med 2011;43(1):60–8 (In eng).
84. van Kimmenade RR, Januzzi JL, Ellinor PT, et al. Utility of amino-terminal pro-brain natriuretic peptide, galectin-3, and apelin for the evaluation of patients with acute heart failure. J Am Coll Cardiol 2006;48(6):1217–24 (In eng).
85. Bayes-Genis A, de Antonio M, Vila J, et al. Head-to-head comparison of 2 myocardial fibrosis biomarkers for long-term heart failure risk stratification: ST2 versus galectin-3. J Am Coll Cardiol 2014; 63(2):158–66 (In eng).
86. Krack A, Sharma R, Figulla HR, et al. The importance of the gastrointestinal system in the pathogenesis of heart failure. Eur Heart J 2005;26(22): 2368–74.
87. Salzano A, Cassambai S, Yazaki Y, et al. The gut axis involvement in heart failure: focus on trimethylamine N-oxide. Heart Fail Clin 2020;16(1):23–31 (In eng).
88. Nagatomo Y, Tang WH. Intersections between microbiome and heart failure: revisiting the gut hypothesis. J Card Fail 2015;21(12):973–80.
89. Koeth RA, Wang Z, Levison BS, et al. Intestinal microbiota metabolism of L-carnitine, a nutrient in red meat, promotes atherosclerosis. Nat Med 2013; 19(5):576–85.
90. Cassambai S, Salzano A, Yazaki Y, et al. Impact of acute choline loading on circulating trimethylamine N-oxide levels. Eur J Prev Cardiol 2019. https://doi.org/10.1177/2047487319831372 (In eng).
91. Suzuki T, Heaney LM, Bhandari SS, et al. Trimethylamine N-oxide and prognosis in acute heart failure. Heart 2016;102(11):841–8.
92. Israr MZ, Bernieh D, Salzano A, et al. Association of gut-related metabolites with outcome in acute heart failure. Am Heart J 2021 Jan 14;234:71–80. https://doi.org/10.1016/j.ahj.2021.01.006.
93. Troseid M, Ueland T, Hov JR, et al. Microbiota-dependent metabolite trimethylamine-N-oxide is associated with disease severity and survival of patients with chronic heart failure. J Intern Med 2015;277(6):717–26.
94. Tang WH, Wang Z, Shrestha K, et al. Intestinal microbiota-dependent phosphatidylcholine metabolites, diastolic dysfunction, and adverse clinical outcomes in chronic systolic heart failure. J Card Fail 2015;21(2):91–6.
95. Schuett K, Kleber ME, Scharnagl H, et al. Trimethylamine-N-oxide and heart failure with reduced versus preserved ejection fraction. J Am Coll Cardiol 2017;70(25):3202–4.
96. Tang WH, Wang Z, Fan Y, et al. Prognostic value of elevated levels of intestinal microbe-generated metabolite trimethylamine-N-oxide in patients with heart failure: refining the gut hypothesis. J Am Coll Cardiol 2014;64(18):1908–14.
97. Suzuki T, Yazaki Y, Voors AA, et al. Association with outcomes and response to treatment of trimethylamine N-oxide in heart failure (from BIOSTAT-CHF). Eur J Heart Fail 2018. https://doi.org/10.1002/ejhf.1338.
98. Hayashi T, Yamashita T, Watanabe H, et al. Gut microbiome and plasma microbiome-related metabolites in patients with decompensated and compensated heart failure. Circ J 2018;83(1):182–92.
99. Yazaki Y, Salzano A, Nelson CP, et al. Geographical location affects the levels and association of trimethylamine N-oxide with heart failure mortality in BIOSTAT-CHF: a post-hoc analysis. Eur J Heart Fail 2019;21(10):1291–4 (In eng).
100. Yazaki Y, Aizawa K, Israr MZ, et al. Ethnic differences in association of outcomes with trimethylamine N-oxide in acute heart failure patients. ESC Heart Fail 2020. https://doi.org/10.1002/ehf2.12777 (In eng).
101. Salzano A, Israr MZ, Yazaki Y, et al. Combined use of trimethylamine N-oxide with BNP for risk stratification in heart failure with preserved ejection fraction: findings from the DIAMONDHFpEF study. Eur J Prev Cardiol 2019. https://doi.org/10.1177/2047487319870355 (In eng).
102. Saccà L. Heart failure as a multiple hormonal deficiency syndrome. Circ Heart Fail 2009;2(2):151–6 (In eng).
103. Salzano A, Cittadini A, Bossone E, et al. Multiple hormone deficiency syndrome: a novel topic in chronic heart failure. Future Sci OA 2018;4(6): FSO311 (In eng).
104. Napoli R, D'Assante R, Miniero M, et al. Anabolic deficiencies in heart failure: ready for prime time? Heart Fail Clin 2020;16(1):11–21 (In eng).
105. Jankowska EA, Biel B, Majda J, et al. Anabolic deficiency in men with chronic heart failure: prevalence and detrimental impact on survival. Circulation 2006;114(17):1829–37 (In eng).
106. Marra AM, Arcopinto M, Salzano A, et al. Detectable interleukin-9 plasma levels are associated with impaired cardiopulmonary functional capacity and all-cause mortality in patients with chronic heart failure. Int J Cardiol 2016;209:114–7.
107. Arcopinto M, Salzano A, Bossone E, et al. Multiple hormone deficiencies in chronic heart failure. Int J Cardiol 2015;184:421–3 (In eng).
108. Salzano A, Marra AM, Ferrara F, et al. Multiple hormone deficiency syndrome in heart failure with preserved ejection fraction. Int J Cardiol 2016;225:1–3 (in English).
109. Jankowska EA, Rozentryt P, Ponikowska B, et al. Circulating estradiol and mortality in men with systolic chronic heart failure. JAMA 2009;301(18): 1892–901 (In eng).

110. Arcopinto M, Salzano A, Giallauria F, et al. Growth hormone deficiency is associated with worse cardiac function, physical performance, and outcome in chronic heart failure: insights from the T.O.S.CA. GHD Study. PLoS One 2017;12(1):e0170058 (In eng).
111. Suskin N, McKelvie RS, Burns RJ, et al. Glucose and insulin abnormalities relate to functional capacity in patients with congestive heart failure. Eur Heart J 2000;21(16):1368–75.
112. Doehner W, Rauchhaus M, Ponikowski P, et al. Impaired insulin sensitivity as an independent risk factor for mortality in patients with stable chronic heart failure. J Am Coll Cardiol 2005;46(6):1019–26.
113. Arcopinto M, Bobbio E, Bossone E, et al. The GH/IGF-1 axis in chronic heart failure. Endocr Metab Immune Disord Drug Targets 2013;13(1):76–91 (In eng).
114. Pasquali D, Arcopinto M, Renzullo A, et al. Cardiovascular abnormalities in Klinefelter syndrome. Int J Cardiol 2013;168(2):754–9 (In eng).
115. Marra AM, Improda N, Capalbo D, et al. Cardiovascular abnormalities and impaired exercise performance in adolescents with congenital adrenal hyperplasia. J Clin Endocrinol Metab 2015;100(2):644–52 (In eng).
116. Salzano A, D'Assante R, Heaney LM, et al. Klinefelter syndrome, insulin resistance, metabolic syndrome, and diabetes: review of literature and clinical perspectives. Endocrine 2018;61(2):194–203 (In eng).
117. Cerbone M, Capalbo D, Wasniewska M, et al. Effects of L-thyroxine treatment on early markers of atherosclerotic disease in children with subclinical hypothyroidism. Eur J Endocrinol 2016;175(1):11–9 (In eng).
118. Arcopinto M, Salzano A, Isgaard J, et al. Hormone replacement therapy in heart failure. Curr Opin Cardiol 2015;30(3):277–84 (In eng).
119. Salzano A, Marra AM, D'Assante R, et al. Growth hormone therapy in heart failure. Heart Fail Clin 2018;14(4):501–15 (In eng).
120. Salzano A, D'Assante R, Lander M, et al. Hormonal replacement therapy in heart failure: focus on growth hormone and testosterone. Heart Fail Clin 2019;15(3):377–91 (In eng).
121. Cittadini A, Marra AM, Arcopinto M, et al. Growth hormone replacement delays the progression of chronic heart failure combined with growth hormone deficiency: an extension of a randomized controlled single-blind study. JACC Heart Fail 2013;1(4):325–30 (In eng).
122. Salzano A, Marra AM, Arcopinto M, et al. Combined effects of growth hormone and testosterone replacement treatment in heart failure. ESC Heart Fail 2019;6(6):1216–21 (In eng).
123. Bossone E, Arcopinto M, Iacoviello M, et al. Multiple hormonal and metabolic deficiency syndrome in chronic heart failure: rationale, design, and demographic characteristics of the T.O.S.CA. Registry. Intern Emerg Med 2018;13(5):661–71 (In eng).
124. Cittadini A, Salzano A, Iacoviello M, et al. Multiple Hormonal and Metabolic Deficiency Syndrome predicts outcome in heart failure. The T.O.S.CA. Registry. Eur J Prev Cardiol 2021. in press.
125. Bozkurt B, Colvin M, Cook J, et al. Current diagnostic and treatment strategies for specific dilated cardiomyopathies: a scientific statement from the American heart association. Circulation 2016;134(23):e579–646 (In eng).
126. Seferović PM, Polovina M, Bauersachs J, et al. Heart failure in cardiomyopathies: a position paper from the heart failure association of the European society of cardiology. Eur J Heart Fail 2019;21(5):553–76 (In eng).
127. Husain H, Velculescu VE. Cancer DNA in the circulation: the liquid biopsy. JAMA 2017;318(13):1272–4.
128. Arroyo AB, de Los Reyes-Garcia AM, Rivera-Caravaca JM, et al. MiR-146a regulates neutrophil extracellular trap formation that predicts adverse cardiovascular events in patients with atrial fibrillation. Arterioscler Thromb Vasc Biol 2018;38(4):892–902.
129. Sanchis J, Garcia-Blas S, Ortega-Paz L, et al. Cell-free DNA and microvascular damage in ST-segment elevation myocardial infarction treated with primary percutaneous coronary intervention. Rev Esp Cardiol (Engl Ed) 2019;72(4):317–23.
130. Xie J, Yang J, Hu P. Correlations of circulating cell-free DNA with clinical manifestations in acute myocardial infarction. Am J Med Sci 2018;356(2):121–9.
131. Jylhava J, Lehtimaki T, Jula A, et al. Circulating cell-free DNA is associated with cardiometabolic risk factors: the Health 2000 Survey. Atherosclerosis 2014;233(1):268–71.
132. De Vlaminck I, Valantine HA, Snyder TM, et al. Circulating cell-free DNA enables noninvasive diagnosis of heart transplant rejection. Sci Transl Med 2014;6(241):241ra77.
133. Macher HC, Garcia-Fernandez N, Adsuar-Gomez A, et al. Donor-specific circulating cell free DNA as a noninvasive biomarker of graft injury in heart transplantation. Clin Chim Acta 2019;495:590–7.
134. Khush KK, Patel J, Pinney S, et al. Noninvasive detection of graft injury after heart transplant using donor-derived cell-free DNA: a prospective multicenter study. Am J Transplant 2019. https://doi.org/10.1111/ajt.15339.
135. Salzano A, Israr MZ, Garcia DF, et al. Circulating cell-free DNA levels are associated with adverse

outcomes in heart failure: testing liquid biopsy in heart failure. Eur J Prev Cardiol 2020. https://doi.org/10.1177/2047487320912375 (In eng).
136. Siong Chan DC, Cao TH, Ng LL. Proenkephalin in heart failure. Heart Fail Clin 2018;14(1):1–11 (In eng).
137. Arbit B, Marston N, Shah K, et al. Prognostic usefulness of proenkephalin in stable ambulatory patients with heart failure. Am J Cardiol 2016;117(8):1310–4 (In eng).
138. Matsue Y, Ter Maaten JM, Struck J, et al. Clinical correlates and prognostic value of proenkephalin in acute and chronic heart failure. J Card Fail 2017;23(3):231–9 (In eng).
139. Ng LL, Squire IB, Jones DJL, et al. Proenkephalin, renal dysfunction, and prognosis in patients with acute heart failure: a GREAT network study. J Am Coll Cardiol 2017;69(1):56–69 (In eng).
140. Emmens JE, Ter Maaten JM, Damman K, et al. Proenkephalin, an opioid system surrogate, as a novel comprehensive renal marker in heart failure. Circ Heart Fail 2019;12(5):e005544 (In eng).
141. Kanagala P, Squire IB, Jones DJL, et al. Proenkephalin and prognosis in heart failure with preserved ejection fraction: a GREAT network study. Clin Res Cardiol 2019;108(8):940–9 (In eng).
142. Nishikimi T, Nakagawa Y. Adrenomedullin as a biomarker of heart failure. Heart Fail Clin 2018;14(1):49–55 (In eng).
143. Nishikimi T, Saito Y, Kitamura K, et al. Increased plasma levels of adrenomedullin in patients with heart failure. J Am Coll Cardiol 1995;26(6):1424–31 (In eng).
144. Jougasaki M, Wei CM, McKinley LJ, et al. Elevation of circulating and ventricular adrenomedullin in human congestive heart failure. Circulation 1995;92(3):286–9 (In eng).
145. Kato J, Kobayashi K, Etoh T, et al. Plasma adrenomedullin concentration in patients with heart failure. J Clin Endocrinol Metab 1996;81(1):180–3 (In eng).
146. von Haehling S, Filippatos GS, Papassotiriou J, et al. Mid-regional pro-adrenomedullin as a novel predictor of mortality in patients with chronic heart failure. Eur J Heart Fail 2010;12(5):484–91 (In eng).
147. Maisel A, Mueller C, Nowak R, et al. Mid-region pro-hormone markers for diagnosis and prognosis in acute dyspnea: results from the BACH (Biomarkers in Acute Heart Failure) trial. J Am Coll Cardiol 2010;55(19):2062–76 (In eng).
148. Xue Y, Taub P, Iqbal N, et al. Mid-region pro-adrenomedullin adds predictive value to clinical predictors and Framingham risk score for long-term mortality in stable outpatients with heart failure. Eur J Heart Fail 2013;15(12):1343–9 (In eng).
149. Goetze JP, Balling L, Deis T, et al. Bioactive adrenomedullin in plasma is associated with biventricular filling pressures in patients with advanced heart failure. Eur J Heart Fail 2020. https://doi.org/10.1002/ejhf.1937 (In eng).
150. Gomes CPC, Schroen B, Kuster GM, et al. Regulatory RNAs in heart failure. Circulation 2020;141(4):313–28 (In eng).
151. Jakob P, Doerries C, Briand S, et al. Loss of angiomiR-126 and 130a in angiogenic early outgrowth cells from patients with chronic heart failure: role for impaired in vivo neovascularization and cardiac repair capacity. Circulation 2012;126(25):2962–75 (In eng).
152. Qiang L, Hong L, Ningfu W, et al. Expression of miR-126 and miR-508-5p in endothelial progenitor cells is associated with the prognosis of chronic heart failure patients. Int J Cardiol 2013;168(3):2082–8 (In eng).
153. Dickinson BA, Semus HM, Montgomery RL, et al. Plasma microRNAs serve as biomarkers of therapeutic efficacy and disease progression in hypertension-induced heart failure. Eur J Heart Fail 2013;15(6):650–9 (In eng).
154. Wohlfahrt P, Melenovsky V, Kotrc M, et al. Association of fibroblast growth factor-23 levels and angiotensin-converting enzyme inhibition in chronic systolic heart failure. JACC Heart Fail 2015;3(10):829–39 (In eng).
155. Ter Maaten JM, Voors AA, Damman K, et al. Fibroblast growth factor 23 is related to profiles indicating volume overload, poor therapy optimization and prognosis in patients with new-onset and worsening heart failure. Int J Cardiol 2018;253:84–90 (In eng).
156. Roy C, Lejeune S, Slimani A, et al. Fibroblast growth factor 23: a biomarker of fibrosis and prognosis in heart failure with preserved ejection fraction. ESC Heart Fail 2020;7(5):2494–507 (In eng).
157. Kanagala P, Arnold JR, Khan JN, et al. Fibroblast-growth-factor-23 in heart failure with preserved ejection fraction: relation to exercise capacity and outcomes. ESC Heart Fail 2020. https://doi.org/10.1002/ehf2.13020 (In eng).
158. Sinning C, Kempf T, Schwarzl M, et al. Biomarkers for characterization of heart failure - Distinction of heart failure with preserved and reduced ejection fraction. Int J Cardiol 2017;227:272–7 (In eng).
159. Nauta JF, Hummel YM, van Melle JP, et al. What have we learned about heart failure with mid-range ejection fraction one year after its introduction? Eur J Heart Fail 2017;19(12):1569–73 (In eng).
160. Paulus WJ, Tschöpe C. A novel paradigm for heart failure with preserved ejection fraction: comorbidities drive myocardial dysfunction and remodeling through coronary microvascular endothelial inflammation. J Am Coll Cardiol 2013;62(4):263–71 (In eng).
161. Sanders-van Wijk S, van Empel V, Davarzani N, et al. Circulating biomarkers of distinct

pathophysiological pathways in heart failure with preserved vs. reduced left ventricular ejection fraction. Eur J Heart Fail 2015;17(10):1006–14 (In eng).

162. Santhanakrishnan R, Chong JP, Ng TP, et al. Growth differentiation factor 15, ST2, high-sensitivity troponin T, and N-terminal pro brain natriuretic peptide in heart failure with preserved vs. reduced ejection fraction. Eur J Heart Fail 2012;14(12):1338–47 (In eng).
163. Tromp J, Westenbrink BD, Ouwerkerk W, et al. Identifying pathophysiological mechanisms in heart failure with reduced versus preserved ejection fraction. J Am Coll Cardiol 2018;72(10): 1081–90 (In eng).
164. Januzzi JL, Troughton R. Are serial BNP measurements useful in heart failure management? Serial natriuretic peptide measurements are useful in heart failure management. Circulation 2013; 127(4):500–7 [discussion 508]. (In eng).
165. Desai AS. Are serial BNP measurements useful in heart failure management? Serial natriuretic peptide measurements are not useful in heart failure management: the art of medicine remains long. Circulation 2013;127(4):509–16 [discussion 516]. (In eng).
166. Motwani JG, McAlpine H, Kennedy N, et al. Plasma brain natriuretic peptide as an indicator for angiotensin-converting-enzyme inhibition after myocardial infarction. Lancet 1993;341(8853): 1109–13 (In eng).
167. Latini R, Masson S, Anand I, et al. Effects of valsartan on circulating brain natriuretic peptide and norepinephrine in symptomatic chronic heart failure: the valsartan heart failure trial (Val-HeFT). Circulation 2002;106(19):2454–8 (In eng).
168. Tsutamoto T, Wada A, Maeda K, et al. Effect of spironolactone on plasma brain natriuretic peptide and left ventricular remodeling in patients with congestive heart failure. J Am Coll Cardiol 2001; 37(5):1228–33 (In eng).
169. Stanek B, Frey B, Hülsmann M, et al. Prognostic evaluation of neurohumoral plasma levels before and during beta-blocker therapy in advanced left ventricular dysfunction. J Am Coll Cardiol 2001; 38(2):436–42 (In eng).
170. Cleland JG, Daubert JC, Erdmann E, et al. The effect of cardiac resynchronization on morbidity and mortality in heart failure. N Engl J Med 2005; 352(15):1539–49 (In eng).
171. Pascual-Figal DA, Domingo M, Casas T, et al. Usefulness of clinical and NT-proBNP monitoring for prognostic guidance in destabilized heart failure outpatients. Eur Heart J 2008;29(8):1011–8 (In eng).
172. Kubánek M, Goode KM, Lánská V, et al. The prognostic value of repeated measurement of N-terminal pro-B-type natriuretic peptide in patients with chronic heart failure due to left ventricular systolic dysfunction. Eur J Heart Fail 2009;11(4): 367–77 (In eng).
173. Zile MR, Claggett BL, Prescott MF, et al. Prognostic implications of changes in N-Terminal Pro-B-Type natriuretic peptide in patients with heart failure. J Am Coll Cardiol 2016;68(22):2425–36 (In eng).
174. Latini R, Masson S, Wong M, et al. Incremental prognostic value of changes in B-type natriuretic peptide in heart failure. Am J Med 2006;119(1): 70. e23–30.
175. Israr MZ, Salzano A, Yazaki Y, et al. Implications of serial measurements of natriuretic peptides in heart failure: insights from BIOSTAT-CHF. Eur J Heart Fail 2020;22(8):1486–90 (In eng).
176. Schuurman AS, Tomer A, Akkerhuis KM, et al. Personalized screening intervals for measurement of N-terminal pro-B-type natriuretic peptide improve efficiency of prognostication in patients with chronic heart failure. Eur J Prev Cardiol 2020. https://doi.org/10.1177/2047487320922639 (In eng).
177. van Boven N, Battes LC, Akkerhuis KM, et al. Toward personalized risk assessment in patients with chronic heart failure: detailed temporal patterns of NT-proBNP, troponin T, and CRP in the Bio-SHiFT study. Am Heart J 2018;196:36–48 (In eng).
178. Januzzi JL, Rehman SU, Mohammed AA, et al. Use of amino-terminal pro-B-type natriuretic peptide to guide outpatient therapy of patients with chronic left ventricular systolic dysfunction. J Am Coll Cardiol 2011;58(18):1881–9 (In eng).
179. Jourdain P, Jondeau G, Funck F, et al. Plasma brain natriuretic peptide-guided therapy to improve outcome in heart failure: the STARS-BNP Multicenter Study. J Am Coll Cardiol 2007;49(16): 1733–9 (In eng).
180. Troughton RW, Frampton CM, Yandle TG, et al. Treatment of heart failure guided by plasma aminoterminal brain natriuretic peptide (N-BNP) concentrations. Lancet 2000;355(9210):1126–30 (In eng).
181. Berger R, Moertl D, Peter S, et al. N-terminal pro-B-type natriuretic peptide-guided, intensive patient management in addition to multidisciplinary care in chronic heart failure a 3-arm, prospective, randomized pilot study. J Am Coll Cardiol 2010; 55(7):645–53 (In eng).
182. Eurlings LW, van Pol PE, Kok WE, et al. Management of chronic heart failure guided by individual N-terminal pro-B-type natriuretic peptide targets: results of the PRIMA (Can PRo-brain-natriuretic peptide guided therapy of chronic heart failure IMprove heart fAilure morbidity and mortality?)

study. J Am Coll Cardiol 2010;56(25):2090–100 (In eng).
183. Karlström P, Alehagen U, Boman K, et al. Brain natriuretic peptide-guided treatment does not improve morbidity and mortality in extensively treated patients with chronic heart failure: responders to treatment have a significantly better outcome. Eur J Heart Fail 2011;13(10):1096–103 (In eng).
184. Shah MR, Califf RM, Nohria A, et al. The STARBRITE trial: a randomized, pilot study of B-type natriuretic peptide-guided therapy in patients with advanced heart failure. J Card Fail 2011;17(8): 613–21 (In eng).
185. Felker GM, Anstrom KJ, Adams KF, et al. Effect of natriuretic peptide-guided therapy on hospitalization or cardiovascular mortality in high-risk patients with heart failure and reduced ejection fraction: a randomized clinical trial. JAMA 2017;318(8): 713–20 (In eng).
186. Januzzi JL, Ahmad T, Mulder H, et al. Natriuretic peptide response and outcomes in chronic heart failure with reduced ejection fraction. J Am Coll Cardiol 2019;74(9):1205–17 (In eng).
187. Felker GM, Hasselblad V, Hernandez AF, et al. Biomarker-guided therapy in chronic heart failure: a meta-analysis of randomized controlled trials. Am Heart J 2009;158(3):422–30 (In eng).
188. Porapakkham P, Zimmet H, Billah B, et al. B-type natriuretic peptide-guided heart failure therapy: a meta-analysis. Arch Intern Med 2010;170(6): 507–14 (In eng).
189. Savarese G, Trimarco B, Dellegrottaglie S, et al. Natriuretic peptide-guided therapy in chronic heart failure: a meta-analysis of 2,686 patients in 12 randomized trials. PLoS One 2013;8(3):e58287 (In eng).
190. Li P, Luo Y, Chen YM. B-type natriuretic peptide-guided chronic heart failure therapy: a meta-analysis of 11 randomised controlled trials. Heart Lung Circ 2013;22(10):852–60 (In eng).
191. Troughton RW, Frampton CM, Brunner-La Rocca HP, et al. Effect of B-type natriuretic peptide-guided treatment of chronic heart failure on total mortality and hospitalization: an individual patient meta-analysis. Eur Heart J 2014;35(23): 1559–67 (In eng).
192. McLellan J, Heneghan CJ, Perera R, et al. B-type natriuretic peptide-guided treatment for heart failure. Cochrane Database Syst Rev 2016;12: CD008966 (In eng).
193. Ouwerkerk W, Zwinderman AH, Ng LL, et al. Biomarker-guided versus guideline-based treatment of patients with heart failure: results from BIOSTAT-CHF. J Am Coll Cardiol 2018;71(4):386–98 (In eng).
194. Miller WL, Hartman KA, Burritt MF, et al. Profiles of serial changes in cardiac troponin T concentrations and outcome in ambulatory patients with chronic heart failure. J Am Coll Cardiol 2009;54(18): 1715–21 (In eng).
195. Miller WL, Hartman KA, Burritt MF, et al. Serial biomarker measurements in ambulatory patients with chronic heart failure: the importance of change over time. Circulation 2007;116(3):249–57 (In eng).

Noninvasive Assessment of Ventricular-Arterial Coupling in Heart Failure

Olga Vriz, MD[a,b,*], Fadl-Elmula M. Fadl Elmula, MD[a], Francesco Antonini-Canterin, MD[c]

KEYWORDS

• Ventricular-arterial coupling • Left ventricular function • Arterial stiffness • Chronic heart failure • Acute heart failure

KEY POINTS

- Ventricular-arterial coupling (VAC) parameters must be considered when evaluating patients with heart failure (HF). These parameters indicate both the condition and the interaction between the arterial system and heart, and can be used as prognostic parameters.
- VAC parameters can be used for patient stratification and tailoring medical therapy.
- Several methods are available for VAC evaluation and each of them can be applied in different clinical scenarios, such as chronic or acute HF.

INTRODUCTION

Ventricular-arterial coupling (VAC) is a concept that was first developed several decades ago. It emerged from the logical notion that the heart and the arterial system are structured to provide adequate pressure and flow to the tissues both at rest and during exercise, as they are anatomically and functionally linked together.[1] The advantage of this concept is that it allows the cardiovascular system to be analyzed as a unique and interconnected system and not as isolated structures.[2] Heart failure (HF) is a common condition in elderly individuals that can present as both an acute or chronic condition. In both cases, HF comprises VAC impairment, marked by a reduced (HFrEF) or preserved ejection fraction (HFpEF), caused or associated with comorbidities such as hypertension, diabetes, obesity, or ischemia. For example, in acute HF it is important to quickly identify rapid hemodynamic changes and choose the best drugs for heart or vascular support (inotropic drugs and/or drugs with a vasodilating or vasoconstricting effect).[3] In chronic HFrEF, it has been demonstrated that left ventricular (LV) remodeling and VAC are important prognostic predictors.[4] In HFpEF the underlying pathology is an increase in LV stiffness, altered diastolic function, and an increase in arterial stiffness, resulting in a more-or-less normal VAC value.[5] In clinical practice, evaluation of VAC found some obstacles that delayed the translation of this concept into clinical practice, such as the invasive assessment of the pressure-volume loop analysis by cardiac catheterization, the lack of simple noninvasive measurements, and the need of similar mathematical terms. In this review, we give more insight into VAC as a means to address HF, and to facilitate its use in clinical practice.

THE CONCEPT OF VENTRICULAR-ARTERIAL COUPLING

The 2 components of VAC are arterial elastance (EA) and end-systolic elastance (EES) of the LV. EA represents afterload, calculated as end-systolic

[a] Heart Centre, King Faisal Specialist Hospital and Research Centre, Zahrawi Street, Al Maather, Al Maazer, Riyadh 12713, Saudi Arabia; [b] Alfaisal University, School of Medicine, Riyadh, Saudi Arabia; [c] Cardiologia Riabilitativa, Ospedale Riabilitativo di Alta Specializzazione, Motta di Livenza, Italy
* Corresponding author. Heart Centre, King Faisal Specialist Hospital and Research Centre, Zahrawi Street, Al Maather, Al Maazer, Riyadh 12713, Saudi Arabia.
E-mail address: olgavriz@yahoo.com

Heart Failure Clin 17 (2021) 245–254
https://doi.org/10.1016/j.hfc.2020.12.003

pressure/stroke volume, whereas left ventricular EES is a relatively load-independent measure of LV chamber performance and stiffness. EES corresponds to the slope of a straight line deriving from the union of end-systolic points of different cardiac cycles from the same heart at different loading conditions. This line represents the intracavitary pressure required to increase the heart volume by 1 unit; this is an expression of maximum ventricular stiffness and is best represented by PV loop (P = pressure, V = volume). The PV loop concept, proposed by Suga and colleagues,[6] represents the total energy of contraction and correlates with myocardial O_2 consumption. LV changes in PV loop include 4 phases: (1) isovolumic relaxation, (2) diastole, (3) isovolumic contraction, and (4) ventricular systole (**Fig. 1**). EES is sensitive to contractility, chamber geometry, and passive LV stiffening.[7] The EA is influenced by peripheral resistances, total vascular compliance, impedance, and heart rate. Cardiac load also can be expressed as the combination of static and pulsatile components: the former is represented by total peripheral resistances that depend on microvascular properties, the latter by the properties of the large vessels such as impedance of the proximal aorta, magnitude and timing of the reflection waves, and total compliance of the arterial system.[8] Normal values at rest, invasively measured, are 2.2 ± 0.8 mm Hg/mL and 2.3 ± 1.0 mm Hg/mL for EA and EES, respectively. When the EA/EES ratio is approximately 1, the LV

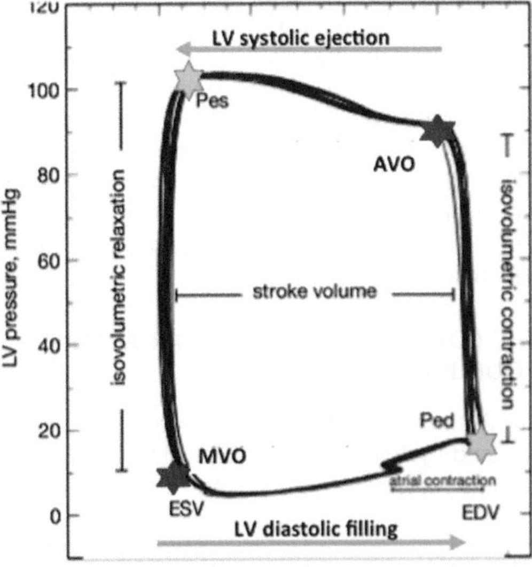

Fig. 1. LV pressure–volume loop. AVO, aortic valve opening; EDV, end diastolic volume; ESV, end systolic volume; MVO, mitral valve opening; Pes, pressure end systole. Red stars: beginning of diastole and systole; blue stars: end of diastole and systole.

and the arterial system are optimally coupled for producing maximum stroke workload. Maximum efficiency is when the ratio is equal to 0.5, when EA is half of EES and the LV produces an EF equal to greater than 60%, which is the normal value for a healthy person. The ratio is in the range of 0.3 to 1.3.[9] Normally the LV and arterial system are optimally coupled either at rest or during exercise. During aging, which is considered a very early stage of HFpEF, arterial and heart stiffening occurs in parallel with preserved optimal coupling. However, the increase in EA limits the capacity of the heart to eject while simultaneously imposing an increased energetic demand amplified by ventricular systolic stiffening.

METHODS OF MEASUREMENT

Table 1 summarizes the noninvasive methods that can be used for the evaluation of VAC in different clinical settings.[10–18] Among the parameters described, in congestive HF the most frequently used method is the echo/Doppler single beat. In addition, 2 new methods are emerging: Wave Intensity (WI) and Myocardial Work (MW).

Echocardiography/Doppler Single Beat Method

The echocardiographic/Doppler's gold standard measurement for the assessment of EA/EES is the so-called single beat method developed by Chen and coworkers.[10] Because the formulas are relatively complex (**Fig. 2**, see **Table 1**), they have been implemented in clinical settings as computerized algorithms, or more lately a calculator,[11] which was specifically designed to allow Chen's algorithm to be deployed at the bedside (iElastance© - Apple iOS App). The operator must enter simple noninvasive parameters that can be collected easily: systolic and diastolic blood pressures, stroke volume, ejection fraction, pre-ejection, and total systolic periods (see **Fig. 2**). This has become the most widely used method because of the software and app's ease-of-use, and the need for only simple echocardiographic parameters that do not require an updated echo-machine. Using this method, patients with HF can be better characterized and assessed during acute changes, such as in acute HF.[19]

Wave Intensity

WI is a hemodynamic index that assesses the working condition of the heart as it interacts with the arterial system; in other words, the interaction between waves traveling from the heart with waves from the periphery. To calculate WI, a blood

Table 1
Noninvasive methods for the evaluation of ventricular-arterial coupling

Echocardiography, App[10,11] Widely used in HF	$EA = (SBP \times 0.9)/SV$ $EES = (DBP - [E_{nd(est)} \times SBP \times 0.9])/E_{nd(est)} \times SV$ $E_{nd(est)} = 0.0275 - 0.165 \times EF + 0.3656 \times (DBP/SBP \times 0.9) + 0.515 \times E_{nd(avg)}$, $E_{nd(avg)} = 0.35695 - 7.2266 \times tNd + 74.249 \times tNd^2 - 307.39 \times tNd^3 + 684.54 \times tNd^4 - 856.92 \times tNd^5 + 571.95 \times tNd^6 - 159.1 \times tNd^7$, where tNd is the ratio of pre-ejection period to total systolic period.	
Wave intensity (WI) Based on: Arterial stiffness Brachial BP.[12,13,20] Clinical use: assessing LV systolic and early diastolic performance from arterial WI. Mostly used for the carotid artery Vendor dependent Linear probe needed Limited studies	WI = (d*P*/d*t*) (d*U*/d*t*) WI has 2 peaks WI1: First peak is found at the very early phase of LV ejection. The magnitude of the first peak reflects LV contractile performance. The magnitude of the first peak is significantly correlated with LV dP/dt. WI2: The second peak is related to the ability of the left ventricle to actively stop aortic blood flow. The magnitude of the second peak reflects the isovolumic relaxation near end-systole. The amplitude of WI2 is correlated with the time constant of LV relaxation.	
LV Pressure-Strain Loop (PSL) Myocardial work Based on Global longitudinal strain (GLS) and Brachial BP.[14] Vendor dependent Limited studies	GCW, global constructive work, work performed by the LV contributing to LV ejection during systole; (mean $\pm$ SD 1896 $\pm$ 308%) GWE, global work efficiency, which is derived from constructive MW/(constructive MW + wasted MW) (these values will not be affected by peak LV pressure); (mean $\pm$ SD 2232% $\pm$ 331%) GWI, global work index, total work within the area of the LV PSL; (mean $\pm$ SD, or median [IQR] 78.5 [53–122.2]) GWW, global work waste, work performed by the LV that does not contribute to LV ejection. (mean $\pm$ SD, or median [IQR] 96 [94–97])	
Systemic arterial compliance (SAC)[23]	SVi/PP	
Valvulo-arterial impedence (Zva)[15]	(SBP + Mean CW gradient across the aortic valve)/SVi	Solid pathophysiological background. Mostly used for stratification in aortic stenosis
Aortic stiffness/Myocardial performance[16,17]	cfPWV/LV GLS Local PWV/LV GLS ($PWV = 1/\sqrt{\rho * DC}$) D = diastolic diameter, C = distensibility coefficient Local = carotid artery	Limited studies Sensitive markers of arterial and myocardial function

Abbreviations: cfPWV, carotid-femoral pulse wave velocity; CW, continous wave doppler; DBP, diastolic blood pressure; (dP/dt)(dU/dt), dP, change in pressure; dt, change in time; dU, change in velocity; EA, arterial elastance; EES, end-systolic elastance; HF, heart failure; IQR, interquartile range; LV, left ventricular; MW, myocardial work; PP, pulse pressure; SBP, systolic blood pressure; SVi, stroke volume index.

pressure waveform in the region of interest is needed; it has been demonstrated that arterial pressure waveforms and arterial changes in the diameter as peak and minimum values are correlated. It can be defined at any part of the circulatory system, although the carotid site is the easiest due to its accessibility. WI is based on a combined color Doppler and echo-tracking system (**Fig. 3**). Mathematically, WI is calculated as the product of the rate of change in blood pressure over time (d*P*/d*t*) and the rate of change in blood flow velocity over time (d*U*/d*t*), and can be expressed as (d*P*/d*t*) (d*U*/d*t*), where d*P*/d*t* and d*U*/d*t* are the derivatives of blood pressure (dP) and velocity (dU) with respect to

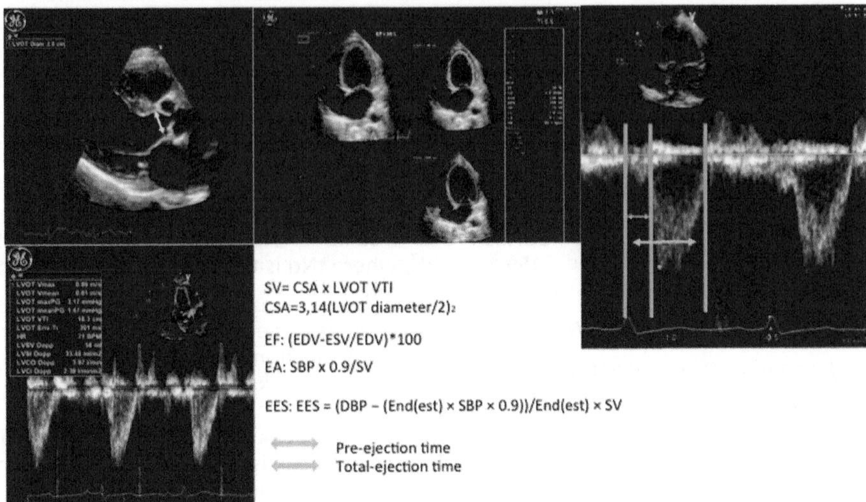

Fig. 2. Echocardiographic parameters used in the Chen formula (see **Table 1** for explanation).

time.[12] During a cardiac cycle, WI presents 2 positive peaks: the first peak (WI1) appears in early ejection, it represents a forward compression wave and its amplitude correlates with increases in cardiac contractility. It is associated with acceleration and increase in aortic pressure generated by the heart contraction. The second peak (WI_2) occurs very close to the end of LV ejection time from end-systole to isovolumetric relaxation and is related to the ability of the LV to actively stop aortic blood flow. The magnitude of the WI2 correlates with LV relaxation performance[13,20] (**Fig. 4**, see **Table 1**).

Myocardial Work

MW is a relatively new method to study LV myocardial systolic function, incorporating LV myocardial deformation and arterial load with promising results.[14] The derived noninvasive pressure-strain loops (PSL) are based on myocardial longitudinal strain analysis and brachial blood pressure (BP) for the estimation of LV pressure. This parameter is supposedly more reliable than strain, which can be affected by afterload, leading to the misinterpretation of true LV contractile function when systolic BP is high.[21] Moreover, it has been shown that noninvasive LV PSL area has a strong correlation with regional myocardial glucose metabolism evaluated by PET.[22] The variables derived from this analysis are global constructive work (GCW); global work efficiency (GWE), constructive MW/(constructive MW + wasted MW); global work index (GWI), total work within the area of the LV PSL; and global

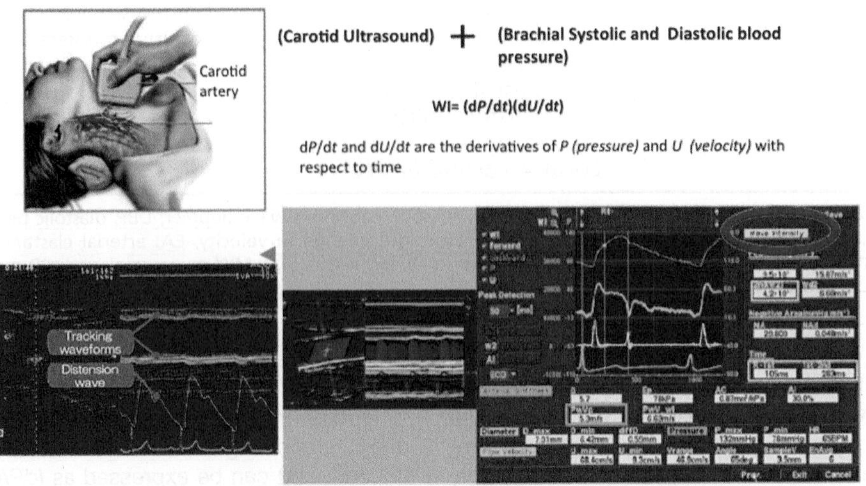

Fig. 3. Calculation of WI from scanning of the carotid artery (*left upper panel*). Output for carotid diameter changings according to BP and (*left lower panel*) and WI values (*right lower panel*).

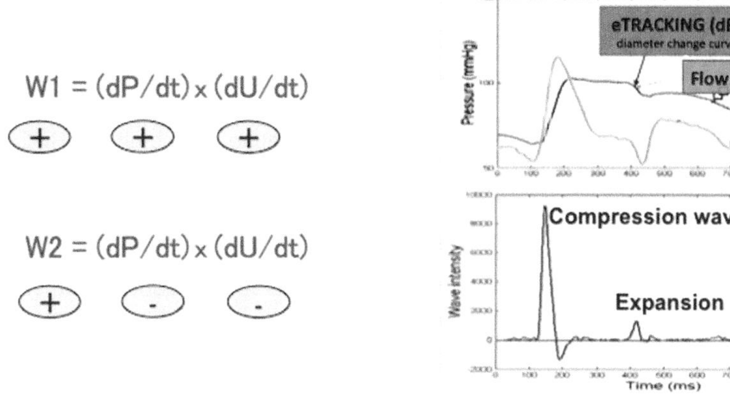

Fig. 4. Definition of WI. Calculation of WI1 and WI2.

work waste (GWW), work performed by the LV that does not contribute to LV ejection (**Fig. 5**, see **Table 1**). It has been shown that MW indices correlate with LVEF and LV size, in addition to strain and BP.[23]

USE OF VENTRICULAR-ARTERIAL COUPLING IN CLINICAL PRACTICE

Chronic Heart Failure

Heart failure with reduced ejection fraction

In HFrEF, cardiac function is primarily reduced (LVEF, SV), ending in systemic tissue hypoperfusion. The physiopathological consequence of this is the activation of the Renin-Angiotensin-Aldosterone system and the sympathetic nervous system, in an attempt to increase vascular volume and arterial load, leading to an increase in arterial elastance (EA). The combination of increased EA and reduced EES, in association with the direct cardiotoxicity due to overactivated sympathetic activity, alongside increased myocardial oxygen demand, creates a vicious circle predisposing the patient to further worsening of cardiovascular function and syndrome progression.

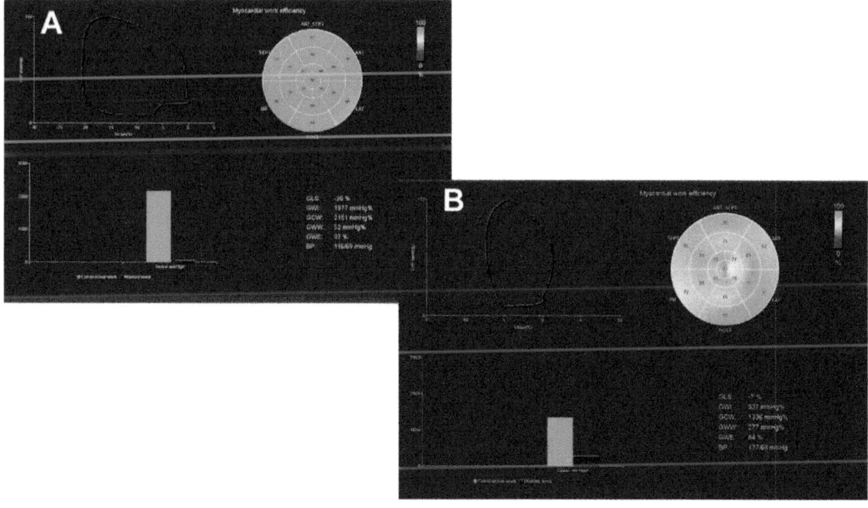

Fig. 5. MW. Traces showing PSLs by LV pressure and speckle-tracking echocardiography. (*A*) Healthy subject. Global longitudinal strain (GLS) −20%, GWI 1977 mm Hg, GCW 2151 mm Hg, GWW 52 mm Hg, GWE 97%, BP 116/69 mm Hg. (*B*) Ischemic heart disease with moderately reduced LV systolic function (LVEF 30%). GLS −7%, GWI 937 mm Hg, GCW 1336 mm Hg, GWW 277 mm Hg, GWE 84%, BP 137/68 mm Hg. GCW, global work efficiency; GWW, global work waste; GWE, global work efficiency GWI, global work index.

Echocardiography/Doppler single beat method The echocardiographic/Doppler single beat method is widely used in research. In the Cardiac Insufficiency Bisoprolol Study in Elderly (CIBIS-ELD),[24] VAC coupling, EA, EES, and their ratio were measured in a group of 887 elderly patients with reduced LVEF (mean EF 41.6% ± 13.5%) before and after 12 weeks of treatment with beta blockers. After 12 weeks, EA decreased, EES remained unchanged, and SV increased with optimal VAC (from 1.7 to 1.5). The same methodology was used by Ky and colleagues,[4] as prognostic parameters in 466 patients with HFrEF (mean EF 27%) who were enrolled and followed-up for all-cause morbidity and mortality. Baseline EA was elevated (1.66 mm Hg/mL), EES was markedly reduced (0.89 mm Hg/mL), and VAC was 2.0. EA and EA/EES were also strongly associated with New York Heart Association functional class. Altogether, EF, EA, and VAC were associated with mortality, heart transplantation, VAD, and hospitalization, suggesting that these parameters could be considered as potential therapeutic targets. On the other hand, EES was not associated with adverse events. According to the investigators, EES alone is not a comprehensive measure of contractile function and the interaction between the ventricle and vascular systems represented by EA/EES has a powerful predictive value. Another suggested application for EA/EES is the management of patients who are candidates for cardiac resynchronization (CRT). Zanon and colleagues[25] reported that a baseline EA/EES ratio of more than 2 could identify those patients who are responders to CRT, in particular those affected by nonischemic cardiomyopathy.

Wave intensity Siniawski and colleagues[26] used local WI parameters on 151 patients with end-stage dilated cardiomyopathy to predict the clinical outcome of those on the waiting list for heart transplantation. The patients were divided into groups with or without events. Among all the variables considered, W1 (<4100 mm Hg/s^3) and $V_{O_{2max}}$ (<14 mL/min) on the stress test were the strongest predictor of events. Vriz and colleagues[27] used local WI as a predictor for clinical events in 62 patients with HFrEF followed for a mean period of 43 months. Cardiovascular mortality was better predicted by W_1 <3900 mm Hg m/s^3 and W_2 <1000 mm Hg m/s^3 and W2 was the strongest predictor of mortality.

Myocardial work MW is a new methodology with promising results. Chen and colleagues[28] used MW in a group of hypertensive patients and in a group affected by dilated cardiomyopathy. In the hypertensive patients, the GCW was increased, represented by an increased PSL area due to the increase in systolic BP. In contrast, patients with dilated cardiomyopathy had a smaller PSL area, reflecting a reduced GCW. Very recently Bouali and colleagues[29] reported their experience in patients with HFrEF treated with Sacubitril/Valsartan and followed for 1 year: GCW and GWW increased significantly during the follow-up period and the receiver operating characteristic (ROC) Operating Curve identified a cutoff value of 910 mm Hg% for GCW as the best predictor of major adverse cardiovascular events. Kaplan-Meier survival curves showed that GCW≤910 mm Hg% was highly associated with poor outcome.

Chronic heart failure with preserved ejection fraction

The typical presentation of HFpEF is characterized by increased LV wall stiffness, impaired diastolic relaxation, and increased arterial stiffness. It is a common condition in elderly individuals, particularly in women, and in those patients with systemic hypertension, diabetes, and obesity. The increase in afterload causes (1) LV remodeling and LV hypertrophy with increase in O2 consumption, and (2) reduced diastolic pressure and reduced coronary perfusion, leading to chronic subendocardial ischemia. LV remodeling and chronic ischemia are responsible for fibrosis and wall stiffness.

Echocardiography/Doppler single beat method The echocardiography/Doppler single beat method has been used widely to evaluate patients with HFpEF. Both EA and EES are increased: patients with HFpEF have a higher resting EA (18%) and EES (20%), compared with healthy controls, resulting in a normal VAC ratio. Women in particular have higher EA and EES values compared with men, either during hypertension without HF symptoms or with HFpEF.[30] Lam at al[30] shed light on the effect of therapy on VAC in general, and in women particularly. Among the hypertensive patients (American College of Cardiology/American Heart Association stage HF B) from the VALIDD and EXCEED trials, women had a higher EA and EEA compared with men either at baseline or at the end of the follow-up period of antihypertensive treatment. Treatment was shown to reduce arterial and LV stiffness, lower VAC, reduce cardiac work, and increase cardiac efficiency, although these changes were smaller in women. Considering the value of the different components of VAC and its ratio, it seems important, especially in women, to start treatment during the very early stages of the disease. The development of post-capillary pulmonary hypertension (PH) is a complication of

HF and exercise increase in pulmonary pressure is a predictive marker of future development of PH. Obokata and colleagues[31] tested the VAC response, pulmonary artery systolic pressure, and the percentage of exercise-induced PH in a group of patients with HF with and without preserved EF. They found that at low-dose exercise (10 W), both groups had a significant increase in EA, EES and decrease in EA/EES, but in patients with HFpEF the decrease in EA/EES was less evident due to the blunted increase in EES. The induced PH was more frequent in HFpEF patients in association with worst EA/EES.

Myocardial work The effect of drug therapy on myocardial fibrosis can also be tested by MW. Galli and colleagues[32] compared a group of patients with hypertrophic cardiomyopathy with a group of healthy subjects. In both groups, LV fibrosis was estimated by cardiac magnetic resonance by qualitative assessment of late gadolinium enhancement and all patients underwent echocardiography MW evaluation. The study found that GCW was a predictor of LV fibrosis at multivariable analysis and a cutoff value of 1623 mm Hg% (area under the curve [AUC] 0.80, 95% confidence interval [CI] 0.66–0.93, $P<.0001$) was able to predict myocardial fibrosis with good sensitivity and fair specificity (82% and 67%, respectively), despite similar LVEF.

Acute heart failure

Acute HF (AHF) is the rapid onset or worsening of the signs and symptoms of HF, resulting in a life-threatening medical condition that requires urgent hospital therapy. AHF may present as a first occurrence (de novo) or, more frequently, as a consequence of acute decompensation of chronic HF. This rapid change could originate from a different primary hemodynamic status caused by primary cardiac dysfunction or precipitated by extrinsic factors, often in patients with chronic HF. Acute myocardial dysfunction (ischemic, inflammatory, or toxic) and acute valve insufficiency are among the most frequent causes of AHF. Acute decompensation of chronic HF can occur without known precipitant factors, but is frequently caused by infection, uncontrolled hypertension, rhythm disturbances, or nonadherence to drug therapy and diet. For these reasons, AHF poses unique diagnostic, monitoring, and management challenges.[33,34] As mentioned previously, AHF can be categorized based on EF, namely HFpEF and HFrEF, and most of the previously suggested methods for VAC assessment can also be applied here. The pathophysiologic alteration of AHF is afterload mismatch with markedly elevated peripheral resistance (SVR) or acute LV dysfunction. Acute changes in afterload may produce a disproportionate transmission of vascular stiffening onto the LV, leading to increased LV end diastolic pressure and ultimately flash pulmonary edema. On the other hand, increase in afterload can determine reduction in systolic function and the increase in SVR is a response consisting of decreased contractility to maintain BP and perfusion of the vital organs. A typical example of acute LV dysfunction is anterior acute myocardial infarction most often combined with significant increase in SVR.

However, the rapid hemodynamic changes in AHF require urgent intervention to correct underlying ventricular-arterial decoupling (VAdC) to restore sufficient organ perfusion. In AHF, the VAC is characterized by increased EA/EES up to threefold or fourfold.[35] In intensive care unit (ICU)/cardiac ICU (CICU) departments, the echocardiography/single beat is the most used method. Trambaiolo and colleagues[3] reported their experience in 48 patients with ischemic ST elevation myocardial infarction and AHF. All patients had primary percutaneous transluminal coronary angioplasty of the culprit lesion and echocardiography that included evaluation of VAC both at baseline and after 24 hours. Patients were treated with levosimendan and norepinephrine (NE). At baseline, patients had significantly higher EA, EES, and similar EA/EES. After 24 hours of therapy, an increase in SV was recorded, likely related to the reduction in EA. High baseline VAC values were predictive of prolonged use for NE. Moreover, an ROC analysis demonstrated a good sensitivity and specificity to predict early mortality (VAC cutoff >1.99; AUC = 0.786, $P = .008$) and 1-year mortality (VAC cutoff >1.68; AUC = 0.769, $P = .002$). In addition to comprehensive echocardiography examination, focus cardiac ultrasound (FoCUS) monitoring for ICU/CICU patients is needed,[36] including repeated assessment of VAC parameters to evaluate hemodynamic changes and tailored treatment. For example, in VAdC caused by increased EA (ie, hypertensive AHF, usually in HFpEF), treatment will require urgent administration of vasodilator agents, and diuretics if congestion exists; whereas for a severe decrease in EES (HFrEF), treatment will require urgent administration of an inotrope agent (and diuretic in the case of congestion) in addition to a trial of cautious administration of vasodilators to keep EA as low as possible to restore normal EA/EES. **Fig. 6** shows patient clinical profiles with AHF based on the presence/absence of congestion and/or hypoperfusion and corresponding VAdC and proposed pharmacologic treatment.

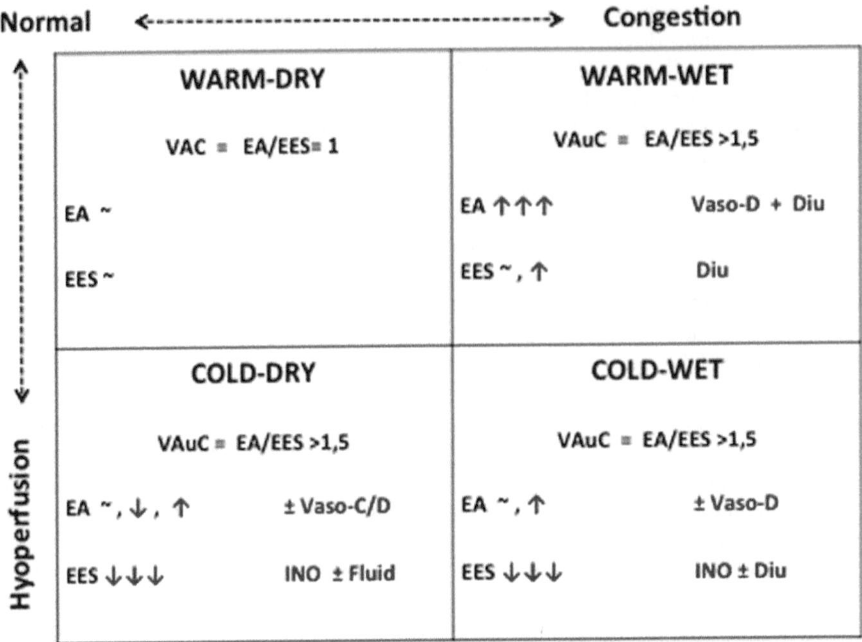

Fig. 6. Clinical profiles of patients with acute HF based on the presence/absence of congestion and/or hypoperfusion and proposed pharmacologic treatment. Diu, diuretic; INO, inotrope; VAdC, ventricular-arterial decoupling; Vaso-D, vasodilator; Vaso-C, vasoconstrictor.

CONCLUSION

Noninvasive assessment of VAC is a promising tool to assess individual hemodynamics and tailor treatment in patients with HF. The echocardiography/Doppler single beat method is becoming increasingly popular using the dedicated app, and clinicians are gaining more experience with this technology. Increased use of newer methods is shedding light on the complex interaction between heart and vessels, and future studies should focus on the different methods available and consider their appropriate use in different settings. This will allow clinicians to better evaluate VAC in patients with HF to determine the therapeutic effect of lifestyle changes and different classes of medications. It is of the utmost importance to start longitudinal studies to obtain robust data and prognostic information derived from these parameters.

SUMMARY

Assessing the interaction between the heart and the arterial system is becoming increasingly common among clinicians as a means to understand the interplay between these 2 systems. This has become possible due to the development of different noninvasive methods, which are more user-friendly, can be deployed at the bedside, or can be used in different clinical settings. It has been shown that VAC and its components have the ability to monitor hemodynamic changes (even in acute situations), and as such have prognostic value and can guide medical therapy. However, although these different tools and parameters show promise, further investigation is needed before introducing them into routine clinical practice.

DISCLOSURES

None of the authors declare any relevant conflict of interest.

REFERENCES

1. Sunagawa K, Sagawa K, Maughan WL. Ventricular interaction with the loading system. Ann Biomed Eng 1984;12:163–89.
2. Kass DA, Kelly RP. Ventriculo-arterial coupling: concepts, assumptions, and applications. Ann Biomed Eng 1992;20:41–62.
3. Trambaiolo P, Bertini P, Borrelli N, et al. Evaluation of ventriculo-arterial coupling in ST elevation myocardial infarction with left ventricular dysfunction treated with levosimendan. J Cardiol 2019;288:1–4.
4. Ky B, French B, May Khan A, et al. Ventricular-arterial coupling, remodeling, and prognosis in chronic heart failure. J Am Coll Cardiol 2013;62:1165–72.
5. Desai AS, Mitchell GF, Fang JC, et al. Central aortic stiffness is increased in patients with heart failure

and preserved ejection fraction. J Card Fail 2009;15: 658–64.
6. Suga H, Hayashi T, Shirahata M, et al. Regression of cardiac oxygen consumption on ventricular pressure-volume area in dog. Am J Physiol 1981; 240:H320–5.
7. Chen CH, Nakayama M, Nevo E, et al. Coupled systolic-ventricular and vascular stiffening with age: implications for pressure regulation and cardiac reserve in the elderly. J Am Coll Cardiol 1998;32:1221–7.
8. Kelly RP, Ting CT, Yang TM, et al. Effective arterial elastance as index of arterial vascular load in humans. Circulation 1992;86:513–21.
9. De Tombe PP, Jones S, Burkhoff D, et al. Ventricular stroke work and efficiency both remain nearly optimal despite altered vascular loading. Am J Physiol 1993;264:H1817–24.
10. Chen CH, Fetics B, Nevo E, et al. Noninvasive single-beat determination of left ventricular end-systolic elastance in humans. J Am Coll Cardiol 2001;38:2028–34.
11. Bertini P. iElastance© - Apple iOS App. Available at: https://itunes.apple.com/it/app/ielastance/id556528864 2019.
12. Harada A, Okada T, Niki K, et al. On-line noninvasive one-point measurements of pulse wave velocity. Heart Vessels 2002;17:61–8.
13. Vriz O, Zito C, di Bello V, et al. Non-invasive one-point carotid wave intensity in a large group of healthy subjects: a ventricular-arterial coupling parameter. Heart Vessels 2016;3:360–9.
14. Manganaro R, Marchetta S, Dulgheru R, et al. Echocardiographic reference ranges for normal non-invasive myocardial work indices: results from the EACVI NORRE study. Eur Heart J Cardiovasc Imaging 2019;20:582–90.
15. Briand M, Dumesnil JG, Kadem L, et al. Reduced systemic arterial compliance impacts significantly LV afterload and functions in aortic stenosis: implications for diagnosis and treatment. J Am Coll Cardiol 2005;46:291–8.
16. Hachicha Z, Dumesnil JG, Bogaty P, et al. Paradoxical low-flow, low-gradient severe aortic stenosis despite preserved ejection fraction is associated with higher afterload and reduced survival. Circulation 2007;115:2856–64.
17. Ikonomidis I, Katsanos S, Triantafyllidi H, et al. Pulse wave velocity to global longitudinal strain ratio in hypertension. Eur J Clin Invest 2019;49:e13049.
18. Wykretowicz A, Schneider A, Krauze T, et al. Pulse wave velocity to the global longitudinal strain ratio in survivors of myocardial infarction. Eur J Clin Invest 2019;49:e13131.
19. Chantler PD, Lakatta EG, Najjar SS. Arterial-ventricular coupling: mechanistic insights into cardiovascular performance at rest and during exercise. J Appl Phys 2008;105:1342–51.
20. Nakayama M, Itoh H, Oikawa K, et al. Preload-adjusted 2 wave-intensity peaks reflect simultaneous assessment of left ventricular contractility and relaxation. Circ J 2005;69:683–7.
21. Ruppert M, Lakatos BK, Braun S, et al. Longitudinal strain reflects ventriculoarterial coupling rather than mere contractility in rat models of hemodynamic overload–induced heart failure. J Am Soc Echocardiogr 2020. https://doi.org/10.1016/j.echo.2020.05.017.
22. Russell K, Eriksen M, Aaberge L, et al. A novel clinical method for quantification of regional left ventricular pressure-strain loop area: a non-invasive index of myocardial work. Eur Heart J 2012;33: 724–33.
23. Manganaro R, Marchetta S, Dulgheru R, et al. Correlation between non-invasive myocardial work indices and main parameters of systolic and diastolic function: results from the EACVI NORRE study. Eur Heart J Cardiovasc Imaging 2020;21:533–41.
24. Dekleva M, Lazic JS, Soldatovic I, et al. Improvement of ventricular-arterial coupling in elderly patients with heart failure after beta blocker therapy: results from the CIBIS-ELD trial. Cardiovasc Drugs Ther 2015;29:287–94.
25. Zanon F, Aggio S, Baracca E, et al. Ventricular-arterial coupling in patients with heart failure treated with cardiac resynchronization therapy: may we predict the long-term clinical response? Eur J Echocardiogr 2009;10:106–11.
26. Siniawski H, Lehmkuhl HL, Dandel M, et al. Prognostic value of wave intensity in patients awaiting heart transplantation. J Basic Appl Phys 2013;2: 95–103.
27. Vriz O, Pellegrinet M, Zito C, et al. One-point carotid wave intensity predicts cardiac mortality in patients with congestive heart failure and reduced ejection fraction. Int J Cardiovasc Imaging 2015; 31:1369–78.
28. Chan J, Edwards NFA, Khandheria BK, et al. A new approach to assess myocardial work by non-invasive left ventricular pressure-strain relations in hypertension and dilated cardiomyopathy. Eur Heart J Cardiovasc Imaging 2019;20:31–9.
29. Bouali Y, Donal E, Gallard A, et al. Prognostic usefulness of myocardial work in patients with heart failure and reduced ejection fraction treated by sacubitril/valsartan. Am J Cardiol 2020;125:1856–62.
30. Gori M, Lam CS, Gupta DK, et al. PARAMOUNT. Sex-specific cardiovascular structure and function in heart failure with preserved ejection fraction. Eur J Heart Fail 2014;16:535–42.
31. Obokata M, Nagata Y, Kado Y, et al. Ventricular-arterial coupling and exercise-induced pulmonary hypertension during low-level exercise in heart failure with preserved or reduced ejection fraction. J Card Fail 2017;23:216–20.

32. Galli E, Vitel E, Schnell F, et al. Myocardial constructive work is impaired in hypertrophic cardiomyopathy and predicts left ventricular fibrosis. Echocardiography 2019;36:74–82.
33. Gheorghiade M, Zannad F, Sopko G, et al. International working group on acute heart failure syndromes. acute heart failure syndromes: current state and framework for future research. Circulation 2005;112:3958–68.
34. Ponikowski P, Voors AA, Anker SD, et al. 2016 ESC Guidelines for the diagnosis and treatment of acute and chronic heart failure: the task force for the diagnosis and treatment of acute and chronic heart failure of the European Society of Cardiology (ESC) developed with the special contribution of the heart failure association (HFA) of the ESC. Eur Heart J 2016;37:2129–200.
35. Fox JM, Maurer MS. Ventriculo-vascular coupling in systolic and diastolic heart failure. Curr Heart Fail Rep 2005;2:204–11.
36. Neskovic AN, Skinner H, Price S, et al. Focus cardiac ultrasound core curriculum and core syllabus of the European Association of Cardiovascular Imaging. Eur Heart J Cardiovasc Imaging 2018;19:475–81.

Novelties in Therapy of Chronic Heart Failure

Sara Doimo, MD*, Daniela Pavan, MD

KEYWORDS

• Chronic heart failure • Preserved ejection fraction • Reduced ejection fraction • Comorbidities • Neurohormonal antagonists • New therapies

KEY POINTS

- The cornerstone of the current therapy for heart failure is the inhibition of the sympathetic nervous system and the renin-angiotensin-aldosterone system.
- Sacubitril/valsartan reduces cardiovascular mortality and hospitalization for heart failure. Furthermore, sacubitril/valsartan prevents ventricular arrhythmias, the deterioration of renal function in diabetics patients, and it leads to better health-related quality of life in patients with heart failure.
- The research for new treatments for comorbidities has recently led to the discovery of new therapeutic approaches in the treatment of heart failure.
- Sodium-glucose cotransporters 2 inhibition has an emerging role in the treatment of heart failure and on cardiovascular outcome.
- New frontiers are open to the development of neurohormonal therapies, antagonists of inflammatory mediators, inotropic agents, and cell-based therapies.

INTRODUCTION

Heart failure (HF) is a clinical syndrome that represents a growing health problem worldwide.

Despite significant advancements in the treatment of HF, the prevalence of HF is about 1% to 2% of the adult population with a 1-year mortality of 7.2% and a 1-year hospitalization rate of 31.9%.[1,2]

Over the years, significant progress has been made in the treatment of reduced ejection fraction (HFrEF), but in patients affected by preserved ejection fraction (HFpEF), the therapies proven to improve outcome in HFrEF have not been demonstrated to be effective. Actually, there is not a specific therapeutic target for patients with HFpEF.[2,3]

This review provides a comprehensive overview of the current advances and the promising therapies in the treatment of chronic HF.

CURRENT TREATMENTS AND EMERGING EVIDENCES

The cornerstone of the current therapy for HF is the inhibition of the sympathetic nervous system and the renin-angiotensin-aldosterone system. The PARADIGM-HF trial with the demonstration of the superiority of angiotensin receptor neprilysin inhibitors (ARNI) sacubitril/valsartan over enalapril in the reduction of cardiovascular mortality (13.3%vs 16.5%; hazard ratio, HR, 0.80 [95% confidence interval, CI, 0.71–0.89]) and hospitalization for HF (12.8% vs 15.6%; HR, 0.79 [95% CI, 0.71–0.89]) in patients with chronic HFrEF represents a breakthrough in the treatment of HF, and it has opened the way for a new line of research for the treatment of HF.[4]

A possible explanation of the effects of sacubitril-valsartan on cardiovascular outcome in patients with HFrEF was provided by the PROVE-HF[5] study in which patients with HFrEF the reduction in NT-pro-brain natriuretic peptide concentration achieved with sacubitril-valsartan was correlated, significantly but weakly, with signs of reverse cardiac remodeling at 1 year.

The results derived from the secondary endpoint of the EVALUATE-HF randomized clinical trial[6] were able to support the findings of PROVE-HF.[5]

Cardio-Cerebro-Vascular Pathophysiology Department, Cardiology Unit, Azienda Sanitaria "Friuli Occidentale", Pordenone, Italy
* Corresponding author.
E-mail address: sarozza@gmail.com

Heart Failure Clin 17 (2021) 255–262
https://doi.org/10.1016/j.hfc.2021.01.006

Among patients with HFrEF, sacubitril/valsartan versus enalapril improved some measures of diastolic function. The primary outcome of EVALUATE-HF was the effect of ARNI on aortic stiffness, but it did not lead to significant results.[6]

The subsequent subanalyses of PARADIGM- HF showed other extracardiac effects of sacubitril/valsartan.[7]

Concerning the effects of ARNI on renal function in comparison with angiotensin-converting enzyme inhibitors (ACEI), Damman and colleagues[8] show superiority of ARNI over ACEI in patients both with and without chronic kidney disease. The decrease in estimated glomerular filtration rate (eGFR) during follow-up was less with sacubitril/valsartan compared with enalapril despite a greater increase in urinary albumin/creatinine ratio with sacubitril/valsartan than with enalapril.

Another analysis concluded that the addition of neprilysin inhibition attenuates the effect of diabetes to accelerate the deterioration of renal function that occurs in patients with chronic HF. In this study, compared with patients treated with enalapril, those treated with sacubitril/valsartan had a slower rate of decline in eGFR.[9]

In addition to this, Desai and colleagues[6] suggested that the risk of severe hyperkalemia is more likely during treatment with enalapril than with sacubitril/valsartan among mineralocorticoid receptor antagonist-treated patients with symptomatic HFrEF.

Several studies evidenced an improvement of glycemia control in diabetic patients.[10,11] The pathophysiological mechanisms, underlying better glycemia control when ARNI is administered, are not fully understood and need further investigation. Currently, it is usually attributed to higher concentration of active peptides, which could not be degraded by inactive neprilysin like brain natriuretic peptide, bradykinin, and glucagon-like peptide-1.[7,12]

The effect of sacubitril/valsartan was also evaluated on the prevention of ventricular arrhythmias or sudden cardiac death. de Diego and colleagues[13] explored the effect of angiotensin-neprilysin inhibition on ventricular arrhythmias compared with angiotensin inhibition in HFrEF patients with an implantable cardioverter-defibrillator (ICD) and remote monitoring. Sacubitril-valsartan significantly decreased nonsustained ventricular tachycardia episodes, sustained ventricular tachycardia, and appropriate ICD shocks.[13] The design of the PARADIGM-HF trial also allowed patients to make a subjective analysis of their health-related quality of life by filling out specific questionnaires. The results demonstrated that sacubitril/valsartan led to better health-related quality of life in surviving patients with HF.[14,15]

In the setting of HFpEF, the efficacy of sacubitril-valsartan on morbidity and mortality was evaluated in the PARAGON-HF trial.[16] In this trial, sacubitril-valsartan was not effective at reducing the incidence of cardiovascular death or hospitalization for HF compared with valsartan. However, in the subgroup analyses, sacubitril-valsartan was associated with a reduction of the primary outcome in women, and it has shown a possible benefit in patients with ejection fraction $\leq$57%.[17,18]

A recently concluded study, the PARALLAX trial[19] (ClinicalTrials.gov Identifier: NCT03066804), evaluated the effect of ARNI on functional capacity in patients with preserved or midrange ejection fraction. In this trial, the primary endpoints were a change from baseline to 12 weeks in plasma N-terminal pro-B-type natriuretic peptide (NT-pro-BNP) and a change in 6-minute walk distance from baseline to 24 weeks. The patients treated with sacubitril/valsartan showed a significant 16.4% greater reduction in NT-pro-BNP than those patients treated with optimal individualized medical therapy after 12 weeks (P<.0001)[19] (**Fig. 1**).

NEW THERAPEUTIC PERSPECTIVES FROM THE TREATMENT OF COMORBIDITIES

Noncardiac comorbidities often complicate the patients with HF, and they are strongly associated with adverse clinical outcomes. Braunstein and colleagues[20] demonstrated that the risk of hospitalization and potentially preventable hospitalization strongly increased with the number of chronic conditions (both P<.0001).

The research for new treatments for comorbidities has recently led to the discovery of new approaches in the treatment of HF (**Table 1**).

The most important advances derive from the new pharmacologic treatments for diabetes.

Diabetes mellitus is a major risk factor for cardiovascular disease, and patients with diabetes have greater than 2 times the risk for developing HF.[21,22]

Recent trials showed an important role of sodium-glucose cotransporters 2 (SGLT2) on cardiovascular outcomes. Inhibition of SGLT2 promotes glycosuria and a catabolic state with lower insulin and increased glucagon levels. Glucagon induces hyperketonemia, and the ketone bodies can be used as substrates of myocardial metabolism and may have a favorable effect on cardiac function.[23,24]

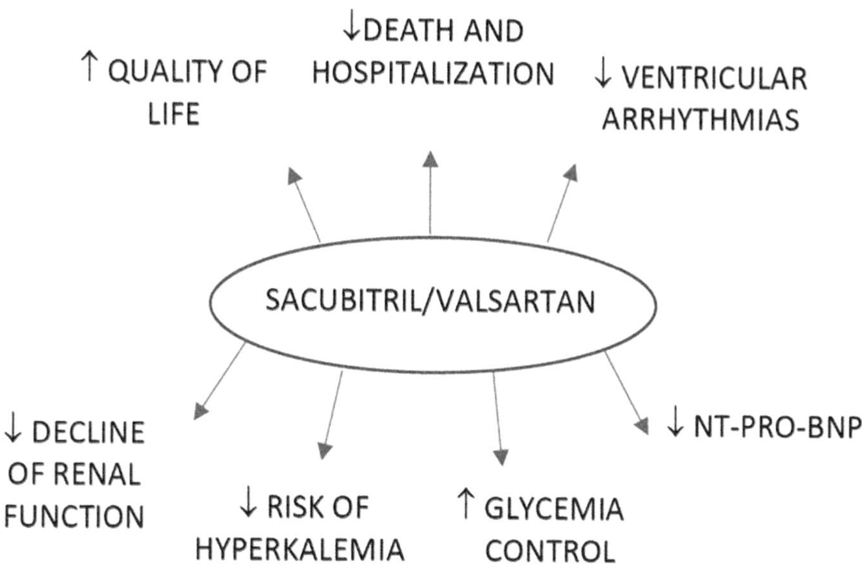

Fig. 1. The effects of sacubitril/valsartan.

Empagliflozin was the first SGLT2 inhibitor to show a relevant impact on cardiovascular outcome in patients with HF in the EMPA-REG OUTCOME trial.[25,26] There were no differences in the rates of myocardial infarction or stroke, but in the empagliflozin group, there were significantly lower rates of death from cardiovascular causes, hospitalization for HF, and death from any cause.

Similar results emerged from other SGLT2 inhibitors. The DECLARE-TIMI 58 trial[27] showed that dapagliflozin is superior to placebo in improving glycemic control and noninferior but not superior for reducing cardiovascular death, myocardial infarction, or ischemic stroke in patients with diabetes and high cardiovascular risk. The CANVAS study[28] demonstrated that the incidence of cardiovascular death, myocardial infarction, or stroke occurred in 26.9 participants per 1000 patient-years of the canagliflozin group versus 31.5 participants per 1000 patient-years of the placebo group (P = .02 for superiority, P<.001 for noninferiority). The benefit for canagliflozin appeared to be similar for patients with HFrEF and those with HFpEF.

Significant results have emerged about the use of SGLT2 in HF derived from 2 recent trials: the EMPEROR reduced trial[29] and the DAPA-HF trial.[30] In the EMPEROR reduced trial,[29] during a median of 16 months, the primary outcome event (cardiovascular death or hospitalization for worsening HF) occurred in 361 of 1863 patients (19.4%) in the empagliflozin group and in 462 of 1867 patients (24.7%) in the placebo group (HR for cardiovascular death or hospitalization for HF, 0.75; 95% CI, 0.65–0.86; P<.001). In the DAPA-HF trial,[30] the primary outcome of cardiovascular death, hospitalization for HF, or urgent HF visit occurred in 16.3% of the dapagliflozin group compared with 21.2% of the placebo group (P<.001). Benefit was consistent across the age spectrum, baseline diuretic use, in diabetics/nondiabetics, across the range of baseline health status, and baseline medication use.

Regarding the role of SGLT2 in HFpEF in patients with diabetes or without diabetes, there are 2 phase 3 ongoing studies: EMPEROR-Preserved with empaglifozin[31] (ClinicalTrials.gov Identifier: NCT03057951) and DELIVER with dapaglifozin[32] (ClinicalTrials.gov Identifier: NCT03619213).

Hyperkalemia is a common complication in patients with nondialysis chronic kidney disease. It is associated with different treatments for HF, and it may preclude the use of neurohormonal antagonists. Hyperkalemia can conduce to weakness, paralysis, arrhythmias, and increased mortality. Patiromer and sodium zirconium cyclosilicate (ZS-9) represent significant pharmacologic progress in the treatment of hyperkalemia.[33]

Patiromer is an oral suspension of nonadsorbed polymer, which binds potassium in the exchange of calcium in the distal colon.[34,35] The PEARL-HF study tested the combined use of patiromer with spironolactone in HF patients receiving standard care but with previous documented hyperkalemia or chronic kidney disease.[36] The use of patiromer was effective at preventing hyperkalemia, and it was especially effective at preventing hyperkalemia among those with eGFR less than 60 mL/min. Patiromer was

Table 1
New therapeutic perspectives and future directions in the treatment of chronic heart failure

SGLT2 Inhibitors (Empagliflozin; Dapagliflozin; Canagliflozin)	Injectable Iron (Ferric Caboxymaltose)	Potassium Binders (Patiromer; ZS-9)	Splanchnic Nerve Blockade	sGC Stimulator (Vericiguat)	Antagonists of Inflammatory Mediators	Selective Cardiac Myosin Activator (Omecamtiv Mecarbil)	Autologous Adult Bone Marrow–Derived Stem/ Progenitor Cells
↓ Cardiovascular death and hospitalization ↑ Glycosuria, uricosuria, and natriuresis ↓ Inflammation and fibrosis ↓ Myocardial remodeling ↓ Arrhythmias	↓ Cardiovascular symptoms ↑ Functional capacity ↑ Quality of life	↓ Iperkaliemia ↑ Patients treated with neurohormonal antagonists	↓ Exercise-induced intracardiac pressure elevations ↑ Cardiac output ↑ Exercise capacity	↑ Antifibrotic effects ↓ Myocardial remodeling ↑ Diastolic relaxation ↓ Cardiovascular death and hospitalization	TNF-α antagonists (etanercept and infliximab): the studies were prematurely discontinued due to lack of clinical benefit Anti-IL-1β-monoclonal antibody (canakinumab): ↓ Adverse cardiac events IL-6 receptor antibody (tocilizumab): ↓ Inflammatory response and primarily percutaneous coronary intervention-related troponin T release in NSTEMI	↑ Systolic ejection time ↑ Cardiac contractility ↑ Measures of right ventricular pulmonary arterial coupling ↓ Cardiovascular events	The use is safe and effective in differentiation capacity and immune modulating properties Low-quality evidence in improving left ventricular ejection fraction over short- and long-term follow- up

well tolerated, except for an increase in gastrointestinal-related adverse events (flatulence, diarrhea, constipation, or vomiting).[34,36]

ZS-9 is a highly selective cation exchanger that entraps potassium in the intestinal tract in exchange for sodium and hydrogen.[33,37] In a multicenter, double-blind, phase 3 trial,[33] patients with hyperkalemia who received ZS-9, as compared with those who received placebo, had a significant reduction in potassium levels at 48 hours, with normokalemia maintained for 12 days of maintenance therapy.

Patiromer and ZS-9 appear to offer some promise for the treatment of hyperkalemia in patients with chronic kidney and cardiac disease, and the use of these agents could improve the number of patients treated with neurohormonal antagonists.

Iron deficiency is one of most common comorbidities in patients with HF. It is associated with reduced exercise capacity and reduced quality of life; moreover, it is an independent factor of death or hospitalizations in patients with chronic HF. The FAIR-HF[38] study has been the first double-blind, placebo-controlled multicenter trial to compare treatment with intravenous ferric carboxymaltose versus placebo among patients with chronic HF and iron deficiency (with or without anemia). In the patients assigned to ferric carboxymaltose, 47% had New York Heart Association functional class I or II at week 24, as compared with 30% of patients assigned to placebo (odds ratio for improvement by 1 class, 2.40; 95% CI, 1.55–3.71), whereas the rates of death, adverse events, and serious adverse events were similar in the 2 study groups.[38]

The only study designed to evaluate the efficacy of ferric carboxymaltose in improving symptoms of HFpEF in patients with iron deficiency is the FAIR-HFpEF trial (ClinicalTrials.gov Identifier: NCT03074591), THE completion of which is estimated for 2021.

The effect of iron deficiency correction on major cardiovascular outcomes is the rationale of 2 ongoing studies, the HEART-FID (ClinicalTrials.gov Identifier: NCT03037931) and THE IRONMAN (ClinicalTrials.gov Identifier: NCT02642562).

FUTURE DIRECTIONS

New frontiers are open to the development of neurohormonal therapies, antagonists of inflammatory mediators, inotropic agents, and cell-based therapies (see **Table 1**).

In chronic HF, cardiopulmonary congestion is the main cause of exercise intolerance and exertional dyspnea. In HF, as a result of a neurohormonal imbalance, the vascular capacitance is decreased, and acute sympathetic nerve activation can result in acute volume redistribution from the abdominal compartment to the heart and lungs, which increases intracardiac pressures and precipitates HF symptoms.[39–41] The sympathetic nervous system controls the splanchnic compartment via branches from the sympathetic thoracic ganglia (T6 through T11), and the splanchnic nerves have been identified as a potential target for treating HF.[41] In a study by Fudim and colleagues[42] that evaluated the safety and efficacy of splanchnic nerve blockade in patients with chronic HFrEF, splanchnic nerve blockade decreased exercise-induced intracardiac pressure elevations with an improvement in cardiac output and a trend toward an improved exercise capacity. However, studies on the long-term effects of this procedure are needed.

The nitric oxide–soluble guanylate cyclase (sGC)-cyclic guanosine monophosphate (cGMP) signaling pathway plays an important role in tissue fibrosis, oxidative stress, and inflammation.[43] Deficiency in sGC-derived cGMP causes both myocardial dysfunction and impaired endothelium-dependent vasomotor regulation, and restoration of sufficient sGC-cGMP signaling has been proposed as a potentially important target in HF therapy.[44]

The effect of a novel sGC stimulator, vericiguat, on cardiovascular outcome in patients with chronic HFrEF has been assessed in the VICTORIA trial.[44] The primary outcome, cardiovascular death or hospitalization for HF, occurred in 35.5% of the vericiguat group compared with 38.5% of the placebo group (HR 0.90, P = .019). Vericiguat was safe and well tolerated and did not require monitoring of renal function or electrolytes.[44]

Currently, there IS no evidence regarding the use of sGC stimulators on HFpEF. The CAPACITY-HFpEF trial[45] and VITALITY-HFpEF trial[46] are evaluating the effect of sGC stimulators on exercise intolerance.

The proinflammatory cytokines, tumor necrosis factor (TNF)-α, interleukin (IL)-1-β, and IL-6, have a crucial role in the pathogenesis of HF. The cytokines suppress contractile function in cardiomyocytes, inducing inflammatory activation in macrophages and stimulating microvascular inflammation.[47]

The TNF-α is the best-studied inflammatory mediator in HF. TNF-α antagonists, etanercept and infliximab, were studied in several trials; however, the studies were prematurely discontinued because of A lack of clinical benefit. The effect of an anti-IL-1β monoclonal antibody canakinumab on cardiovascular outcome (hospitalizations and HF-related death) has been evaluated in the CANTOS trial, involving 10,061 patients with previous myocardial infarction and a high-sensitivity

C-reactive protein level of 2 mg or more per liter. This study showed that canakinumab was effective at preventing adverse cardiac events over a median of 3.7 years.[48,49]

IL-6 plays an important function in inflammatory response in different diseases; therefore, it is one of THE principal therapeutic targets in several conditions. A double-blind, placebo-controlled trial enrolled 117 patients with non-ST-elevation myocardial infarction (NSTEMI), showing that IL-6 receptor antibody, tocilizumab, attenuated the inflammatory response and primarily percutaneous coronary intervention-related troponin T release in NSTEMI patients.[50]

Currently, traditional inotropic agents improve cardiac contractility but are associated with myocardial ischemia, arrhythmias, and mortality. A novel selective cardiac myosin activator, omecamtiv mecarbil, activates the sarcomere proteins directly, resulting in prolonged systolic ejection time and increased cardiac contractility. In the phase 2 COSMIC-HF trial[51] in patients with chronic HF and reduced systolic function, 20 weeks of omecamtiv mecarbil treatment was associated with improvement in several measures of right ventricular function together with improvement in measures of right ventricular pulmonary arterial coupling. A phase 3 study, the GALACTIC-HF trial,[52] will determine if treatment with omecamtiv mecarbil, when added to standard of care, is well tolerated and superior to placebo in reducing the risk of cardiovascular death or HF events in subjects with chronic HFrEF.

A promising approach in the treatment of chronic HF is the use of autologous adult bone marrow–derived stem/progenitor cells. A recent systematic review and meta-analysis suggested that mesenchymal stem cells as a regenerative therapeutic approach for HF is safe and effective by virtue of their self-renewal potential, vast differentiation capacity, and immune modulating properties.[53] However, the results of the studies are not univocal for the use of this therapy in HF. A Cochrane critical evaluation of clinical evidence on the safety and efficacy of stem cells as a treatment of chronic HF found low-quality evidence in improving left ventricular ejection fraction over short- and long-term follow-up.[54]

For these reasons, further studies are needed to determine the evidence-based indications of the use of autologous adult bone marrow-derived stem/progenitor cells in HF.

SUMMARY

In recent decades, considerable advances have been made in the treatment of HF. The main target of HF therapy is the inhibition of the sympathetic nervous system and the renin-angiotensin-aldosterone system. The angiotensin receptor blockers represent a breakthrough in the treatment of HF with a demonstrated effect on reduction of cardiovascular events. However, new perspectives are derived from the latest drugs developed for diabetes, iron deficiency, and hyperkalemia. New frontiers are also opened to the development of neurohormonal therapies, antagonists of inflammatory mediators, inotropic agents, and cell-based treatments.

CLINICS CARE POINTS

Significant progress has been made in the treatment of heart failure with reduced ejection fraction, in particular, in the development of neurohormonal therapies, but for the patients affected by heart failure with preserved ejection fraction, there is currently no evidence of an effective therapy that can improve the cardiovascular outcome. Further studies are needed to identify possible therapeutic targets for heart failure with preserved ejection fraction and to verify the long-term effects of the recently discovered drugs.

DISCLOSURE

The author has nothing to disclose.

REFERENCES

1. Savarese G, Lund LH. Global public health burden of heart failure. Card Fail Rev 2017;3:7–11.
2. Chioncel O, Lainscak M, Seferovic PM, et al. Epidemiology and one-year outcomes in patients with chronic heart failure and preserved, mid-range and reduced ejection fraction: an analysis of the ESC Heart Failure Long-Term Registry. Eur J Heart Fail 2017;19:1574–85.
3. Ponikowski P, Voors AA, Anker SD, et al. 2016 ESC Guidelines for the Diagnosis and Treatment of Acute and Chronic Heart Failure: the Task Force for the diagnosis and treatment of acute and chronic heart failure of the European Society of Cardiology (ESC). Developed with the special contribution of the Heart Failure Association (HFA) of the ESC. Eur J Heart Fail 2016;18:891–975.
4. McMurray JJV, Packer M, Desai AS, et al. Angiotensin-neprilysin inhibition versus enalapril in heart failure. N Engl J Med 2014;371:993–1004.
5. Januzzi JLJ, Prescott MF, Butler J, et al. Association of change in N-terminal pro-B-type natriuretic

peptide following initiation of sacubitril-valsartan treatment with cardiac structure and function in patients with heart failure with reduced ejection fraction. JAMA 2019;322:1–11.

6. Desai AS, Solomon SD, Shah AM, et al. Effect of sacubitril-valsartan vs enalapril on aortic stiffness in patients with heart failure and reduced ejection fraction: a randomized clinical trial. JAMA 2019; 322:1–10.
7. Książczyk M, Lelonek M. Angiotensin receptor/neprilysin inhibitor-a breakthrough in chronic heart failure therapy: summary of subanalysis on PARADIGM-HF trial findings. Heart Fail Rev 2020; 25:393–402.
8. Damman K, Gori M, Claggett B, et al. Renal effects and associated outcomes during angiotensin-neprilysin inhibition in heart failure. JACC Heart Fail 2018;6:489–98.
9. Packer M, Claggett B, Lefkowitz MP, et al. Effect of neprilysin inhibition on renal function in patients with type 2 diabetes and chronic heart failure who are receiving target doses of inhibitors of the renin-angiotensin system: a secondary analysis of the PARADIGM-HF trial. Lancet Diabetes Endocrinol 2018;6:547–54.
10. Seferovic JP, Claggett B, Seidelmann SB, et al. Effect of sacubitril/valsartan versus enalapril on glycaemic control in patients with heart failure and diabetes: a post-hoc analysis from the PARADIGM-HF trial. Lancet Diabetes Endocrinol 2017;5:333–40.
11. Kristensen SL, Preiss D, Jhund PS, et al. Risk related to pre-diabetes mellitus and diabetes mellitus in heart failure with reduced ejection fraction: insights from prospective comparison of ARNI with ACEI to determine impact on global mortality and morbidity in heart failure trial. Circ Heart Fail 2016; 9:e002560.
12. Willard JR, Barrow BM, Zraika S. Improved glycaemia in high-fat-fed neprilysin-deficient mice is associated with reduced DPP-4 activity and increased active GLP-1 levels. Diabetologia 2017;60:701–8.
13. de Diego C, González-Torres L, Núñez JM, et al. Effects of angiotensin-neprilysin inhibition compared to angiotensin inhibition on ventricular arrhythmias in reduced ejection fraction patients under continuous remote monitoring of implantable defibrillator devices. Heart Rhythm 2018;15:395–402.
14. Lewis EF, Claggett BL, McMurray JJV, et al. Health-related quality of life outcomes in PARADIGM-HF. Circ Heart Fail 2017;10:e003430.
15. Chandra A, Lewis EF, Claggett BL, et al. Effects of sacubitril/valsartan on physical and social activity limitations in patients with heart failure: a secondary analysis of the PARADIGM-HF trial. JAMA Cardiol 2018;3:498–505.
16. Solomon SD, McMurray JJV, Anand IS, et al. Angiotensin–neprilysin inhibition in heart failure with preserved ejection fraction. N Engl J Med 2019; 381:1609–20.
17. Solomon SD, Vaduganathan M, Claggett L, et al. Sacubitril/valsartan across the spectrum of ejection fraction in heart failure. Circulation 2020;141: 352–61.
18. Murphy SP, Ibrahim NE, Januzzi JLJ. Heart failure with reduced ejection fraction: a review. JAMA 2020;324:488–504.
19. Wachter R, Shah SJ, Cowie MR, et al. Angiotensin receptor neprilysin inhibition versus individualized RAAS blockade: design and rationale of the PARALLAX trial. ESC Hear Fail 2020;7:856–64.
20. Braunstein JB, Anderson GF, Gerstenblith G, et al. Noncardiac comorbidity increases preventable hospitalizations and mortality among Medicare beneficiaries with chronic heart failure. J Am Coll Cardiol 2003;42:1226–33.
21. Sarwar N, Gao P, Seshasai SRK, et al. Diabetes mellitus, fasting blood glucose concentration, and risk of vascular disease: a collaborative meta-analysis of 102 prospective studies. Lancet 2010;375: 2215–22.
22. Arnold SV, Echouffo-Tcheugui JB, Lam CSP, et al. Patterns of glucose-lowering medication use in patients with type 2 diabetes and heart failure. Insights from the Diabetes Collaborative Registry (DCR). Am Heart J 2018;203:25–9.
23. Butler J, Hamo CE, Filippatos G, et al. The potential role and rationale for treatment of heart failure with sodium-glucose co-transporter 2 inhibitors. Eur J Heart Fail 2017;19:1390–400.
24. Seferović PM, Fragasso G, Petrie M, et al. Sodium-glucose co-transporter 2 inhibitors in heart failure: beyond glycaemic control. The position paper of the Heart Failure Association of the European Society of Cardiology. Eur J Heart Fail 2020;22(9):1495–503.
25. Pellicori P, Ofstad AP, Fitchett D, et al. Early benefits of empagliflozin in patients with or without heart failure: findings from EMPA-REG OUTCOME. ESC Hear Fail 2020;7(6):3401–7.
26. Zinman B, Wanner C, Lachin JM, et al. Empagliflozin, cardiovascular outcomes, and mortality in type 2 diabetes. N Engl J Med 2015;373:2117–28.
27. Wiviott SD, Raz I, Bonaca MP, et al. Dapagliflozin and cardiovascular outcomes in type 2 diabetes. N Engl J Med 2019;380:347–57.
28. Neal B, Perkovic V, Matthews DR. Canagliflozin and cardiovascular and renal events in type 2 diabetes. N Engl J Med 2017;377:2099.
29. Packer M, Anker SD, Butler J, et al. Cardiovascular and renal outcomes with empagliflozin in heart failure. N Engl J Med 2020;383(15):1413–24.
30. Jackson AM, Dewan P, Anand IS, et al. Dapagliflozin and diuretic use in patients with heart failure and reduced ejection fraction in DAPA-HF. Circulation 2020;142:1040–54.

31. Anker SD, Butler J, Filippatos GS, et al. Evaluation of the effects of sodium-glucose co-transporter 2 inhibition with empagliflozin on morbidity and mortality in patients with chronic heart failure and a preserved ejection fraction: rationale for and design of the EMPEROR-Preserved Trial. Eur J Heart Fail 2019; 21:1279–87.
32. Nassif ME, Kosiborod M. Effects of sodium glucose cotransporter type 2 inhibitors on heart failure. Diabetes Obes Metab 2019;21(Suppl 2):19–23.
33. Packham DK, Rasmussen HS, Lavin PT, et al. Sodium zirconium cyclosilicate in hyperkalemia. N Engl J Med 2015;372:222–31.
34. Pitt B, Anker SD, Bushinsky DA, et al. Evaluation of the efficacy and safety of RLY5016, a polymeric potassium binder, in a double-blind, placebo-controlled study in patients with chronic heart failure (the PEARL-HF) trial. Eur Heart J 2011;32:820–8.
35. Sciatti E, Dallapellegrina L, Metra M, et al. New drugs for the treatment of chronic heart failure with a reduced ejection fraction: what the future may hold. J Cardiovasc Med (Hagerstown) 2019;20: 650–9.
36. Buysse JM, Huang I-Z, Pitt B. PEARL-HF: prevention of hyperkalemia in patients with heart failure using a novel polymeric potassium binder, RLY5016. Future Cardiol 2012;8:17–28.
37. Stavros F, Yang A, Leon A, et al. Characterization of structure and function of ZS-9, a K+ selective ion trap. PLoS One 2014;9:e114686.
38. Anker SD, Comin Colet J, Filippatos G, et al. Ferric carboxymaltose in patients with heart failure and iron deficiency. N Engl J Med 2009;361:2436–48.
39. Fudim M, Hernandez AF, Felker GM. Role of volume redistribution in the congestion of heart failure. J Am Heart Assoc 2017;6:e006817.
40. Fudim M, Yalamuri S, Herbert JT, et al. Raising the pressure: hemodynamic effects of splanchnic nerve stimulation. J Appl Physiol 2017;123:126–7.
41. Fudim M, Jones WS, Boortz-Marx RL, et al. Splanchnic nerve block for acute heart failure. Circulation 2018;138:951–3.
42. Fudim M, Boortz-Marx RL, Ganesh A, et al. Splanchnic nerve block for chronic heart failure. JACC Heart Fail 2020;8:742–52.
43. Zheng X, Zheng W, Xiong B, et al. The efficacy and safety of soluble guanylate cyclase stimulators in patients with heart failure: a systematic review and meta-analysis. Medicine (Baltimore) 2018;97: e12709.
44. Armstrong PW, Roessig L, Patel MJ, et al. A multicenter, randomized, double-blind, placebo-controlled trial of the efficacy and safety of the oral soluble guanylate cyclase stimulator: the VICTORIA Trial. JACC Heart Fail 2018;6:96–104.
45. Udelson JE, Lewis GD, Shah SJ, et al. Rationale and design for a multicenter, randomized, double-blind, placebo-controlled, phase 2 study evaluating the safety and efficacy of the soluble guanylate cyclase stimulator praliciguat over 12 weeks in patients with heart failure with preserved ejection fraction (CAPACITY HFpEF). Am Heart J 2020;222:183–90.
46. Butler J, Lam CSP, Anstrom KJ, et al. Rationale and design of the VITALITY-HFpEF Trial. Circ Heart Fail 2019;12:e005998.
47. Hanna A, Frangogiannis NG. Inflammatory cytokines and chemokines as therapeutic targets in heart failure. Cardiovasc Drugs Ther 2020;34(6):849–63.
48. Ridker PM, Everett BM, Thuren T, et al. Antiinflammatory therapy with canakinumab for atherosclerotic disease. N Engl J Med 2017;377:1119–31.
49. Ridker PM, MacFadyen JG, Thuren T, et al. Residual inflammatory risk associated with interleukin-18 and interleukin-6 after successful interleukin-1β inhibition with canakinumab: further rationale for the development of targeted anti-cytokine therapies for the treatment of atherothrombosis. Eur Heart J 2020;41: 2153–63.
50. Kleveland O, Kunszt G, Bratlie M, et al. Effect of a single dose of the interleukin-6 receptor antagonist tocilizumab on inflammation and troponin T release in patients with non-ST-elevation myocardial infarction: a double-blind, randomized, placebo-controlled phase 2 trial. Eur Heart J 2016;37: 2406–13.
51. Teerlink JR, Felker GM, McMurray JJV, et al. Chronic Oral Study of Myosin Activation to Increase Contractility in Heart Failure (COSMIC-HF): a phase 2, pharmacokinetic, randomised, placebo-controlled trial. Lancet 2016;388:2895–903.
52. Teerlink JR, Diaz R, Felker GM, et al. Omecamtiv mecarbil in chronic heart failure with reduced ejection fraction: rationale and design of GALACTIC-HF. JACC Heart Fail 2020;8:329–40.
53. Shen T, Xia L, Dong W, et al. A systematic review and meta-analysis: safety and efficacy of mesenchymal stem cells therapy for heart failure. Curr Stem Cell Res Ther 2020. https://doi.org/10.2174/1574888X15999200820171432.
54. Fisher SA, Doree C, Mathur A, et al. Stem cell therapy for chronic ischaemic heart disease and congestive heart failure. Cochrane Database Syst Rev 2016;12:CD007888.

Exercise-Based Cardiac Rehabilitation Programs in Heart Failure Patients

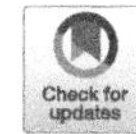

Alessandro Patti, MD[a], Laura Merlo, MD[a], Marco Ambrosetti, MD[b], Patrizio Sarto, MD[a,*]

KEYWORDS

- Exercise training • Cardiac rehabilitation • Heart failure • Exercise prescription
- Cardiopulmonary testing • Peak V_{O_2}

KEY POINTS

- Exercise training is recommended by major societies' guidelines for patients with heart failure.
- Exercise training improves exercise capacity and quality of life, and reduces symptoms of depression in patients with heart failure. Moreover, it can improve survival and reduce the risk for hospitalizations.
- Exercise-based cardiac rehabilitation can be offered with different modalities, such as continuous interval or aerobic training, resistance and inspiratory muscle training.
- The intervention has to be tailored taking into account the patient's cardiovascular conditions and functional capacity.
- To date, the adherence to exercise-based programs is scarce, due to socioeconomic factors, patients' characteristics and lack in referral.

INTRODUCTION

One of the main clinical features that characterize heart failure (HF) is the limited exercise tolerance. Patients with HF often experience dyspnea and fatigue at relatively low workloads, and diminished physical work capacity.[1] In the past, conventional common sense has led physicians to advise patients with HF to avoid physical exertion (to reduce the occurrence of symptoms and a potential worsening of the disease). Nevertheless, in the past decades a change of attitude has slowly permeated the medical practice due to evidence illustrating the benefits of physical exercise on myocardial function, symptoms, functional capacity, quality of life (QOL), and hospitalizations of these patients.[1,2] The present review describes the evidence supporting the use of exercise training in the management of patients with HF and the main types of exercise training programs commonly included in these patients' exercise prescriptions.

EFFECTS OF EXERCISE TRAINING

Molecular Effects

Exercise training (ET) is known to be an effective measure for the control of several cardiovascular (CV) risk factors, such as increased body mass index, hypertension, insulin resistance, and reduced high-density lipoprotein cholesterol.[3] However, these effects seem to account only for part of the benefits induced by regular ET, whereas up to 40% is thought to be related to other factors.[4]

In this context, it is important to underline the anti-inflammatory role of ET in reducing the blood levels of several proinflammatory cytokines, such as tumor necrosis factor alpha, interleukin-6 and their soluble receptors, and apoptotic mediators, such as Fas and Fas ligand.[5,6]

Moreover, the generation of reactive oxygen species during exercise could serve as a molecular pathway to activate important antioxidant enzymes, such as mitochondrial superoxide

[a] Sports Medicine Unit, AULSS 2, Via Castellana 2, 31100 Treviso, Italy; [b] Cardiological Rehabilitation Unit, ASST Crema, Presidio S. Marta, Viale Monte Grappa 15, 26027 Rivolta d'Adda (CR), Italy
* Corresponding author.
E-mail address: patrizio.sarto@aulss2.veneto.it

Heart Failure Clin 17 (2021) 263–271
https://doi.org/10.1016/j.hfc.2021.01.007

dismutase and inducible nitric oxide synthase that may mediate, at least in part, the exercise-induced cardioprotection against ischemia-reperfusion injury.[7,8] Similar effects have been demonstrated for the increase in the expression of inducible health-shock protein 70, which can be related to ET.[9,10]

Regular exercise has also been shown to improve endothelial function and flow-mediated vasodilatation in patients with HF. In fact, it improves both basal endothelial nitric oxide formation and agonist-mediated endothelium-dependent vasodilatation of the skeletal muscle and prevents the production of vasoconstrictor prostanoids and free radicals, possibly contributing to the improvement of exercise capacity.[11,12] In addition to that, ET can enhance endothelial progenitor cells (a cellular lineage implied in postischemic neoangiogenesis and endothelial repair) in patients with HF, promoting endothelial repair and contributing to the improvement in endothelial function.[13,14]

Skeletal Myopathy and Sarcopenia

Malnutrition, physical inactivity, low muscle blood flow, inflammation and oxidative stress, apoptosis, and other changes at the molecular and hormonal level all contribute to skeletal muscle dysfunction and wasting in patients with HF.[15,16] These changes can result in the development of a skeletal myopathy, which not only is induced by cardiac failure, but contributes itself to the progression of the disease and is responsible for the occurrence of clinical symptoms.[15]

In this context, ET can result in an increase in the oxidative capacity of the muscle, secondary to an increase in the total volume density of mitochondria. This change can improve the peak oxygen consumption (V_{O_2}) and the ventilatory threshold.[17] The importance of this adaptation consists of delaying the onset of the anaerobic metabolism, reducing the "anaerobic burden" during effort and leading to an increase in exercise tolerance. Moreover, resistance training has been demonstrated to be a positive stimulus on muscle mass, muscle quality and physical performance in patients with HF.[18]

"Central" Effects

In parallel with the aforementioned changes at the molecular level, ET can result in several adaptations at the cardiac and neurohumoral level. In their meta-analysis, Haykowsky and colleagues[19] reported a statistically significant improvement in left ventricular ejection fraction (LVEF) of 2.6% in patients with HF performing ET compared with nonexercising controls, mirrored by a reduction in end-diastolic and end-systolic volumes of 11.5 and 12.9 mL, respectively.

Moreover, ET helps counteracting the increase in sympathetic tone, which is typical of patients with HF, reducing sympathetic outflow, increasing baroreflex sensitivity and heart rate variability and reducing circulating levels of catecholamines, angiotensin II, vasopressin, and atrial and brain natriuretic peptide.[20,21] These effects are observable both at rest and during exercise.[22]

In patients with HF with preserved LVEF, ET appeared to be safe and conferred improvements in cardiorespiratory fitness and QOL, without significantly impacting the diastolic or systolic function.[23,24] It has been hypothesized that the improvements in peak V_{O_2} can derive from muscular or microvascular adaptations that result in increased peak exercise arterial-venous oxygen difference without a change in peak exercise cardiac output, central arterial stiffness, and peripheral arterial endothelial function.[25]

Effects on Functional Capacity

Taken together, the adaptations to ET described previously favorably affect exercise tolerance and exercise capacity in patients with HF. In fact, improvements in peak V_{O_2} after ET can range from 13% to 31%. A meta-analysis of 57 studies involving patients with reduced ejection fraction reported an average increase in peak V_{O_2} of 17%. Considering 8 studies that included 70% of patients taking beta-blockers and angiotensin-converting enzyme inhibitors (ACE-i), the unadjusted median change was comparable (15%) and superior to that of nonexercising controls (1%).[22,26]

In addition to that, previous evidence reported superior effects of high-intensity interval training (HIIT) compared with continuous moderate-intensity training alone, with improvements of peak V_{O_2} up to 48%.[26,27] Even though, a recent meta-analysis that included 11 studies found no difference in the improvement of cardiopulmonary exercise testing (CPET) parameters comparing interval with continuous training. An improvement of LVEF and left ventricular end-diastolic diameter was noted after interval training.[28] Further evidence will help to elucidate the effects of this modality, compared with continuous aerobic ET, on functional capacity in patients with HF.[29]

Finally, strength training is also effective in improving functional capacity of patients with HF. In fact, it has been demonstrated that it improves muscle strength, aerobic capacity, and QOL, serving as a complementary tool to aerobic ET or as an alternative strategy for patients unable to perform aerobic ET.[30,31]

Outcome

The positive impact of physical activity on patients with HF has been described also for clinical endpoints. In fact, in patients with symptomatic HF, physical inactivity has been shown to be associated with higher all-cause and cardiac mortality, while even modest exercise is associated with survival benefit.[32]

A recently updated meta-analysis by the Cochrane Collaboration Group pointed out how exercise-based cardiac rehabilitation may make little or no difference in all-cause mortality in the short term but may improve all-cause mortality in the long term (>12 months) compared with no exercise controls. Moreover, cardiac rehabilitation probably reduces the risk of all-cause hospital admissions and may reduce HF-specific hospital admissions in the short term.[33]

Another recent individual participant data meta-analysis evaluated the endpoints of all-cause and HF-related mortality and hospitalizations in patients with HF undergoing ET. The pooled time-to-event estimates were found to be in favor of patients undergoing ET but had wide confidence intervals and were not statistically significant.[34] Similar results are described in the Cardiac Rehabilitation Outcome Study in HF.[35]

The largest trial on ET in patients with HF was the HF: A Controlled Trial Investigating Outcomes of Exercise Training (HF-ACTION). In this study, a mild but significant decrease in both all-cause mortality and HF hospitalizations was found after adjustment for major prognostic baseline factors and HF etiology.[36]

Effects on Quality of Life and Depression

There is large agreement on the positive effects of ET on QOL and depression metrics. Several studies reported an increase in QOL in patients with HF undergoing ET. In the HF-ACTION trial, patients undergoing ET showed greater improvements in the Kansas City Cardiomyopathy Questionnaire than controls. Comparable results were subsequently confirmed by meta-analyses.[35,37–40] An improvement in depression was also reported for patients with HF after ET: a meta-analysis of 16 randomized trials, including mostly patients with HF with reduced LVEF (HFrEF), found that ET reduced symptoms of depression, with an antidepressant effect, which was consistent in patients younger than and older than 65 years.[41]

Cost-Effectiveness

The benefits in term of survival and hospitalizations gained with ET, paralleled with the relatively low costs of an ET intervention, seem to translate in a little systematic benefit in terms of overall medical resources, as testified by a cost-analysis of the HF-ACTION trial.[42] These results support previous evidence that found ET cost-effective in patients with HF.[43] Similarly, cost-effectiveness of supervised ET in the management of HF was confirmed in a model developed by Kühr and colleagues[44] from the perspective of the Brazilian health care system. Comparable results have been confirmed also for home-based cardiac rehabilitation.[45]

INDICATIONS FOR REFERRAL TO AN EXERCISE TRAINING PROGRAM

ET is currently included in the major societies' guidelines and recommendations for the management of HF.[29,46–48] In the European Society of Cardiology (ESC) guidelines, properly designed exercise is recommended for all patients with HF (regardless of LVEF). Recommendations are to encourage regular exercise to improve functional capacity, symptoms, and QOL in all patients with HF and also to reduce the risk of HF hospitalization (for patients with stable HF with reduced EF).[29,47] ET is recommended for patients with stable New York Heart Association (NYHA) class I-III HF, and should be initiated only in clinically stable individuals after medical therapy for HF has been optimized. ESC guidelines define stable patients as treated patients with symptoms and signs that have remained generally unchanged for at least 1 month.[47] Contraindications to initiating an exercise program include hypotension or hypertension at rest or during exercise, unstable cardiac disease, deteriorating symptoms of HF, myocardial ischemia despite therapy (exercise may be permitted up to ischemic threshold), or severe and suboptimally treated pulmonary disease.[49] The Canadian guidelines provide similar recommendations, and specify between flexibility exercises (recommended in all patients with HF), aerobic exercises (recommended in patients with NYHA I-III HF and only for selected populations of patients with recently diagnosed HF or NYHA IV HF under supervision of an expert team) and isometric/resistance exercise (only recommended for patients with NYHA I-III HF).[48] Clinical stability is defined by Canadian guidelines as no change in NYHA functional class, no hospitalizations for HF, and no major CV events or procedures during the previous 6 weeks.[25]

EXERCISE TRAINING PROGRAMS

The ET program should be individualized for each patient, including aerobic training, strength training, flexibility, and/or inspiratory training. It seems reasonable that combined programs could be the best choice for patients without contraindications.[50,51]

An individualized exercise prescription should be based on physical evaluation findings, risk stratification, comorbidities, and patient and program goals. The general key components should be frequency of the training sessions, intensity of the exercises, duration of the exercises, modalities, and progression.[52]

Preliminary Evaluation

There is currently no agreement on a universal exercise prescription for patients with HF. All exercise programs should be preceded by an accurate screening for contraindications to exercise including medical history, physical examination, resting electrocardiogram (ECG), a symptom-limited exercise test, and echocardiography.[2] Medical history should assess CV diagnoses and prior CV procedures (including assessment of the LVEF), comorbidities, symptoms of CV disease, medications, CV risk profile, and educational barriers and preferences. Physical examination should assess cardiopulmonary systems, post-CV procedure wound, orthopedic and neuromuscular status, and cognitive function. In addition to these evaluations, an evaluation of QOL is advised. Exercise testing should be performed after clinical stabilization and optimization of medical therapy with assessment of the respiratory gas exchanges (CPET) and include heart rate, rhythm, signs, symptoms, ST-segment changes, and exercise capacity. The test should be repeated if the clinical condition changes. Patient's education concerning medical adherence, nutritional evaluation with nutritional advices or dietary prescriptions, psychosocial management, and physical activity counseling are also warranted.[52] Further examinations can be added as appropriate.[2] Before starting cardiac rehabilitation, clinical stabilization of the patient must be achieved. Correction of CV risk factors and optimization of pharmacologic therapy appear thus of crucial importance.[2,49]

Continuous Aerobic Training

Continuous aerobic ET is commonly the core component of the exercise prescriptions for patients with HF and can include different training modalities, such as cycling, walking, jogging, or rowing, according to the patient's preferences and capabilities.[25] The gold-standard method for exercise intensity assessment is symptom-limited cardiopulmonary exercise testing. In this case, the exercise intensity can be prescribed relative to peak V_{O_2}, the V_{O_2} reserve (difference between the basal and the peak V_{O_2}) or the anaerobic threshold (when clearly detected).[2]

In general, the target intensity is considered to be 40% to 80% of peak V_{O_2}, with a lower range (40%–50%) as starting point and a higher range (50%–80%) as target intensity, to be reached progressively.[2,52,53]

The recent ESC guidelines on sports cardiology and exercise suggest to maintain a lower intensity (<40% of peak V_{O_2}) in patients in NYHA functional class III, according to perceived symptoms and clinical status during the first 1 to 2 weeks.[49]

Other common methods to assess exercise intensity are the heart rate reserve (HRR, difference between the basal and peak heart rate [HR]), and the rate of perceived exertion (RPE) on the Borg scale. In these cases, the target intensity should be set between 40% and 70% of the HRR or 10/20 to 14/20 of the Borg RPE.[2]

The target frequency of the ET sessions should be 3 to 5 sessions per week (optimally daily), and the duration of each session should be 20 to 60 minutes.[49] These goals can be reached with progression and more deconditioned patients can start with 10-minute to 20-minute sessions twice a week.[2,52] The progression in the ET programs should be made first in the duration of the exercise sessions, then in their frequency and lastly in the intensity of the exercises.[2,26] Warm-up and cool-down must be included in each exercise session.

Aerobic Interval Training

In patients with HF, interval training periods can take the form of walking, cycling, rowing, swimming or other forms of exercise, according to the patient's characteristics and capabilities.[54]

Low-intensity programs may be used at the initial stages of high-risk patients with HFrEF whereas HIIT may be applied to selected low-risk stable patients.[29]

Low-intensity interval training can be performed on an electrically braked cycle ergometer, with hard segments of 30 seconds (at 50% of the power output achieved during a ramp test or a 10 W $\times$ 1 incremental test) and recovery periods of 60 seconds. The duration of the segments can be adjusted according to the patient's capabilities to different ratios (for example 20/70 seconds or 10 seconds/80 seconds).[2] Depending on the work/recovery interval chosen, ~10 to 12 work phases can be performed per 15 to 30-minute training sessions. The intensity of the phases can be adjusted at the beginning/end of each session to serve as warm-up or cool-down, and must be adapted to the patient's progresses.[2]

Approaches to HIIT have typically involved 2-minute to 4-minute periods at an intensity equivalent to at least 80% to 95% of peak Vo_2, followed by a similar duration of lower-intensity ET such as 40% to 50% of peak Vo_2 or a passive recovery.[2,54] Warm-up and cool-down periods of 5 to 10 minutes should be included at low-intensity (for example 40%–50% of peak Vo_2 during warm-up and 30%–40% of peak Vo_2 during cool-down). It has been suggested to perform 3 to 4 repeat intervals and increase to 4 to 6 intervals after adapting to the ET regimen.

Patients who are highly deconditioned or susceptible to rhythm abnormalities have not been considered candidates for interval ET.[54]

Resistance Training

Resistance training has been proposed as a complementary intervention to endurance aerobic training. It is suggested to perform such type of exercise 2 to 3 times per week.[52,53] The training intensity has to be set relative to the 1 repetition maximum (1-RM, eg, the maximum weight that an individual can lift only once), taking into account the size of the working muscle and relation between the duration of the muscle contraction and the rest period. Even though the 1-RM is generally determined through a maximal strength test, for patients with HF it is more safe to perform a graded stress test (in order to avoid Valsalva maneuver), setting the training intensity at a level at which the patient can perform 10 repetitions without abdominal straining or symptoms. It is suggested to provide medical supervision during the initial sessions of resistance training, with an individualized introduction to the program and adaptation of the exercises.[2] Resistance training should be performed after a patient acquires tolerance to aerobic training.[26]

A good example of progression in resistance training is represented by a 3-step model. First, an instruction phase must be performed, with slow exercises conducted with very low resistance (<30% 1-RM) until the patient is confident with the course of the movements. In the following phase, "resistance-endurance" training can be started with a high number of repetitions (12–25) and a low intensity (30%–40% 1-RM). The last phase should introduce "strength" training, with a higher intensity (40%–60% 1-RM).[2]

A generalized prescription for ET can include 10 to 15 repetitions per set to moderate fatigue,1 to 3 sets of 8 to 10 different upper and lower body exercises. The modality of exercise can vary (calisthenics, elastic bands, cuff/hand weights, dumbbells, free weights, wall pulleys or weight machines).[52] In patients with moderate risk, stress perception should be at a maximum RPE of 15.[2]

Warm-up and cool-down must be included in each exercise session.

Inspiratory Training

Inspiratory muscle training can improve exercise capacity and QOL of patients with HF. Moreover, it has been described how a subgroup of patients with inspiratory muscle weakness (defined as a maximal inspiratory mouth pressure during quasi-static maneuver of <70% of predicted) may benefit the most from this type of intervention.[2,55,56] The suggested modality is to start at 30% of the maximal inspiratory mouth pressure and readjust intensity every 7 to 10 days up to 60%. Training duration should be 20 to 30 min/d with a frequency of 3 to 5 session/week for a minimum of 8 weeks. The modalities are varied and can include isocapnic hyperpnea, incentive spirometry, resistive pressure threshold load, and computer-controlled biofeedback trainers.[2]

SPECIAL POPULATIONS

Implantable Cardioverter Defibrillator

The use of ET in patients with an implantable cardioverter defibrillator (ICD) is safe and not associated with an increased risk of shocks, while it is associated with an increase in aerobic capacity.[57,58] Moreover, ET can have positive effects on anxiety in patients with an ICD and can reduce the fear of exercise.[59]

It has been suggested to perform a symptom-limited CPET in all patients with an ICD to evaluate the chronotropic response to exercise, the presence of exercise-induced arrhythmias, HR in case of onset of an arrhythmia, the effectiveness of pharmacologic HR control and the risk of reaching an HR in the ICD intervention zone. ET in these patients should be initially supervised, under HR monitoring and the exercise prescription should be addressed to avoid activities with an intrinsic risk (for example swimming or climbing heights) that may result in a risk of harm to the patient in case of a transitory loss of consciousness due to an ICD discharge. Moreover, exercise prescription and/or ICD programming should be arranged to keep the maximal HR 20 beats below the ICD intervention zone.[2] Avoiding a physical trauma to the device, including activities with pronounced arm/shoulder movements, is also sensible. It has been proposed to restrict upper body resistance exercise until 6 weeks after implantation to prevent dislodgement of newly implanted device leads and healing of the defibrillator site.[59] The staff caring for patients with an ICD should be exhaustively informed about the medical condition of the patient and the ICD settings. In case of an ICD intervention an evaluation of the causes is recommended, followed by possible modifications to the ICD setting, therapy or exercise regimen as appropriate.[2]

SETTING

Supervised Versus Home-Based Programs

During the initial phases and for more frail or unstable patients, ET should be supervised to monitor the individual response and tolerability, or potential signs and symptoms that may indicate the need to modify the therapy. The supervision should include physical examination, monitoring of HR, blood pressure, and rhythm before, during, and after ET. A first supervised phase is important also for the education of the patient and for close control of adherence to the prescribed therapies. With the target of keeping the gained benefits over time, a home-based program will be an important prosecution of the path, ideally with a gradual transition.[2,53] This modality of training has proved to be as safe and effective as center-based rehabilitation in low-risk and clinically stable patients. Initial exercise testing and patient education remain recommended for these patients.[2,50] In addition to the aforementioned options, the possibility to address patients to selected local gymnasiums of the territory has also been described. In this context, specifically trained instructors should follow these patients ensuring compliance to the exercise prescription and monitoring individual progression and responses to ET, referring these data to the prescribing physician for follow-up or reevaluations.[60]

ADHERENCE

Patients with HF can be considered adherent to an exercise program if they meet 80% of the recommended dose. Although most studies do not indicate adherence as primary outcome, in the review by Deka and colleagues[61] reported adherence to ET protocols varied between 30% and 110%. In the HF-ACTION trial, only 31.5% of the patients enrolled completed 36 supervised training sessions, and only approximately 40% of patients in the exercise group reported weekly training volumes at or above the recommended 90 minutes per week at month 3, or 120 minutes per week from month 3 to month 12, possibly explaining the lower than expected increments in peak V_{O_2} observed in the trial.[62]

The reasons for the low adherence to ET programs must be researched at a multifactorial level, including socioeconomic factors, patients' characteristics and physician effectiveness in educating and referring patients to ET. With regard to the latter factor, it is of interest to note that in a recent study by Golwala and colleagues,[63] referral of patients with HF to cardiac rehabilitation was only 10.4% at discharge after hospitalization for HF. Future research of effective strategies to improve adherence to ET in these patients is thus warranted, and exercise prescription or referral to ET should become common practice inside the hospital and outpatient settings.

SUMMARY

In conclusion, ET has beneficial effects at multiple levels in patients with HF and is recommended by major societies' guidelines. This type of intervention improves exercise capacity, QOL, and reduces symptoms of depression in these patients. Moreover, it can improve survival and reduce the risk for hospitalizations. Exercise-based cardiac rehabilitation can be offered with different modalities, such as continuous or interval aerobic training, resistance, and inspiratory muscle training. There is no agreement on a universal type of exercise prescription that can suit all patients, the intervention has thus to be individualized after an accurate evaluation of the patient's CV conditions and functional capacity. Despite the multiple benefits of ET, these patients lack in adherence to exercise-based programs. This can be due to socioeconomic factors, patients' characteristics, and also to lack in referral from the physician in charge.

CLINICS CARE POINTS

- Exercise training significantly improves exercise capacity and quality of life in patients with heart failure and has shown modest effects on all-cause and heart failure-specific mortality and hospitalization.
- Aerobic exercise training is recommended for stable patients with heart failure (New York Heart Association class I-III) and should be initiated after medical therapy for heart failure has been optimized.
- Resistance exercise training may be complementary to aerobic exercise training with the purpose of preventing or reversing muscle mass loss.
- Exercise training appears safe also in patients with an implantable cardioverter defibrillator and is not associated with increased risk of shocks.

DISCLOSURE

The authors have no conflicts of interest to report.

REFERENCES

1. Kokkinos PF, Choucair W, Graves P, et al. Chronic heart failure and exercise. Am Heart J 2000;140(1):21–8.
2. Piepoli MF, Conraads V, CorrÁ U, et al. Exercise training in heart failure: From theory to practice. A consensus document of the Heart Failure Association and the European Association for Cardiovascular Prevention and Rehabilitation. Eur J Heart Fail 2011;13(4):347–57.
3. Kasiakogias A, Sharma S. Exercise: The ultimate treatment to all ailments? Clin Cardiol 2020;43(8):817–26.
4. Thijssen DHJ, Maiorana A, O'Driscoll G, et al. Impact of inactivity and exercise on the vasculature in humans. Eur J Appl Physiol 2010;108:845–75.
5. Adamopoulos S, Parissis J, Karatzas D, et al. Physical training modulates proinflammatory cytokines and the soluble Fas/soluble Fas ligand system in patients with chronic heart failure. J Am Coll Cardiol 2002;39(4):653–63.
6. Smart NA, Steele M. The effect of physical training on systemic proinflammatory cytokine expression in heart failure patients: a systematic review. Congest Heart Fail 2011;17(3):110–4.
7. Ji LL, Gomez-Cabrera MC, Vina J. Exercise and hormesis: activation of cellular antioxidant signaling pathway. Ann N Y Acad Sci 2006;1067(1):425–35.
8. Powers SK, Sollanek KJ, Wiggs MP, et al. Exercise-induced improvements in myocardial antioxidant capacity: the antioxidant players and cardioprotection. Free Radic Res 2014;48(1):43–51.
9. Martin JL, Mestril R, Hilal-Dandan R, et al. Small heat shock proteins and protection against ischemic injury in cardiac myocytes. Circulation 1997;96(12):4343–8.
10. Liu Y, Lormes W, Wang L, et al. Different skeletal muscle HSP70 responses to high-intensity strength training and low-intensity endurance training. Eur J Appl Physiol 2004;91(2–3):330–5.
11. Hambrecht R, Fiehn E, Weigl C, et al. Regular physical exercise corrects endothelial dysfunction and improves exercise capacity in patients with chronic heart failure. Circulation 1998;98(24):2709–15.
12. Varin R, Mulder P, Richard V, et al. Exercise improves flow-mediated vasodilatation of skeletal muscle arteries in rats with chronic heart failure: role of nitric oxide, prostanoids, and oxidant stress. Circulation 1999;99(22):2951–7.
13. Sarto P, Balducci E, Balconi G, et al. Effects of exercise training on endothelial progenitor cells in patients with chronic heart failure. J Card Fail 2007;13(9):701–8.
14. Pearson MJ, Smart NA. Effect of exercise training on endothelial function in heart failure patients: a systematic review meta-analysis. Int J Cardiol 2017;231:234–43.
15. Josiak K, Jankowska EA, Piepoli MF, et al. Skeletal myopathy in patients with chronic heart failure: significance of anabolic-androgenic hormones. J Cachexia Sarcopenia Muscle 2014;5(4):287–96.
16. Yin J, Lu X, Qian Z, et al. New insights into the pathogenesis and treatment of sarcopenia in chronic heart failure. Theranostics 2019;9(14):4019–29.
17. Hambrecht R, Niebauer J, Fiehn E, et al. Physical training in patients with stable chronic heart failure: Effects on cardiorespiratory fitness and ultrastructural abnormalities of leg muscles. J Am Coll Cardiol 1995;25(6):1239–49.
18. Lena A, Anker MS, Springer J. Muscle wasting and sarcopenia in heart failure—the current state of science. Int J Mol Sci 2020;21(18):1–27.
19. Haykowsky MJ, Liang Y, Pechter D, et al. A meta-analysis of the effect of exercise training on left ventricular remodeling in heart failure patients. the benefit depends on the type of training performed. J Am Coll Cardiol 2007;49(24):2329–36.
20. Braith RW, Welsch MA, Feigenbaum MS, et al. Neuroendocrine activation in heart failure is modified by endurance exercise training. J Am Coll Cardiol 1999;34(4):1170–5.
21. Gademan MGJ, Swenne CA, Verwey HF, et al. Effect of exercise training on autonomic derangement and neurohumoral activation in chronic heart failure. J Card Fail 2007;13(4):294–303.
22. Keteyian SJ. Exercise training in congestive heart failure: risks and benefits. Prog Cardiovasc Dis 2011;53(6):419–28.
23. Taylor RS, Davies EJ, Dalal HM, et al. Effects of exercise training for heart failure with preserved ejection fraction: a systematic review and meta-analysis of comparative studies. Int J Cardiol 2012;162(1):6–13.
24. Sheng L, Christopher AM M. Exercise training in patients with heart failure and preserved ejection fraction: a meta-analysis of randomized control trials. Physiol Behav 2016;176(1):100–6.
25. Haykowsky MJ, Daniel KM, Bhella PS, et al. Heart failure: exercise-based cardiac rehabilitation: who, when, and how intense? Can J Cardiol 2016;32(10):S382–7.
26. Ades PA, Keteyian SJ, Balady GJ, et al. Cardiac rehabilitation exercise and self-care for chronic heart failure. JACC Hear Fail 2013;1(6):540–7.
27. Keteyian SJ. High intensity interval training in patients with cardiovascular disease: a brief review of physiologic adaptations and suggestions for future research. J Clin Exerc Physiol 2013;2(1):13–9.
28. Cornelis J, Beckers P, Taeymans J, et al. Comparing exercise training modalities in heart failure: A systematic review and meta-analysis. Int J Cardiol 2016;221:867–76.
29. Ambrosetti M, Abreu A, Corrà U, et al. Secondary prevention through comprehensive cardiovascular

rehabilitation: From knowledge to implementation. 2020 update. A position paper from the Secondary Prevention and Rehabilitation Section of the European Association of Preventive Cardiology. Eur J Prev Cardiol 2020. https://doi.org/10.1177/2047487320913379.

30. Jewiss D, Ostman C, Smart NA. The effect of resistance training on clinical outcomes in heart failure: A systematic review and meta-analysis. Int J Cardiol 2016;221:674–81.
31. Giuliano C, Karahalios A, Neil C, et al. The effects of resistance training on muscle strength, quality of life and aerobic capacity in patients with chronic heart failure — A meta-analysis. Int J Cardiol 2017;227:413–23.
32. Doukky R, Mangla A, Ibrahim Z, et al. Impact of physical inactivity on mortality in patients with heart failure. Physiol Behav 2017;176(12):139–48.
33. Long L, Ir M, Bridges C, et al. Exercise-based cardiac rehabilitation for adults with heart failure (Review). Cochrane Database Syst Rev 2019;1(1). https://doi.org/10.1002/14651858.CD003331.pub5. www.cochranelibrary.com.
34. Taylor RS, Walker S, Ciani O, et al. Exercise-based cardiac rehabilitation for chronic heart failure: The EXTRAMATCH II individual participant data meta-analysis. Health Technol Assess (Rockv) 2019; 23(25):1–97.
35. Bjarnason-Wehrens B, Nebel R, Jensen K, et al. Exercise-based cardiac rehabilitation in patients with reduced left ventricular ejection fraction: The Cardiac Rehabilitation Outcome Study in Heart Failure (CROS-HF): A systematic review and meta-analysis. Eur J Prev Cardiol 2020;27(9):929–52.
36. O'Connor CM, Whellan DJ, Lee KL, et al. Efficacy and safety of exercise training in patients with chronic heart failure HF-ACTION randomized controlled trial. JAMA 2009;301(14):1439–50.
37. Flynn KE, Piña IL, Whellan DJ, et al. Effects of exercise training on health status in patients with chronic heart failure HF-ACTION randomized controlled trial. JAMA 2009;301(14):1451–9.
38. Davies EJ, Moxham T, Rees K, et al. Exercise training for systolic heart failure: Cochrane systematic review and meta-analysis. Eur J Heart Fail 2010;12(7):706–15.
39. Taylor RS, Sagar VA, Davies EJ, et al. Exercise-based rehabilitation for heart failure. Cochrane Database Syst Rev 2014;2017(10). https://doi.org/10.1002/14651858.CD003331.pub4.
40. Taylor RS, Walker S, Smart NA, et al. Impact of exercise rehabilitation on exercise capacity and quality-of-life in heart failure: individual participant meta-analysis. J Am Coll Cardiol 2019;73(12):1430–43.
41. Tu RH, Zeng ZY, Zhong GQ, et al. Effects of exercise training on depression in patients with heart failure: A systematic review and meta-analysis of randomized controlled trials. Eur J Heart Fail 2014; 16(7):749–57.
42. Reed SD, Whellan DJ, Li Y, et al. Economic evaluation of the HF-ACTION randomized controlled trial: an exercise training study of patients with chronic heart failure. Circ Cardiovasc Qual Outcomes 2011;3(4):374–81.
43. Georgiou D, Chen Y, Appadoo S, et al. Cost-effectiveness analysis of long-term moderate exercise training in chronic heart failure. Am J Cardiol 2001; 87(8):984–8.
44. Kühr EM, Ribeiro RA, Rohde LEP, et al. Cost-effectiveness of supervised exercise therapy in heart failure patients. Value Heal 2011;14(5 SUPPL):S100–7.
45. Taylor RS, Sadler S, Dalal HM, et al. The cost effectiveness of REACH-HF and home-based cardiac rehabilitation compared with the usual medical care for heart failure with reduced ejection fraction: a decision model-based analysis. Eur J Prev Cardiol 2019;26(12):1252–61.
46. Yancy CW, Jessup M, Bozkurt B, et al. 2013 ACCF/AHA guideline for the management of heart failure: A report of the American College of Cardiology Foundation/American Heart Association task force on practice guidelines. Circulation 2013;128(16): 240–327.
47. Ponikowski P, Voors AA, Anker SD, et al. 2016 ESC Guidelines for the diagnosis and treatment of acute and chronic heart failure. Eur Heart J 2016;37(27): 2129–2200m.
48. Ezekowitz JA, O'Meara E, McDonald MA, et al. 2017 Comprehensive update of the Canadian Cardiovascular Society guidelines for the management of heart failure. Can J Cardiol 2017;33(11):1342–433.
49. Pelliccia A, Sharma S, Gati S, et al. 2020 ESC Guidelines on sports cardiology and exercise in patients with cardiovascular disease. Eur Heart J 2020; 1–80. https://doi.org/10.1093/eurheartj/ehaa605.
50. Labate V, Guazzi M. Past, present, and future rehabilitation practice patterns for patients with heart failure. The European Perspective. Heart Fail Clin 2015; 11(1):105–15.
51. Van Iterson EH, Olson TP. Therapeutic targets for the multi-system pathophysiology of heart failure: exercise training. Curr Treat Options Cardiovasc Med 2017;19(11). https://doi.org/10.1007/s11936-017-0585-8.
52. Balady GJ, Williams MA, Ades PA, et al. Core components of cardiac rehabilitation/secondary prevention programs: 2007 update - A scientific statement from the American Heart Association Exercise, Cardiac Rehabilitation, and Prevention Committee, the Council on Clinical Cardiology; the Councils on Cardiovascular Nursing, Epidemiology and Prevention, and Nutrition, Physical Activity, and Metabolism; and the American Association of Cardiovascular

and Pulmonary Rehabilitation. Circulation 2007; 115(20):2675–82.

53. Piepoli MF, Corrà U, Adamopoulos S, et al. Secondary prevention in the clinical management of patients with cardiovascular diseases. Core components, standards and outcome measures for referral and delivery: A policy statement from the Cardiac Rehabilitation Section of the European Association for Cardiovascular Prevention & Rehabilitation. Eur J Prev Cardiol 2014;21(6):664–81.
54. Arena RA, Myers JN, Forman DE, et al. Should high-intensity-aerobic interval training become the clinical standard in heart failure? Heart Fail Rev 2013;18(1): 95–105.
55. Ribeiro JP, Chiappa GR, Neder AJ, et al. Respiratory muscle function and exercise intolerance in heart failure. Curr Heart Fail Rep 2009;6(2):95–101.
56. Montemezzo D, Fregonezi GA, Pereira DA, et al. Influence of inspiratory muscle weakness on inspiratory muscle training responses in chronic heart failure patients: a systematic review and meta-analysis. Arch Phys Med Rehabil 2014;95(7):1398–407.
57. Isaksen K, Morken IM, Munk PS, et al. Exercise training and cardiac rehabilitation in patients with implantable cardioverter defibrillators: A review of current literature focusing on safety, effects of exercise training, and the psychological impact of programme participation. Eur J Prev Cardiol 2012; 19(4):804–12.
58. Steinhaus DA, Lubitz SA, Noseworthy PA, et al. Exercise interventions in patients with implantable cardioverter-defibrillators and cardiac resynchronization therapy: a systematic review and meta-analysis. J Cardiopulm Rehabil Prev 2019;39(5):308–17.
59. Ul Haq MA, Goh CY, Levinger I, et al. Clinical utility of exercise training in heart failure with reduced and preserved ejection fraction. Clin Med Insights Cardiol 2015;9:1–9.
60. Sarto P, Merlo L, Astolfo P, et al. Comprehensive therapeutic program for cardiovascular patients: Role of a sports medicine unit in collaboration with local gymnasiums. J Cardiovasc Med 2009;10(1): 27–33.
61. Deka P, Pozehl B, Williams MA, et al. Adherence to recommended exercise guidelines in patients with heart failure. Heart Fail Rev 2017;22(1):41–53.
62. Maeyer C, Beckers P, Vrints CJ, et al. Exercise training in chronic heart failure. Ther Adv Chronic Dis 2013;4(3):105–17.
63. Golwala H, Pandey A, Ju C, et al. Temporal trends and factors associated with cardiac rehabilitation referral among patients hospitalized with heart failure: findings from Get With The Guidelines-Heart Failure Registry. J Am Coll Cardiol 2015;66(8): 917–26.

Role of Cardiac Rehabilitation After Ventricular Assist Device Implantation

Concetta Di Nora, MD[a,*], Federica Guidetti, MD[b], Ugolino Livi, MD[a], Francesco Antonini-Canterin, MD[c]

KEYWORDS

- Ventricular assist device • Cardiac rehabilitation • Cardiopulmonary test

KEY POINTS

- Ventricular assist device (VAD) has rapidly emerged as a durable and safe therapy for patients with end-stage heart failure.
- Cardiac rehabilitation should be recognized as one fundamental component to improve outcome in patients with heart failure not only candidate to VAD therapy but also carrying the VAD system.
- The exercise training should be individualized in VAD patients considering the patient's condition, the previous functional capacity, left ventricular assist device parameters, comorbidities, and possible complications after surgery.
- Before starting a cardiac rehabilitation program, it is necessary to have specific information about the uncommon characteristics of these patients (ie, no arterial pulse is detectable) and the peculiarity of the VAD system.

INTRODUCTION

The word "rehabilitation" originates from the Latin *rehabilitare*: "re-" means "again," "-ation" means "do," and *habilitare* means "to fit" or "to qualify." Rehabilitation has come to mean the process of recovery of the patient's abilities and restoration, as rehabilitation into society of a social life. The core of rehabilitation is the *therapeutic exercise*, which was defined by the American Heart Society as the "coordinated sum of interventions required to ensure the best physical, psychological, and social conditions so that patients with chronic or post-acute cardiovascular disease may, by their own efforts, preserve or resume optimal functioning in society and, through improved health behaviours, slow or reverse progression of disease."[1,2]

Patients with heart failure (HF) suffered by a complex syndrome, where the filling of the ventricle or ejection of the blood from the ventricle is impaired. The classical symptoms of HF are *dyspnea* and *fatigue*, which may limit exercise tolerance, and *fluid retention*, leading to pulmonary congestion and peripheral edema.[3] In this contest, exercise capacity decreases for many reasons, one of them is the insufficient oxygen transfer due to reduced cardiac output and anemia.[4]

Ventricular assist device (VAD) has rapidly emerged as a durable and safe therapy for patients with end-stage HF. The effectiveness of therapeutic exercise in patients with HF has been

[a] Department of Cardiothoracic Science, Azienda Sanitaria Universitaria Integrata di Udine, Italy; [b] Department of Cardiology, University Heart Center, University Hospital Zurich, Zurich, Switzerland; [c] Cardiac Prevention and Rehabilitation Unit, Highly Specialized Rehabilitation Hospital, Motta di Livenza, Italy

* Corresponding author. Department of Cardiothoracic Science, Azienda Sanitaria Universitaria Integrata di Udine, Hospital S. Maria della Misericordia, Udine, Italy.
E-mail address: concetta.dinora@gmail.com

Heart Failure Clin 17 (2021) 273–278
https://doi.org/10.1016/j.hfc.2021.01.008

reported recently,[5,6] and exercise should be recognized as one fundamental component within a comprehensive plan to improve overall outcome in patients with HF not only candidate to VAD therapy but also carrying the VAD system.[7]

DISCUSSION

Ventricular Assist Device—A New Chance for Patients with Heart Failure

According to the most recent HF guidelines published by the American College of Cardiology and American Heart Association,[8] VAD implantation is indicated for patients who have stage D HF with reduced ejection fraction. Considering the INTERMACS scale (Interagency Registry for Mechanically Assisted Circulatory Support), which divides advanced HF (New York Heart Association [NYHA] score III–IV) into 7 different risk levels, most of the patients receiving VADs are INTERMACS classes 2 (36.4%) or 3 (29.9%).[9] There are different types of VADs according to the heart chamber mainly supported: left ventricular assist device (LVAD), right ventricle (RVAD), or both chambers (BiVAD). Generally, RVADs and BiVADs are mostly used in hospital, as bridge-to-transplant (BT) or bridge-to-recovery supports, with few chances of discharge home (**Fig. 1**). Conversely, LVAD, originally conceived only for BT indication, is currently also used with the aim of being destination therapy (DT), thanks to recent significant advancements in medical management and technology.[10] Moreover, the REMATCH (Randomized Evaluation of Mechanical Assistance for the Treatment of Congestive Heart Failure) trial by Rose and colleagues[11,12] first demonstrated the potential of using VADs as a durable DT platform with superior survival outcomes compared with conventional medical therapy alone. Smaller and more durable, their early results demonstrated significantly improved survival and complication profiles. Furthermore, therapeutic benefits of LVAD implantation also extend to functional capacity and quality of life; as far as randomized clinical trial have consistently demonstrated that ≈80% of patients belong to NYHA functional class I or II symptoms at 24 months postimplantation.[13]

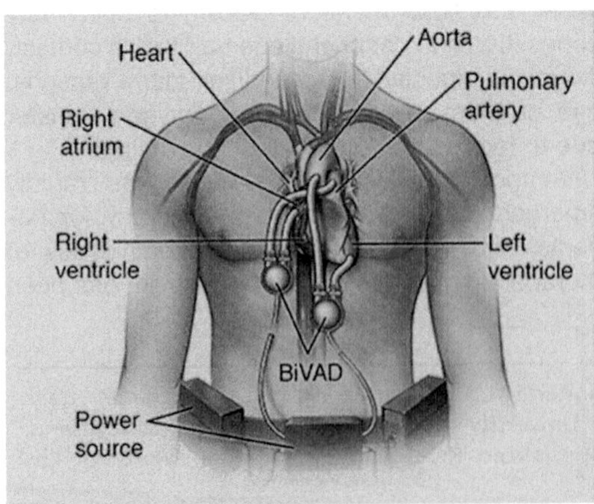

Fig. 1. An example of biventricular assist device. The external support has been guaranteed by 2 external pumps, one for the left ventricle and one for the right ventricle, as shown.

Left Ventricular Assist Device—Looking Inside

Nowadays, continuous-flow LVADs use new-generation rotary blood pumps that are designed to provide extended circulatory support. They consist of an internal LVAD *blood pump* with a percutaneous lead that connects the pump to an *external system controller* and a *power source* (batteries or line power) (**Fig. 2**). Continuous-flow LVADs consist of 3 basic components:

1. An *inflow cannula* from the LV apex that draws blood into the device;
2. An *impeller* that moves the blood forward in parallel with native cardiac output;
3. An *outflow cannula* that returns blood back into the proximal aorta or descending aorta.

There are different types of continuous-flow LVADs, but all of them share important functional characteristics, the most important of which is the continuous unloading of the LV throughout the cardiac cycle, thus this mechanism diminishes or eliminates the arterial pulse. Moreover, whether the LV has a contractile reserve, its contraction generates pressure capable of overcoming systemic arterial pressure, so the aortic valve will open, and the total cardiac output will be supplemented by native LV ejection. This is a valuable sign of improving after LVAD implantation.

Patient Selection for Left Ventricular Assist Device Support

On top of heart transplantation, where some systematic diseases have not been an absolute contraindication anymore,[14,15] the selection of patients for VAD implantation may vary greatly for a lot of aspects, beyond the native cardiomyopathy. Furthermore, candidates for LVAD support will present with comorbidities that vary in severity, depending on the extent and duration of HF.[16] The acceptance of candidates for LVAD support and the timing of device implant need to be determined by careful consideration of potential risks and benefits. The highest risk of death after LVAD implant is before hospital discharge. Thus,

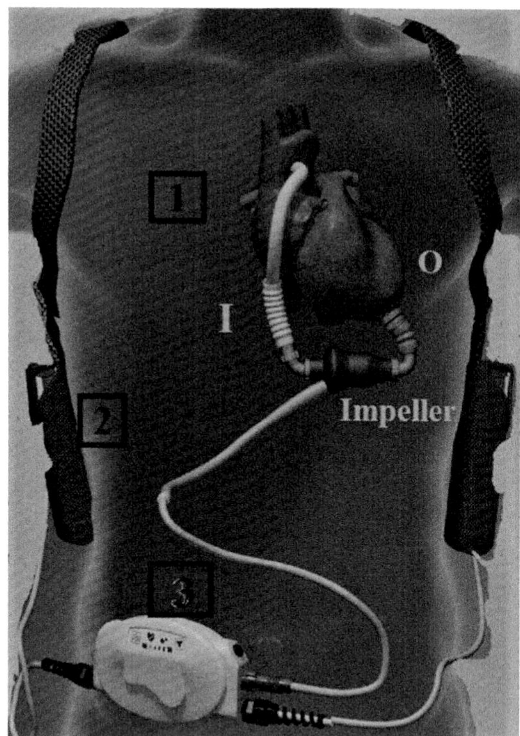

Fig. 2. An example of left ventricular assist device. *Number 1* shows the internal component of the VAD, with the *I* for the inflow cannula, the *impeller*, and the *O* for the outflow cannula. *Number 2* shows the power sources, whereas *number 3* shows the external system controller.

patient selection and the *timing of implant* are 2 of the major determinants of success.[17] For these reasons, the need of a cardiac rehabilitation (CR) program is imperative in this setting. Preimplant optimization of comorbid conditions is particularly important in minimizing the incidence and severity of postoperative adverse events and for enhancing survival. The most influential preimplant measures are improving the nutritional status and enhancing the body through physical activity, so the rehabilitative programs are crucial for these aims.[18]

Functional Capacity in Left Ventricular Assist Device Patients

Cardiopulmonary exercise test (CPET) is considered the gold standard in assessing the physiologic response to exercise, and it is the best tool to assess functional capacity in patients with HF; although, its role in LVAD patients seems still controversial.[19] Hence, as demonstrated by several studies, the maximum oxygen uptake (Vo_2 peak) remains considerably limited in LVAD patients, ranging from 11 to 20 mL/kg/min, corresponding to 40% to 50% of predicted exercise capacity.[20,21] After LVAD implantation, the contribution of native LV contractility is complex: at rest, the device provides most of the cardiac output, whereas, during exercise, a variable contribution of the native heart has been described depending on right and LV contractile reserve interplay. However, LVAD patients seem to exhibit a different relationship between submaximal and maximal exercise capacity when compared with subjects with HF.[22,23] This difference might indicate that LVAD therapy is more effective in improving mild physical activities, such as walking, rather than enhancing intense exertion. For all these reasons, before starting the CR program, a CPET, sometimes replaced by a 6-minute walk test, should be performed in every LVAD patient to estimate the initial functional capacity. As previously demonstrated, the limiting factors of both peak and submaximal exercises were influenced by parameters underlying patients' general condition and by cardiac related factors.[24] Hence, in the study by Fresiello and colleagues,[25] the LVAD timing, LVAD pulsatility index, diabetes, creatinine, and urea have been discussed as some of the predictors of submaximal exercise test. Moreover, previous studies have reported the crucial role of chronotropic response in determining exercise performance.[26] Interestingly, in LVAD patients performing peak exercise, heart rate can help the right side in accommodating a higher cardiac output, as well as the left side if the aortic valve starts to open.[27,28] Further investigations should be conducted to better clarify whether β-blocker dosage can affect inotropic and chronotropic response and in turn exercise, bearing in mind the importance of β-blocker therapy in stimulating myocardial recovery also in LVAD patients.[29]

Considering these premises, it is noteworthy that the exercise training should be individualized along to a series of factors, such as the patient's condition, the previous functional capacity, LVAD parameters, comorbidities, and possible complications after surgery. Moreover, a longer rehabilitation intervention followed by a maintenance program of regular physical activity is suggestable to obtain the best results along time.[30]

Ventricular Assist Device—New Frontiers in the Cardiac Rehabilitation

The increasing number of patients treated with LVAD have provided new challenges to the staff in exercise-based CR programs. However, the benefits of CR in VAD patients are enormous.

The first aim of CR in VAD-supported patients is obviously to progressively reduce their physical and functional impairments, so that they will be able to resume meaningful daily activities. Thus, exercise improves myocardial contractility, heart rate variability, and skeletal muscle functions.[31,32] Symptom burden, the disabling consequences of HF, and the treatment regimen affect the daily lives of patients with HF and contribute to a decreased quality of life. In LVAD patients, the decrease in the capacity to exercise was explained with prolonged bed rest and skeletal muscle alterations. It has been reported that when the hemodynamics of a patient are stable after LVAD implantation, some physical rehabilitation may begin with the aim of restoring a minimum of mobility independence.[33,34] Some studies have also reported that after rehabilitation LVAD patients improved in anxiety, depression, and QoL, and caregivers reduced their strain.[35] The ability of LVAD patients to achieve a minimum level of physical fitness after CR seems to be associated with improved long-term survival, as reported in a study in which patients who walked more than 300 m on a 6-minute walk test conducted for more than 2 months after device implantation presented a significantly lower risk for future all-cause mortality.[36] However, it should be noted that most of the studies had no control group, probably because each study aimed at detecting CR effects instead of the efficacy of a given rehabilitative treatment over another. Moreover, it is obvious that the population of LVAD patients is still representing a narrow context if compared with other cohorts more numerous. Finally, recent publications have identified limitations of the current infrastructure to manage this complex group of patients. This is true even among highly experienced and high-volume VAD centers, emphasizing the impact of non-HF comorbidities on outcomes after VAD therapy.[37,38]

CLINICS CARE POINTS

Cardiac Rehabilitation in Left Ventricular Assist Device Patients—Tips and Tricks

Before starting a complete CR program, it is noteworthy to have some important information about the specific setting of these patients[39–41]:

1. In preparing exercise prescriptions, clinicians should consider a variety of factors: *safety factors* (clinical history, risk stratification and exercise risk, and any cognitive or psychological impairment that may impede adherence to exercise limits), *associated factors* (vocational and avocational requirements, orthopedic limitations, premorbid state before onset, current activities, and personal health and fitness goals), and *noncardiac considerations*.
2. During exercise, mean arterial blood pressure shows an initial increase, correlated with the level of metabolic equivalents achieved. However, at higher intensities of exertion, peripheral vasodilation may progressively develop and lead to symptomatic hypotension, especially when the limited maximal output of LVAD is associated with limited contribution of the native heart to global circulatory output.
3. Maintenance of an "optimal" circulating volume is critical during CR; thus, it is relevant to check the fluid status before starting the physical activities and every time necessary. It is fundamental to avoid both symptomatic hypotension, as well as suction effects induced by the device on the interventricular septum.
4. To be aware of episodes of orthostatic hypotension, mainly due to the presence of a profound cardiac dysautonomia, which may persist at least during the first few months after the beginning of circulatory support.
5. Mean blood pressure should range between 70 and 90 mm Hg: hypertension could affect the LVAD capacity to pump the blood forward, causing a reduced exercise performance.
6. Devices and drivelines should be intensively managed during physical activities to avoid catastrophic accidents.

SUMMARY

Although the available experience and evidence in CR of LVAD patients is still limited, it seems that LVAD patients may undergo exercise-based rehabilitation without major problems and obtaining the best results along time. Specific surveillance measures must be encouraged in this setting to avoid drastic consequences, such as traumatism of the LVAD components or drivelines. Moreover, giving the complexity of these patients, a comprehensive approach is desirable, which includes psychological health, attenuation of risk factors, and social support on top of exercise training.

DISCLOSURE

Nothing.

REFERENCES

1. Cardiac rehabilitation programs. A statement for healthcare professionals from the American Heart Association. Circulation 1994;3:1602–10.

2. Taylor RS, Brown A, Ebrahim S, et al. Exercise based rehabilitation for patients with coronary heart disease: systematic review and meta-analysis of randomized controlled trials. Am J Med 2004;10: 682–92.
3. Pina IL, Apstein CS, Balady GJ, et al. Exercise and heart failure: a statement from the American Heart Association Committee on Exercise, Rehabilitation, and Prevention. Circulation 2003;8:1210–25.
4. Giannuzzi P, Temporelli PL, Corra U, et al. Antiremodeling effect of long-term exercise training in patients with stable chronic heart failure: results of the Exercise in Left Ventricular Dysfunction and Chronic Heart Failure (ELVD-CHF) trial. Circulation 2003;5: 554–5.
5. Pollock ML, Franklin BA, Balady GJ, et al. AHA Science Advisory. Resistance exercise in individuals with and without cardiovascular disease: benefits, rationale, safety, and prescription. Circulation 2000; 7:828–33.
6. Hunt SA, Baker DW, Chin MH, et al. ACC/AHA guidelines for the evaluation and management of chronic heart failure in the adult: executive summary. Circulation 2001;24:2996–3007.
7. Reedy JE, Swartz MT, Lohmann DP, et al. The importance of patient mobility with ventricular assist device support. ASAIO J 1992;3:M151–3.
8. Yancy CW, Jessup M, Bozkurt B, et al. 2017 ACC/AHA/HFSA Focused Update of the 2013 ACCF/AHA Guideline for the Management of Heart Failure: A Report of the American College of Cardiology/American Heart Association Task Force on Clinical Practice Guidelines and the Heart Failure Society of America. J Card Fail 2017;8:628–51.
9. Stevenson LW, Pagani FD, Young JB, et al. INTERMACS profiles of advanced heart failure: the current picture. J Heart Lung Transplant 2009;28:535–41.
10. Buchholz S, Guenther SPW, Michel S, et al. Ventricular assist device therapy and heart transplantation: Benefits, drawbacks, and outlook. Herz 2018;5: 406–14.
11. Rose EA, Moskowitz AJ, Packer M, et al. The REMATCH trial: rationale, design, and end points. Randomized Evaluation of Mechanical Assistance for the Treatment of Congestive Heart Failure. Ann Thorac Surg 1999;3:723–30.
12. Lietz K, Long JW, Kfoury AG, et al. Outcomes of left ventricular assist device implantation as destination therapy in the post-REMATCH era: implications for patient selection. Circulation 2007;116:497–505.
13. Ando M, Garan AR, Takayama H, et al. A continuous-flow external ventricular assist device for cardiogenic shock: Evolution over 10 years. J Thorac Cardiovasc Surg 2018;1:157–65.e1.
14. Di Nora C, Miani D, D'Elia AV, et al. Heart transplantation in Danon disease: Long term single centre experience and review of the literature. Eur J Med Genet 2020;2:1036–45.
15. Di Nora C, Paldino A, Miani D, et al. Heart Transplantation in Kearns-Sayre Syndrome. Transplantation 2019;12:e393–4.
16. Matlock DD. Destination unknown: the ventricular assist device and the advance of technology. J Am Geriatr Soc 2012;1:154–5.
17. Kormos RL, Teuteberg JJ, Siegenthaler MP, et al. Pre-VAD implant risk factors influence the onset of adverse events (AEs) while on VAD. J Heart Lung Transplant 2009;28:S153.
18. Ueno A, Tomizawa Y. Cardiac rehabilitation and artificial heart devices. J Artif Organs 2009;12:90–7.
19. Jung MH, Gustafsson F. Exercise in heart failure patients supported with a left ventricular assist device. J Heart Lung Transplant 2015;34:489–96.
20. Hasin T, Topilsky Y, Kremers WK, et al. Usefulness of the Six-Minute Walk Test after continuous axial flow left ventricular device implantation to predict survival. Am J Cardiol 2012;9:1322–8.
21. Kerrigan DJ, Williams CT, Ehrman JK, et al. Cardiac rehabilitation improves functional capacity and patient-reported health status in patients with continuous-flow left ventricular assist devices: the Rehab-VAD randomized controlled trial. JACC Heart Fail 2014;6:653–65.
22. Loyaga-Rendon RY, Plaisance EP, Arena R, et al. Exercise physiology, testing, and training in patients supported by a left ventricular assist device. J Heart Lung Transplant 2015;34:1005–16.
23. Martina J, de Jonge N, Rutten M, et al. Exercise hemodynamics during extended continuous flow left ventricular assist device support: the response of systemic cardiovascular parameters and pump performance. Artif Organs 2013;37: 754–62.
24. Lilliu M, Onorati F, Luciani GB, et al. The determinants of functional capacity in left ventricular assist device patients: many actors with not well defined roles. J Cardiovasc Med 2020;7:472–80.
25. Fresiello L, Jacobs S, Timmermans P, et al. Limiting factors of peak and submaximal exercise capacity in LVAD patients. PLoS One 2020;7:e0235684.
26. Dimopoulos S, Diakos N, Tseliou E, et al. Chronotropic incompetence and abnormal heart rate recovery early after left ventricular assist device implantation. Pacing Clin Electrophysiol 2011;34: 1607–14.
27. Adamopoulos S, Corra' U, Laoutaris ID, et al. Exercise training in patients with ventricular assist devices: a review of the evidence and practical advice. A position paper from the Committee on Exercise Physiology and Training and the Committee of Advanced Heart Failure of the Heart Failure Association of the European Society of Cardiology. Eur J Heart Fail 2019;21:3–13.

28. Camboni D, Lange TJ, Ganslmeier P, et al. Left ventricular support adjustment to aortic valve opening with analysis of exercise capacity. J Cardiothorac Surg 2014;9:93.
29. Keteyian SJ, Kitzman D, Zannad F, et al. Predicting maximal HR in heart failure patients on β-blockade therapy. Med Sci Sports Exerc 2012;44(3):371–6.
30. Compostella L, Russo N, Setzu T, et al. A practical review for cardiac rehabilitation professionals of continuous-flow left ventricular assist devices: historical and current perspectives. J Cardiopulm Rehabil Prev 2015;5:301–11.
31. Dimopoulos SK, Drakos SG, Terrovitis JV, et al. Improvement in respiratory muscle dysfunction with continuous-flow left ventricular assist devices. J Heart Lung Transplant 2010;29:906–8.
32. Kerrigan DJ, Williams CT, Ehrman JK, et al. Muscular strength and cardiorespiratory fitness are associated with health status in patients with recently implanted continuous-flow LVADs. J Cardiopulm Rehabil Prev 2013;33:396–400.
33. Ades PA, Keteyian SJ, Balady GJ, et al. Cardiac rehabilitation exercise and self-care for chronic heart failure. JACC Heart Fail 2013;6:540–7.
34. Alsara O, Reeves RK, Pyfferoen MD, et al. Inpatient rehabilitation outcomes for patients receiving left ventricular assist device. Am J Phys Med Rehabil 2014;10:860–8.
35. Abshire M, Dennison Himmelfarb CR, Russell SD. Functional status in left ventricular assist device-supported patients: a literature review. J Card Fail 2014;20:973–83.
36. Prichard RA, Juul M, Gazibarich G, et al. Six-minute walk distance predicts VO2 (max) in patients supported with continuous flow left ventricular assist devices. Int J Artif Organs 2014;37(7):539–45.
37. Dunlay SM, Park SJ, Joyce LD, et al. Frailty and outcomes after implantation of left ventricular assist device as destination therapy. J Heart Lung Transplant 2014;33:359–65.
38. Cowger JA, Stulak JM, Shah P, et al. Impact of center left ventricular assist device volume on outcomes after implantation: an INTERMACS analysis. J Am Coll Cardiol 2017;5:691–9.
39. Myers TJ, Bolmers M, Gregoric ID, et al. Assessment of arterial blood pressure during support with an axial flow left ventricular assist device. J Heart Lung Transplant 2009;5:423–7.
40. Gross C, Marko C, Mikl J, et al. LVAD pump flow does not adequately increase with exercise. Artif Organs 2019;43(3):222–8.
41. Garan N, Nahumi J, Han P, et al. Chronotropic incompetence may impact exercise capacity in patients supported by left ventricular assist device. J Heart Lung Transplant 2013;32(4):S93.

Role of New Technologies in Supporting the Treatment of Complex Patients

Leopoldo Pagliani, MD, PhD*, Nicolosi Elisa, MD, Rivaben Dante Eduardo, MD, Dal Corso Lorenza, MD, Di Naro Agnese, MD, Francesco Antonini-Canterin, MD

KEYWORDS

- e-health • Heart failure • Implantable devices • Remote telemonitoring • Telemedicine
- Rehabilitation

KEY POINTS

Pearls

- Improving the level of interaction between the territory and operators.
- Reducing the need for travel, often problematic in the case of fragile users.
- Ensuring a significant reduction in costs.
- Ensuring greater equity of access to care.
- Ensuring better management of chronic cases thanks to continuous and multidisciplinary management and, in some specific cases, prompt intervention.

Pitfalls

- Creating extra medical work.
- Risk of not training operators in new practices.
- Poor clinical engagement with patients and families.
- The proliferation of for-profit telemedicine companies with different languages and tools.

PROBLEM DIMENSION

Heart failure (HF) is a common syndrome and is the most important cause of hospitalization for patients greater than 65 years of age. It affects 2% to 3% of the general population and, if considering only the elderly, 10% to 15%. The aging of the general population and the improvement of treatment in the acute phase of cardiovascular diseases will cause a 25% increase from 2010 to 2030, which inevitably will cause an increase in direct and indirect costs of care (+215% approximately). In the United States, for example, annual health costs related to HF are expected to rise from $24.7 billion to $77.7 billion, while indirect costs due to comorbidities and mortality are expected to rise from $9.7 billion to $17.4 billion.[1–7]

HF is a widespread condition with significant consequences in patients' well-being and mortality. Its impact on health services is significant, mostly on hospital care. Assistance to patients suffering HF is at different levels: general practitioners, specialist outpatient clinics, and hospitalizations. Even though hospital care becomes necessary for the most serious cases, it also can be potentially avoidable or reduced though careful management of people suffering from chronic HF. Because HF is a condition destined to increase, it is essential to find and highlight possible areas of improvement by monitoring the burden linked to the disease, care pathways, and outcomes.

On the occasion of the European Day of Heart Failure, the European Society of Cardiology highlighted that the number of people who are affected

Cardiology Unit, High Specialization Rehabilitation Hospital Motta di Livenza, Via Padre Bello 3c, Motta di Livenza, Treviso 31045, Italy
* Corresponding author.
E-mail addresses: leopoldo.pagliani@unipd.it; leopoldo.pagliani@ospedalemotta.it

Heart Failure Clin 17 (2021) 279–287
https://doi.org/10.1016/j.hfc.2021.01.009
1551-7136/21/

by HF in the world is approximately 22 million, of whom 14 million are Europeans.[8]

According to recent estimates, in less than 10 years, the number of chronic hearth failure (CHF) patients will reach the 30 million. The increase in the spread related to this pathology certainly is due to improvement of patient survival from ischemic heart disease and myocardial infarction as consequences of more successful treatments but also to the general lengthening of the average life span. The prevalence of SCC increases exponentially with age: it is less than 1% in people up to 60 years; it becomes 2% in people between ages 60 and 70; it rises to 5% in people between ages 70 and 80; and it is greater than 10% after the age of 80. The median age of onset of HF is 77 years for men and 83 years for women.

The absorption of health resources caused by this widespread pathology is relevant, and it frequently leads to repeated hospitalizations of the same subject. The 16% of patients discharged alive are registered again in a hospital within 3 months after the first hospitalization, 30% within 6 months, and greater than 40% within 1 year.

The therapeutic approach to HF has changed profoundly in the past 20 years, thanks to the transposition into clinical practice of the results of numerous and important clinical trials. The prognosis for people suffering from HF, however, is still burdened by an important load of mortality and morbidity. Hospitalization for HF is an indicator of a very high risk of death or rehospitalization. With record-linkage techniques, subsequent hospitalizations for HF and eventual death (with date and cause) have been identified. After the first hospitalization for HF, the probability of a new hospitalization for the same cause is high: 16% of total discharged have a new hospitalization within 3 months, 30% within 6 months, and greater than 40% within a year. The in-hospital mortality is approximately 17%; it exceeds 40% after 1 year from the date of admission of hospitalization for HF; and it reaches 60% within 3 years. Mortality increases with the age of the population, but at the same time, even at younger ages, mortality is high (3-year mortality rate of 36% in individuals aged up to 64 years and 46% among those aged 65 years to 74 years). These data fully justify the comparison of HF with a malignant tumor.[9]

POTENTIAL OF TELEMEDICINE IN THE ADVANCED REHABILITATION SETTING OF HEART FAILURE

The term, *telemedicine* (*TM*), lends itself to multiple definitions. The one that has become historic was developed in 1990 by a Commission of experts of the European Community. According to the Commission, TM is "the integration, monitoring and management of patients, as well as the education of patients and staff, using systems that allow ready access to expert advice and patient information, regardless of where the patient or the information resides."[10] The same principles underlie the definition given 7 years later by the World Health Organization, which describes TM as "the provision of health services, when distance is a critical factor, for which it is necessary for operators to use information and telecommunications technologies in order to exchange useful information for the diagnosis, treatment and prevention of diseases and to guarantee continuous information to health care providers and support research and evaluation of treatment."[11] A further authoritative definition of the term TM was given by the Food and Drug Administration, which qualifies TM as "the provision of health care and patient counseling services and the remote transmission of health information using telecommunications technologies, which include: clinical prevention, diagnosis and therapy, counseling and follow-up services, remote patient monitoring, rehabilitation services and patient education. Ultimately, telemedicine and everything that, thanks to telematics, is practiced remotely, such as: remote diagnosis, teaching/professional updating, remote data/image processing, doctor/doctor consultation, doctor/nurse etc."[12] Therefore, the many applications of telediagnosis, teledidactics, teleconsultation, teleservice, and telemonitoring (TLM) are distinguished in this article. In particular, the term, TLM, means a class of TM services useful for people who are chronically ill, goal of which is to remotely monitor the patient's health conditions, recording and sending biological signals and significant clinical parameters to the competent professional.[13,14]

International registries have clearly shown that many of the stages of instability in HF patients can be avoided if the follow-up pathway is improved during both the vulnerable postdischarge and the medium-term to long-term phases. The new remote control techniques of vital signs, and of health status in general, can help prevent HF instability (reduced coronary perfusion; uncontrolled hypertension; brady-tachyarrhythmias; various comorbidities, such as anemia; infections; deterioration of function; and poor compliance with drug and nondrug therapy) by stimulating early therapeutic interventions and/or appropriate behavioral changes.

TM, and in general the set of health technologies that go under the name of eHealth, identifies any digital exchange of health information and re-elaborates them in order to support and optimize the care process remotely, thus ensuring maximum home safety and the best quality of life to citizens. The same article includes tools designed to promote adherence and persistence to therapeutic and behavioral measures, such as text messaging reminders.

A classic structure of a TLM home model should take into consideration not only the clinical but also the socio-assistance needs of the patients, based on their characteristics (frailty, multiple comorbidities, high clinical complexity, and reduced mobility) with an integrated approach. The devices should transmit the signal to a single control unit placed at home (with low impact for the patient and his family) and from this to the server, of through secure protocols. This happens without the need for telephone contact between the patient and the operator. The transmission of data from sensors connected to the patient directly to a remote control is a valid alternative for patients not bound to treatments exclusively at their own home. The availability of a personal computer or tablet and a Wi-F network can offer the patient the possibility to communicate via videoconference with the socio-assistance team, anywhere they are.

In some solutions, the continuous management of flows and the verification of data transmission and quality of alarms, or of any possible malfunctions are arranged by a call center.

Among the most common devices used for the HF patients are the pulse oximeter, the scale, the sphygmomanometer, the electrocardiogram (ECG) with 1 or more leads, the motion/fall detector of the patient, and the call device for assistance requests. If deemed useful, any environmental sensor (temperature, humidity, water, and gas) can be installed. If necessary, a videoconference connection can be established with the client.

The transition from a simple technology (eg, the telephone) to a sophisticated one (multiparametric TLM) is accompanied by higher costs, which create greater difficulty in demonstrating a substantial benefit of the intervention in terms of cost-effectiveness From 2007 to 2013, numerous meta-analyses[15–22] were published, attempting to demonstrate that TLM interventions are associated with a significant reduction of events during follow-up. The randomized studies available in the literature were selected, often monocentric, with endpoints, such as mortality and hospitalization for HF, generally with a short observation period (only 6–12 months). In 2011, Inglis and colleagues[18] published a meta-analysis separating studies that used a structured telephone interview and a TLM TM system (digital/broadband/satellite/wireless or Bluetooth transmission of physiologic data [eg, ECG blood pressure, weight, pulse oximetry, respiratory rate, and other data]). The effect of the 2 interventions was similar regarding hospitalizations for HF.

On the contrary, the TLM was more effective on mortality than the structured telephone interview alone.

The message of the pioneering studies dates a decade back[23,24] and seems to suggest a neutral effect of TLM techniques on the main events during follow-up of both acute and stable HF patients, thus confirming other data from European multicenter studies published in previous years.[25–27] In more recent meta-analyses,[21] however, the remote assistance methods in the various randomized studies were compared again, and the result was that, despite the negative results of the latest trials, both the simple telephone support and the TLM system were associated with a significant clinical benefit in terms of both hospitalization and mortality reduction.

TM takes place remotely, without physical contact with patients, and requires an efficient health care organization and highly experienced staff who know the needs and characteristics of a person's disease, comorbidities, and social problems. In the past, often those who were appointed to follow the TLM did not know the patient well; in other cases, the work organization was not sufficient or inadequate resources managed the data that arrived at the coordinating center. The outpatients already followed and well known to the HF centers, often in New York Heart Association classes III to IV, frequently with geographic and socio-economic barriers, are much more suitable to be followed in a remote TLM program. It also should be considered, as in the German study, that if patients already are followed-up periodically by a dedicated clinic within an efficient hospital-territory network, it becomes difficult to obtain a substantial difference with the TLM program; thus, study results may be negative. The Home or Hospital in Heart Failure study[25] is a good example of this concept; when the analysis was restricted to Italian centers (responsible for 50% of enrollments) that had much more experience in using the TLM system; the differences in the primary endpoint of hospitalization for HF and total mortality became largely significant in favor of the TLM.

Among the various forms of TM, of particular interest are teleradiology, telecardiology, teleassistance of respiratory patients, telerehabilitation, and teleconsultation. For the development of these technologies, it is necessary to guarantee the following:

- Reliable connectivity
- Sensitive data
- Training of patients
- Caregivers
- Health professionals
- Synergy between health organizations and universities for the development of the technology

From a technical point of view, the system is composed of 3 main modules[28]:

1. A multiaccess and multiprofile Web platform for the enrollment, capable of defining activity plans and monitoring patients
2. A mobile device application (app) to guide patients in self-measurement of their vital parameters in accordance with the personalized measurement plan though Bluetooth sensors, which also guide the transmittal to the platform. The app is equipped with a user-friendly graphic interface to guide patients with audiovisual reminders of the measurements to be carried out and provide immediate feedback on their outcome. The acquisition of data though Bluetooth medical sensors is completely automatic, as is the immediate transmission of the data collected to the Web platform.
3. An app to support health care workers during their home visits to patients. The app can manage multiple patients within the same health care facility. Once logged in using personal credentials, the doctor sees the list of patients and the trend of the vital parameters measured. The doctor can manage the events reported by the system and make changes to the activity plan. In addition, the app allows to record access to basic, specialist and hospital medicine as well as store generic notes regarding the patient.

TELEMEDICINE: TECHNOLOGICAL AND ORGANIZATIONAL ASPECTS

A growing section of TM is mobile health (mHealth), which uses mobile devices (mobile phones, smartphones, tablets, PDAs, and wearable sensors) and widespread communication technologies (SMS and e-mail) for remote health status monitoring.[29]

Due to their advanced technology, smartphones can be considered pocket computers that allow the acquisition of information from various sources. Other devices can be worn, attached to the skin, or even ingested in order to quantify any physiologic activity or change (type of exercise, heart rate, sleep, and drug intake).

The interesting aspect of these devices is that the knowledge of the acquired data allows the patient to take an increasingly active role in the management of his/her chronic disease[30]; therefore, these innovations increasingly are welcome by patients. If in the past the access to the Internet was possible only via computer, thus excluding those categories of people who were not familiar with it (elderly or people with lower income/education), now mobile phones are within the reach of the vast majority of the population.[31–33] This has led to the creation of countless apps related to the health world. In the near future, mobile technology can become a useful resource capable of facilitating curative interventions in the health care field, which also can guarantee an excellent cost/effectiveness ratio.[34,35]

The future prospect is to fortify the personal health record (PHR), an electronic record of individual health information, compliant with interoperability standards recognized at least at national level, which can be enriched from various sources while remaining under the control of the individual, who may possibly share it. There are many critical elements in the PHR implementation, however: on 1 side it includes a strong authentication system to guarantee the privacy of individuals; on the other side, there must be attention on the information content. It is difficult to manage the quantity and the quality of the data in the absence of certified information or in the presence of potential conflicts of interest. In addition, there may be legal implications because the responsibility of doctors in cases of misdiagnosis, based on inaccurate data provided by patients, still is not clear.[36] Only a few applications have been scientifically validated and certified as medical devices and, even among the best studied, there often is no comparison with a control group.[37–39]

Standard of a Health Training Project for Doctors and Nurse

The launch of a TM service in a hospital generally is caused by a lack of dedicated human resources; usually, there is a redistribution of resources from other services and dedicated to telemedicine as a part time.

It, therefore, is necessary to identify and train existing human resources; then, create new human resources proportional to the growth of the service; and insert the concept of development and training of human resources in all professional dynamics in which telemedicine can be applied.

Regarding the specific activity, the challenge is to evaluate and adapt the characteristics of the professionals already present and create new intermediate figures.

In most of the projects dedicated to rehabilitative TM in HF, cardiology specialists are aged between 35 years and 60 years and have at least 5 years of experience in a coronary intensive care unit, with substantial knowledge of the main information technology operating systems, as sharing the main lines heart disease guide.

It will be useful to arrange the sending of quarterly update data (discharge diagnoses of all patients sent to the emergency department and reports of patients who went to an emergency department after a teleconsultation that did not require it). Then, a clinical debriefing will have to be performed to verify incorrect reports and/or patient approach problems and the interventions recorded and error analysis data archived.

The introduction of new technologies easily can be integrated into the work carried out by nurses, provided that ad hoc training programs and appropriate quality controls on the work performed are carried out.

The need for new management models arises from the progressive aging of the population, from reduction of mortality in the acute phase of heart disease and, therefore, from an increase in chronic diseases, with subsequent increase in costs for national health services. The management of the patient in areas through TM seems to be an effective and efficient method to assist patients with chronic diseases. With this new service, new professionals are born: they must be organized and trained.

Training shall include an ECG entry test and constant guided ECG reporting.

The nurse then needs to share the main guidelines for heart disease and explain the main operational flow charts concerning the main symptoms (heart rate, dyspnea, and so forth).

LEGAL AND REGULATORY ASPECTS

If telecardiology means the possibility of sending information about the cardiopathic patient remotely, thus facilitating the therapeutic and assistance treatment, it follows that on 1 side new targets for continuous and more effective assistance to the patient are opened up, but on the other side, the various health professionals involved must assume responsibilities that must be clarified from a medicolegal point of view.

In an activity in which the barriers of space and time are overcome by telecommunication techniques, competence no longer is reduced to the simple relationship between the patient and the doctor or the nurse, but it is expanded to involving more people, such as the general practitioner, any doctor from other hospitals, the cardiologist (coming from a highly specialized cardiology center), and finally the professional nurse, who assumes, in some respects, the real key role of the whole therapeutic-assistance project.

In order to allow to the professional nurse to have operational autonomy, however, it is not enough that the nurse possesses all the formal and substantial requisites to carry out activity: the nurse must obtain both general and a specific consent to operate directly from the patient. This consent is what makes the nurse action lawful.

Generic informed consent is the patient's authorization to be included in a telecardiology program, whereas the specific consent is the patient's authorization given to all the professional nurse's activity, such as collecting and sending clinical data as well as direct therapeutic and assistance services.

Therefore, it will be essential that the consent form prepared for telecardiology services contains a brief but detailed information on the meaning and usefulness of the telecardiology program and also include the patient's authorization for autonomous, home-based activities established by the telematic monitoring program.

The formulation of the diagnostic judgment and of the choice of therapeutic treatment are strictly up to the cardiologist, but the execution of the therapy again becomes largely the responsibility of the professional nurse, except in those cases requiring direct intervention by the cardiologist or the hospitalization of the patient.

In this phase of the activity, however, there are risks for nurses of possibly trespassing their role. Should any complications or adverse events occur as a result of an excessively autonomous nurse's decisions, even in the diagnostic-therapeutic field, these may lead to legal implications. The absence of legislation on the matter is a gap that can lead to the danger of an uncontrollable application of telecardiology.

Until a few decades ago, the treatment of health data mostly was carried out in the context of the trustworthy relationship between the patient and the treating physician though paper or even mnemonic methods. The introduction of information and communication technologies has changed this framework profoundly, determining the legislation to protect clients with respect to the processing of their health data.[40] The creation of software capable of processing clinical data, of electronic archives capable of collecting a large amount of such data, and of networks capable of allowing their transmission in real time entails enormous advantages from medical and scientific points of view, because it now is possible to find, process, and compare health-related information in a few seconds. This development, however, has increased the number of subjects who actually hold health data. It also increased the speed of transmission of such data and the amount of information electronically stored (often not in the national territory). These improvements have led to an exponential exposure of sensitive data to the dangerous breach of confidentiality, which could imply the infringement of the dignity and of the fundamental rights of the patient.

In other words, the validity of the use of new technologies in the medical science shall in no way lead to neglecting the centrality of the patient and the primary goal of medicine itself.

The bureaucratic formalities to be adapted, with the aim of recognizing services provided from a distance, do not represent the only regulatory obstacle to the growth of TM. TM systems involve the possibilities not only of patients communicating with their health care professional but also transmitting data related to the measurements that a patient makes remotely through self-analysis tools in order to allow a doctor to prescribe the treatment. This process involves the remote collection of sensitive patient data, which then are stored in a database that the doctor can access remotely. This collection and processing of personal data pose significant legal problems to

- The subjects who operate as data controllers (hospitals or health authorities)
- The security measures to be adopted to protect from unauthorized access to the data collected in the database
- Which purposes the data collected can be used for and that must be expressly accepted by the patient in written form

Refundability and Elements of Economic Recognition

The TM must propose itself to national health services in an innovative way and with respect to the reimbursement model, in order to allow the administrations to correctly and dynamically plan and allocate costs as well as to directly correlate them with the evidence of the benefits brought to the system. The tariff definition for the TM services is considered essential: TM is a treatment modality that improves the effectiveness, efficiency, and appropriateness of the system; therefore, not including it in the services of the national health services reduces any efficiency and increases waste. As a short-term proposal, it is suggested to define a reimbursement of benefits by analogy, unique throughout the national territory. Looking ahead, it will be necessary to define new reimbursement models linked to chronic diseases.

FUTURE PERSPECTIVES

All the national and international epidemiologic investigations recently conducted reveal 2 things:

1. HF patients are on the rise.
2. There is a marked increase in costs caused by hospitalizations.

Nonetheless, there still is little use of the recent, innovative telematic disease management methods that could help coordinate patient management.

In this context, TM could achieve a turning point in the management of chronic HF.[41]

In the future, the key points of where to intervene, to develop and implement the new models of remote surveillance, can be represented by

- The insertion of the patient into a management model for chronic diseases through integrated communication systems and TLM activities already present in the model of care but which sometimes highlight implementation difficulties, such as patient, family, and caregiver education
- Close monitoring follow-up of the patient
- Careful and adequate adherence to the pharmacologic path and its changes, according to the needs of the pathology
- Inclusion of a true case manager able to combine the needs of a patient with chronic pathology in a context of multiple comorbidities

The choices of the ideal patient and the type of TM program are critical, because there are many aspects to be considered: age, severity and phase of the HF (with particular attention to the postdischarge transition phase), multiple associated pathologies, degree of self-sufficiency and cognitive responsiveness, family background, and presence of a caregiver.

The adoption of a reference figure for the patient, such as a case manager, will be considered essential. This professional, who coordinates social and health services, will ensure continuity of care. Advanced training must be required to carry out this role. In the future, it would be desirable to adopt and recognize the figure of the case manager in all the realities of health services in order to ensure a new organization model that accompanies and enhances the client in the in-home care path.

Decision support systems intended as software, which make it possible to increase the effectiveness of the analysis of health professionals, doctors, nurses, and sometimes even caregivers and patients, will be increasingly present. The system will rely on a database or on a neural network, helping users make better decisions, and will connect with busines intelligence tools.

In the future, any interventions will have to be personalized and not implemented according to rigid welfare models. The technology through the app and smartphone systems on the Internet will facilitate the transmission and sharing of data significantly. Some aspects, however, remain mandatory. Parametric input will be required to judge the signs of instability from different points of view (eg, by integrating weight/heart rate/blood pressure/brain natriuretic peptide and parameters from defibrillation and cardiac resynchronization therapy devices, when available). Patients admitted to the TM program must be trained in the data transmission procedure with the highest possible adherence, according to a tailor-made management program within a system that also includes the case manager, the specialist(s), and the dedicated nursing staff to the care of the HF. The algorithms and intervention protocols must be customized in relation to the characteristics of the disease, the comorbidities, the neurologic and frailty aspects, and the presence of support from the caregivers; The Internet of You systems (IoY), will play a central role. The home and mobile TLM services can now count on the potential of the IoY as the true evolution in the health sector. IoY technologies (wearable and environmental) automatically send the collected data to the PHR, allowing doctors to interact with patients virtually and in real time.

IoY also can integrate customizable algorithms for monitoring and interpreting patient behaviors during their normal daily activities, allowed though wireless monitoring with automatic learning techniques to supervise.

- The time spent, frequency, and compliance with daily standards of domestic activities (taking medicines, preparation of meals, physical activity, and so forth)
- Processing vital signs in real time
- Correlating the multiparameter environmental, behavioral, and health monitoring with clinical history
- Identifying, through the application of appropriate models, early diagnosis and incipient destabilization of the clinical picture, generating the necessary support for clinical decision[42]

Therefore, clinical innovation will consist of the possibility of collecting personalized information both of vital parameters (body sensor) and of the environmental context (ambient sensor) related to the clinical history of each patient, thus allowing minimal invasive remote controls, early diagnosis of instability, and more effective follow-up.

CLINICS CARE POINTS

- Technological innovation can contribute to a reorganization of health care, in particular by supporting the modification of the focus of health care from the hospital to the environment, through innovative care models centered on the citizen and facilitating access to services.
- A harmonization of the application models of TM is necessary as a prerequisite for the interchangeability of TM services and as a requirement for the transition from an experimental logic to a structured logic of widespread use of TM services, especially in chronic disease.
- The rehabilitation and follow-up of HF are a fundamental test for using and centralizing the role of new technologies in the treatment of cardiovascular diseases.

DISCLOSURE

Nothing to disclose.

REFERENCES

1. Schaufelberger M, Swedberg K, Köster M, et al. Decreasing oneyear mortality and hospitalization rates for heart failure in Sweden: data from the Swedish Hospital Discharge Registry 1988 to 2000. Eur Heart J 2004;25:300–7.
2. Jhund PS, Macintyre K, Simpson CR, et al. Long-term trends in first hospitalization for heart failure and subsequent survival between 1986 and 2003: a population study of 5.1 million people. Circulation 2009;119:515–23.
3. Tavazzi L, Senni M, Metra M, et al. INHF (Italian Network on Heart Failure) Outcome Investigators. Multicenter prospective observational study on acute and chronic heart failure: one-year follow-up results of IN-HF (Italian Network on Heart Failure) outcome registry. Circ Heart Fail 2013;6:473–81.
4. Cleland JG, Swedberg K, Follath F, et al. EuroHeart Failure survey programme - a survey on the quality of care among patients with heart failure in Europe: Part 1: patient characteristics and diagnosis. Eur Heart J 2003;24:442–63.
5. Gheorghiade M, Zannad F, Sopko G, et al. International Working Group on Acute Heart Failure

Syndromes. Acute heart failure syndromes: current state and framework for future research. Circulation 2005;112:3958–68.
6. Rudiger A, Harjola VP, Müller A, et al. Acute heart failure: clinical presentation, one-year mortality and prognostic factors. Eur J Heart Fail 2005;7:662–70.
7. Adams KF Jr, Fonarow GC, Emerman CL, et al. Characteristics and outcomes of patients hospitalized for heart failure in the United States: rationale, design, and preliminary observations from the first 100 000 cases in the Acute Decompensated Heart Failure National Registry (ADHERE). Am Heart J 2005;149:209–16.
8. European Society of Cardiology (ESC). Heart failure association (HFA) of the ESC. Rome (Italy): European Heart Failure Days: press release; 2015.
9. Stewart S, MacIntyre K, Hole DJ, et al. More 'malignant' than cancer? Five-year survival following a first admission for heart failure. Eur J Heart Fail 2001; 3(3):315–22.
10. O 'Rourke M, et al. Report to the Commission for the European Community. The Advanced Informatics in Medicine (AIM) Program 1990.
11. WHO A. Health telematics Policy in support of WHO's health for AllStrategy for Global health development. Genova (Switzerland): Report of the WHO Group Consultation on Health Telematics; 1997.
12. Food and Drug Administration (FDA). Definition of telemedicine. Available at: www.fda.gov. Accessed: June 25, 2015.
13. Italian Ministry of Health, Telemedicine - national guidelines, State-Regions Agreement, 2014.
14. GiordaniG, et al. Observatory and projects on telemedicine applications. Notebooks Arsenàl.IT 2008.
15. Polisena J, Tran K, Cimon K, et al. Home telemonitoring for congestive heart failure: a systematic review and meta-anal- ysis. J Telemed Telecare 2010;16: 68–76.
16. Clark RA, Inglis SC, McAlister FA, et al. Telemonitoring or structured telephone support programmes for patients with chronic heart failure: systematic review and meta-analysis. BMJ 2007;334:942.
17. Clarke M, Shah A, Sharma U. Sys- tematic review of studies on telemoni- toring of patients with congestive heart failure: A meta-analysis. J Telemed Telecare 2011;17:7–14.
18. Inglis SC, Clark RA, McAlister FA, et al. Which components of heart failure programmes are effective? A systematic review and meta-analysis of the outcomes of structured telephone support or telemonitoring as the primary component of chronic heart failure management in 8323 patients: Abridged Cochrane Review. Eur J Heart Fail 2011; 13:1028–40.
19. Seto E. Cost comparison between telemonitoring and usual care of heart failure: a systematic review. Telemed J E Health 2008;14:679–86.
20. Pandor A, Gomersall T, Stevens JW, et al. Remote monitoring after recent hospital discharge in patients with heart failure: a systematic review and network metaanalysis. Heart 2013;99:1717–26.
21. Kotb A, Cameron C, Hsieh S, et al. Comparative effectiveness of different forms of telemedicine for individuals with heart failure (HF): a systematic review and network meta-analysis. PLoS One 2015; 10:e0118681.
22. Chaudhry SI, Mattera JA, Curtis JP, et al. Telemonitoring in patients with heart failure. N Engl J Med 2010;363:2301–9.
23. Koehler F, Winkler S, Schieber M, et al. Impact of remote telemedical management on mortality and hospitalizations in ambulatory patients with chronic heart failure: The Telemedical Interventional Monitoring in Heart Failure study. Circulation 2011;123: 1873–80.
24. Ferrante D, Varini s, Macchia A, et al. GENICA Investigators. Long-term re- sults after a telephone intervention in chronic heart failure: DIAL (Randomized Trial of Phone Intervention in Chronic Heart Failure) follow-up. J Am Coll Cardiol 2010;56:372–8.
25. Mortara A, Pinna GD, Johnson P, et al. HHH Investigators. Home telemonitor- ing in heart failure patients: the HHH study (Home or Hospital in Heart failure). Eur J Heart Fail 2009;11:312–8.
26. Whellan DJ, Ousdigian KT, Al-Khatib SM, et al, PARTNERS Study Investigators. Combined heart failure device diagnostics identify patients at higher risk of subse quent heart failure hospitalizations: results from PARTNERS HF (Program to Access and review Trending information and eval- uate correlation to symptoms in Patients With heart failure) study. J Am Coll Cardiol 2010;55:1803–10.
27. Giordano A, Scalvini S, Paganoni AM, et al. Home-based telesurveillance program in chronic heart failure: effects on clinical status and implications for 1-year progno- sis. Telemed J E Health 2013;19:605–12.
28. Klersy C, De Silvestri A, Gabutti G, et al. A meta-analysis of re- mote monitoring of heart failure patients. J Am Coll Cardiol 2009;54:1683–94.
29. Demiris G, Afrin LB, Speedie S, et al. Patient-centered applications: use of information technology to promote dis- ease management and wellness: a white paper by the AMIA Knowledge in Motion Working Group. J Am Med Inform Assoc 2008;15:8–13.
30. Brennan PF, Strombom I. Improving health care by understanding patient pref- erences: the role of computer technology. J Am Med Inform Assoc 1998;5:257–62.
31. Smith A. Mobile access 2010. Available at: http://www.pewinternet.org/files/old-me- dia//Files/Reports/2010/PIP_Mobile_Ac- cess_2010.pdf. Accessed May 5, 2016.
32. Pew Research Internet. Project: cell phone and smartphone ownership demo- graphics 2014.

Available at: http://www.pewinternet.org/data-trend/mobile/cell-phone-and-smart-phone-ownership-demographics/. Accessed May 5, 2016.
33. Rock Health. Digital Health Funding 2015 Midyear Review. Available at: https://rockhealth.com/reports/digital-health-2015-midyear/. Accessed May 5, 2016.
34. mHealth App Developer Econom- ics 2014: The State of the Art of mHealth App Publishing. research2guidancewebsite. Available at: http://research2guidance.com/r2g/research- 2guidance-mHealth-App-Developer-Eco- nomics-2014.pdf. Accessed May 5, 2016.
35. Burke LE, Ma J, Azar KM, et al. Current science on consumer use of mo- bile health for cardiovascular disease pre- vention: a scientific statement from the American Heart Association. Circulation 2015; 132:1157–213.
36. Desai AS, Stevenson LW. Connect- ing the circle from home to heart-fail- ure disease management. N Engl J Med 2010;363:2364–7.
37. Patrick K, Raab F, Adams MA, et al. A text message-based intervention for weight loss: randomized controlled trial. J Med Internet Res 2009;11:e1.
38. Whittaker R, Borland R, Bullen C, et al. Mobile phone-based interventions for smoking cessation. Cochrane Database Syst Rev 2009;(4):CD006611.
39. Nakamura N, Koga T, Iseki H. A me- ta-analysis of remote patient monitoring for chronic heart failure patients. J Telemed Telecare 2014;20:11–7.
40. REGULATION (EU) 2016/679 OF THE EUROPEAN PARLIAMENT AND OF THE COUNCIL of 27 April 2016 on the protection of natural persons with regard to the processing of personal data and on the free movement of such data, and repealing Directive 95/46/EC (General Data Protection Regulation).
41. Scalvini S, Giordano A. Heart fail- ure: optimal post-discharge management of chronic heart failure. Nat Rev Cardiol 2012;10:9–10.
42. Di Lenarda A, Casolo G, Gulizia MM, et al. The future of telemedicine for the management of heart failure patients: a Consensus Document of the Italian Association of Hospital Cardiologists (A.N.M.C.O), the Italian Society of Cardiology (S.I.C.) and the Italian Society for Telemedicine and eHealth (Digital S.I.T.). Eur Heart J Suppl 2017;19(Suppl D): D113–29.

Cardiac Resynchronization Therapy in Patients with Heart Failure: What is New?

Giuseppe Palmiero, MD[a,b,*], Maria Teresa Florio, MD[c], Marta Rubino, MD[b], Martina Nesti, MD[d], Michal Marchel, MD, PhD[e], Vincenzo Russo, MD, PhD[f]

KEYWORDS

• Cardiac resynchronization therapy • Heart failure • Multimodality imaging

BACKGROUND

Cardiac resynchronization therapy (CRT) is an established treatment of patients with medically refractory, mild-to-severe systolic heart failure (HF), impaired left ventricular (LV) function, and wide QRS complex. The pathologic activation sequence observed in patients with abnormal QRS duration and morphology results in a dyssynchronous ventricular activation and contraction, leading to cardiac remodeling, worsening systolic and diastolic function, and progressive HF.[1]

Over the last 20 years, several clinical trials[2–5] have firmly established that CRT produces consistent improvements in quality of life, functional status, and exercise capacity while also providing strong evidence for reverse remodeling and diminished functional mitral regurgitation, resulting in reductions in both HF hospitalizations and all-cause morbidity and mortality.

Despite the well-documented benefits of CRT, about ~30% of system recipients do not improve their HF symptoms.[6]

The aim of the present review is to explore the current CRT literature, focusing our attentions on the promising innovation in this field.

INDICATIONS TO CARDIAC RESYNCHRONIZATION THERAPY

The evidence of electrical dyssynchrony on 12-lead electrocardiography (ECG) is a prerequisite for CRT response and is usually established by prolonged QRS duration (≥120 ms) and/or left bundle branch block (LBBB) morphology. Then, QRS analysis is the cornerstone in current recommendation for patient selection in CRT[7,8]: a prolonged QRS duration (≥150 ms) and an LBBB QRS morphology, reflecting a significant intraventricular conduction delay, are strong indications (class I, A) for CRT implantation in patients with HF with reduced ejection fraction (HFrEF), which remains symptomatic despite optimal medical therapy (OMT), whereas weaker recommendations are reserved for patients with QRS less than 150 ms and non-LBBB morphology (class IIb, B). In patients with HF with LBBB and QRS duration ranging from 120 to 129 ms, there is less agreement, especially in patients with a QRS duration less than 129 ms and New York Heart Association (NYHA) functional class II symptoms: in this subgroup of patients, the European Heart Rhythm Association (EHRA) guidelines[8]

Funding: "This research received no external funding."
[a] Department of Cardiology, AORN Ospedali dei Colli - Monaldi Hospital, Naples, Italy; [b] Inherited and Rare Cardiovascular Diseases Unit, Department of Translational Medical Sciences, University of Campania "Luigi Vanvitelli", Naples, Italy; [c] Division of Internal Medicine, University of Campania "Luigi Vanvitelli", Naples, Italy; [d] Cardiovascular and Neurology Department, Ospedale San Donato, Arezzo, Italy; [e] 1st Department of Cardiology, Medical University of Warsaw, Warsaw, Poland; [f] Department of Translational Medical Sciences, University of Campania "Luigi Vanvitelli", Naples, Italy
* Corresponding author. Department of Cardiology, AORN Ospedali dei Colli - Monaldi Hospital, Naples, Italy.
E-mail address: g.palmiero@hotmail.it

Heart Failure Clin 17 (2021) 289–301
https://doi.org/10.1016/j.hfc.2021.01.010

recommend the CRT implantation (class IIb, B), whereas the Heart Failure Association (HFA) guidelines[7] do not recommend it (class III), accepting the results from Echo-CRT study that showed no CRT benefit in otherwise eligible patients with a QRS duration less than 130 ms.[9]

Nevertheless, QRS characteristics as a surrogate of electrical dyssynchrony fails to reflect the mechanical pattern within any single heart. Patients with broad QRS and LBBB but without mechanical dyssynchrony have been described, indicating that the electromechanical correlation is variable even in the presence of broad LBBB.[10] On the other hand, approximately 30% of patients with a normal QRS duration have mechanical dyssynchrony and could potentially have same benefit from CRT.[11]

INDICATIONS TO CARDIAC RESYNCHRONIZATION THERAPY IN SPECIAL POPULATIONS

Patients Needing Antibradycardia Pacing

Right ventricular (RV) pacing may cause delayed LV activation similar to the pattern observed in LBBB[12] and may thus lead to deterioration in HF symptoms.[13] CRT is recommended in patients with reduced LV ejection fraction (LVEF) and an indication for ventricular pacing due to high-degree atrioventricular (AV) block; moreover, it may be considered patients with HF who develop worsening of LV function due to high percentage of conventional RV pacing may be considered for an upgrade to CRT (class IIb, B). The BIOPACE study[14] comparing conventional dual-chamber pacing with CRT in patients with high-degree AV block and near-normal LV function failed to show any significant improvement in mortality and hospitalizations by CRT. Thus, CRT should be reserved to patients with some degree of LV dysfunction.

Patients with Atrial Fibrillation

Atrial fibrillation (AF) is a frequent comorbidity in patients with HF; however, only one of the major CRT trials included AF patients.[5] Meta-analytic evidence suggests that AF patients derive a similar benefit from CRT as sinus rhythm patients with regard to EF reduction but have a less functional response and remain at a higher risk of nonresponse and death.[15] Thus, CRT is indicated in AF patients with reduced LV function if they have an indication for ventricular pacing (including patients undergoing AV node ablation) regardless of functional NYHA class (class I, A) and should be considered in patients with NYHA class III–IV HF, LVEF less than or equal to 35%, and QRS greater than or equal to 130 ms (class IIa, B), provided a strategy to ensure biventricular capture is in place or the patient is expected to return to sinus rhythm.

Patients with Hypertrophic Cardiomyopathy

About 5% of patients with hypertrophic cardiomyopathy (HCM) develop LV systolic dysfunction and congestive HF due progressive myocardial fibrosis.[16] In the subset of patients with HCM with systolic ventricular impairment and dyssynchrony, CRT was associated with reverse remodeling of the left atrium and ventricle,[17,18] and it may be considered for alleviating the HF symptoms.[19,20] Small cohort studies have also examined CRT as a treatment of LV outflow tract obstruction, but its superiority over conventional RV pacing is not established.[21,22]

Patients with Neuromuscular Disorders

LV systolic dysfunction represents the most common involvement in patients with dystrophinopathies,[23,24] comprising both Duchenne muscular disease (DMD) and Becker muscular disease (BMD), and is noticed in about 14.6% of myotonic dystrophy type I patients (DM1).[25] Because conduction system disease and the need for right ventricular pacing frequently accompany severe LV dysfunction in advanced stage of neuromuscular disease, CRT may be an option in selected cases.[26] To date, there are only a few case reports of benefit with CRT in patients with DMD,[27] BMD,[28] and DM1[29,30] with LV systolic dysfunction and electromechanical dyssynchrony.

Elderly Patients

Pivotal clinical trials in CRT did not set upper age limits for enrollment; however, because of enrollment of predominately younger patients, these studies were not specifically designed or powered to assess outcomes in elderly patients. A substudy of the Multicenter Trial-Cardiac Resynchronization Therapy (MADIT-CRT) demonstrated that elderly patients (≥75 years) benefit from preventive CRT-D similar to younger patients, significantly reducing the composite endpoint of death and HF with no increase in complication rates.[31] Some observational studies investigating the clinical and echocardiographic outcomes in octogenarians receiving CRT for advanced HF showed similar clinical benefits as younger patients.[32–34] Advanced age should not be the sole reason for avoiding preventive CRT-D therapy in elderly patients with CHF.

Transthyretin Cardiac Amyloidosis

Cardiac amyloidosis is an infiltrative cardiomyopathy caused by extracellular deposition of misfolded precursor proteins.[35] Transthyretin cardiac amyloidosis (ATTR-CA) is common among the elderly and represents a possible cause of HF with preserved EF (HFpEF).[36] Moreover, due to the progressive nature of the disease, many advanced stage patients are classified in HFrEF category. Prolonged intraventricular delay with or without LBBB morphology is common in ATTR-CA due to the infiltration of conduction pathway by amyloid deposits. This means that many ATTR-CA patients meet the criteria for CRT implantation. Donnellan and colleagues[37] have evaluated in a recent study the efficacy of CRT in ATTR-CA and its impact on survival. Thirty consecutive patients with ATTR-CA who underwent CRT implantation are matched based on age, sex, LVEF, NYHA functional class, and ATTR-CA stage with 30 patients with ATTR-CA who did not receive CRT device. In conclusions, CRT is associated with improved survival and improvements in HF symptoms and LVEF in ATTR-CA. The beneficial effects of CRT were greater in appropriately selected patients who meet guideline criteria. However, given the poor prognosis of ATTR-CA with reduced LVEF, the utility of CRT in this setting is still controversial.

REMOTE MONITORING IN CARDIAC RESYNCHRONIZATION THERAPY

Remote monitoring (RM) has become a new standard of care in the follow-up of patients with cardiac implantable devices (CIEDs). The strategy of remote CIEDs monitoring and interrogation, combined with at least annual in-person evaluation, is actually recommended over a calendar-based schedule of in-person CIED evaluation alone.[38] A daily RM has been shown to reduce all-cause mortality and a combined endpoint including cardiovascular (CV) mortality and CV hospitalization, mainly driven by the prevention of HF exacerbation,[39] and this suggests that patients with more severe HF may gain a greater clinical benefit of RM; moreover, the beneficial effect of RM on survival is more likely in patients with more depressed LVEF, who generally have a high mortality risk.

According to HFA Guidelines,[7] daily multiparameter RM may be considered in patients with symptomatic HF treated with implantable cardioverter defibrillator/CRT-Ds, who have reduced LVEF despite OMT. RM offers an opportunity to improve follow-up efficiency by monitoring technical function and disease-specific parameters, in particular to modify the progression of HF, which is a source of considerable patient morbidity and mortality and cost for health care.

THE PROBLEM OF "NON-RESPONDERS" TO CARDIAC RESYNCHRONIZATION THERAPY

The main goal of CRT is restoring synchrony of LV by multisite pacing in order to induce LV reverse remodeling (LVRR) and, consequently, to improve clinical patient's outcome. Nevertheless, as mentioned, about 30% of patients with HF treated with CRT according to the current guidelines does not respond adequately due to lack of LVRR and/or poor clinical outcome. This subgroup is classified as *"non-responder"* although no unifying definition of response to CRT exists.[6] Nonresponse to CRT seems to be multifactorial and attributable to inadequate patient selection, inappropriate delivery, or LV lead position. CRT outcomes could be improved using a multidisciplinary, protocol-driven CRT optimization clinic as part of a HF disease management program.[40]

Novel advanced multimodality imaging promises to support electrocardiography in redefining the individual's candidacy for CRT and guiding the correct lead positioning in the coronary sinus in order to achieve device optimization and provide a sustained CRT response. The response to CRT is commonly evaluated in terms of LVRR (LV end-systolic volume [LVESV] reduction of 15% or more compared with baseline) that is associated with better long-term outcome after CRT and considered the best predictor of mortality and HF-related hospitalization in this setting.[41]

Patient Selection

The patient selection is of pivotal importance for increasing the rate of CRT response. Nonischemic disease, wider QRS, LBBB morphology, and female gender are well-known prognostic factors for response.[8] However, as stated previously, QRS duration and morphology does not predict always a prolonged LV activation time correlated to CRT response. Novel electrocardiographic and multimodality imaging techniques are currently changing the classical scenarios in patient selection for CRT (**Table 1**).

Role of electrocardiography

Novel noninvasive ECG mapping technique has showed to be useful in identifying patients with abnormally late-activating regions of the LV and, therefore, susceptible to CRT. *Vectorcardiography-derived* QRS_{area},[42] consisting in a 3-dimensional (3D) vector loop derived mathematically from a standard digital ECG, has proved to be

Table 1
Parameters used to improve the cardiac resynchronization therapy response

Before Implantation	During Implantation	After Implantation
Patient selection: • Cause of CMP • QRS length • QRS morphology • Sex • Myocardial scar	LV lead position Quadripolar lead Multipolar pacing Multisite pacing His bundle pacing	Device optimization: • AV interval • VV interval • FOI • Biventricular pacing Pharmacologic therapy Physical activity

Abbreviations: CMP, cardiomyopathy; FOI, fusion-optimized intervals; VV, interventricular.

superior to classical QRS analysis of duration and morphology in predicting LVRR assessed by echocardiography in the MARC study. Moreover, the *high-resolution noninvasive electrocardiographic imaging* shows in many studies to be superior to LBBB in predicting acute hemodynamics and long-term clinical response to CRT.[43]

Role of echocardiography

Classical echocardiographic assessment of CRT candidates comprises evaluation of LV regional and global function and the evaluation of cardiac mechanical dyssynchrony.

Assessment of LV global function is pivotal in the candidacy for CRT: the LVEF calculation is included in all international guidelines recommendation; moreover, the measurement of LVESV, as stated, defines the echocardiographic response to CRT after 3 to 6 months of device implantation.[41]

On the other hand, the definition of cardiac dyssynchrony with ultrasounds is still debated. The echocardiography ability in measuring mechanical dyssynchrony and predicting CRT response better than electrocardiography has been investigated in many single-center studies in the past, showing promising data and suggesting a potential role in improving patient selection for CRT.

The mechanical dyssynchrony has been classically established by various echocardiographic modalities, including conventional M-mode, tissue Doppler imaging (TDI), myocardial deformation analysis, and 3D echocardiography. Echocardiographic evaluation of dyssynchrony involves assessment of atrioventricular, interventricular, and intraventricular dyssynchrony.

Atrioventricular dyssynchrony assessment has showed limited value in predicting CRT response. However, significant atrioventricular dyssynchrony, assessed by pulsed-wave (PW) Doppler of transmitral flow is currently implied for atrioventricular delay optimization after device implantation. The classical parameter used is the LV filling ratio (LVFT/RR), obtained by dividing the LV diastolic filling time (the sum of E- and A-wave duration) with the RR interval duration. An LVFT/RR less than 40% identified significant atrioventricular dyssynchrony and, in this setting, short-AV and long-AV delays can be identified from the PW transmitral flow pattern.[44]

Interventricular dyssynchrony is defined by asynchronous activation of LV and RV and indicated by the delay greater than 40 ms between LV and RV preejection time measured by PW-Doppler or by a delay less than 56 ms between the onset of systolic motion between RV free wall basal segment versus the most delayed basal LV segment measured by TDI.[45,46]

Interventricular dyssynchrony has been evaluated by several different echocardiographic techniques. Conventional echocardiographic parameters have been abandoned because they are nonapplicable in patients with previous myocardial infarction.[47] The main tissue velocity imaging (TDI) dyssynchrony parameters are represented by the *standard deviation (SD) of time-to-peak myocardial systolic velocities* from 12 LV segments and the *basal septal-to-lateral delay*,[48] expressed as the difference between the time-to-peak myocardial systolic velocities of the basal septum and the lateral wall. However, TDI is affected by a major limitation given by its angle dependency. This limitation has been overcome by 2D speckle-tracking echocardiography (2D-STE), which could evaluate myocardial mechanisms in multidimensional fashion (longitudinal, radial, and circumferential strain). Moreover, deformation imaging can distinguish between active contraction and passive motion due to tethering of adjacent myocardial regions. Circumferential strain by 2D-STE proved to be the best strain analysis in predicting CRT response in terms of LVRR,[49] whereas global longitudinal strain by 2D-STE is a powerful predictor of response to CRT. Moreover, a peculiar LV rotational mechanics, consisting in a significant rotational delay between the anteroseptal and the posterior apical segments, showed to be an independent predictor of LVRR by CRT at 6-month follow-up.[50]

However, the measure of mechanical dyssynchrony to aid in patient selection failed, as showed by the multicenter PROSPECT trial.[51] The PROSPECT study, a large prospective multicenter trial investigating the performance of the most promising conventional and advanced echocardiographic parameters against the classical ECG characteristics, could not demonstrate an additional value of these echocardiographic measures of dyssynchrony in predicting CRT response. It has been postulated that those poor results may be attributable to possible inadequate LV lead position (no data were reported about that), the complexity of dyssynchrony parameters evaluated, and the presence of significant interobserver variability. The same results were obtained in the EchoCRT study, a randomized controlled trial in which the STE was compared with QRS in mechanical dyssynchrony measurement.[9] Moreover, the EchoCRT studies showed that CRT increases mortality among patients with a reduced EF and mechanical dyssynchrony but a QRS duration less than 130 msec.[9] Other parameters, before, during, and after implantation, can be useful to improve the CRT response. In ischemic patients the presence of myocardial scar is the main reason of nonresponse,[52,53] and recent studies tried to describe new scores to assess it.[54,55]

However, novel parameters measuring mechanical dyssynchrony assessed by echocardiography are showing some promise. Subsequent evidence has shown that the septal flash, or its appearance/increase after infusion of low doses of dobutamine in CRT-candidate patients, is predictive of LVRR after CRT, as well as apical rocking.[56] Moreover, the apical rocking seems to be associated with both echocardiographic and clinical response to CRT, and the presence of both septal flash and apical rocking in CRT candidates is associated with increased long-term survival.[57] Risum and colleagues examined the role of potentially reversible strain patterns in the selection of CRT candidates. Typical LBBB longitudinal deformation pattern shows early shortening of basal or midventricular segments in the septal wall and early stretching in basal or midventricular segments in the lateral wall, early septal peak shortening, and lateral wall peak shortening after aortic valve closure. Delayed segments do not fully contribute to end-systolic function, resulting in increased LVESV. This phenomenon has been mainly observed in patients with QRS greater than or equal to 150 ms, and it was strongly associated with effective CRT response.[58] Instead, the absence of a typical LBBB longitudinal strain pattern seems to be correlated with a bad prognosis after CRT.[59] In the MUSIC study, the *strain delay index* (the difference between end-systolic strain, measured at aortic valve closure, and peak strain across LV segments) was significantly correlated with LVRR after CRT.[60]

Mechanical dyssynchrony may be also observed in patients with a narrow QRS. Yu and colleagues[61,62] assumed that QRS length was not indispensable for indicating CRT. Nevertheless, as stated, the Echo-CRT trial shows that in patients with HFrEF and a QRS less than 130 ms, CRT does not reduce death and hospitalization rate and may increase mortality.[9] Furthermore, CRT may be useful in patients with intermediate QRS duration (120–149 ms) and echo-assessed mechanical dyssynchrony. However, mechanical dyssynchrony in patients with HFrEF without electrical dyssynchrony seems to be primarily related to changes in LV regional function and loading conditions and does not represent an appropriate target for CRT. Real-time 3D (RT3D) echocardiography seems to be a promising new tool in this setting. A recent evidence found a correlation between RT3D findings and LVRR: a *systolic dyssynchrony index* greater than or equal to 5.6% was indeed predictive for acute response to CRT.[63] 3D speckle tracking imaging is a recently investigated approach in providing simultaneous strain and volume measurements: global and segmental myocardial efficiency is reduced in dyssynchronous LV because systolic myocardial shortening, as well as diastolic lengthening, does not synchronize with chamber volume changes. Analysis of strain–volume loops may provide more accurate measurements for predicting CRT efficacy.[64]

More recently, some studies have explored the role of novel myocardial work estimated by pressure-strain loops (PSLs) analysis in predicting cardiac outcome of patients with HF undergoing CRT. Galli and colleagues[65] showed in a retrospective study that reduction in constructive work (CW), assessed by PSLs, was the only independent predictor of mortality at 6-month follow-up of 166 CRT-candidates implanted with classical recommendations. Moreover, the addition of CW to a model including age, coronary artery disease, SF, and CRT response determined a powerful increase in model power prediction of cardiac death.

Role of cardiac magnetic resonance

In the recent years cardiac magnetic resonance (CMR) became a gold standard in cardiac imaging, with late gadolinuim enhancement (LGE) giving information on tissue characterization. This plays an important role in clinical evaluation to CRT indications; in fact LGE can provide information on etiopathogenesis and possible management of ventricular arrhythmias and sudden cardiac death. Moreover, CMR with LGE promises to improve the response rate, improving, in the first step, the selection of candidates. Recent literature supports the prognostic value of CMR scar to predict arrhythmia-free survival. Not only the extension of scar and its mass but also other features such as heterogeneity of myocardial tissue around the scar (ie, prevalence of border zone over dense scar) are important; these aspects have the power to predict ventricular arrhythmias.[66] In 2018, the GAUDI-CRT study, published by Acosta and colleagues,[67] described the role of CMR scar in CRT-P or CRT-D indications. In the period of "tailored medicine" where we have highly sophisticated and costly device therapies (CRT) to cure our patients, CMR gives us a detailed assessment of myocardial fibrosis extension and heterogeneity, and they seem to be much more cost-effective. Moreover, CMR can give information not only on tissue characterization but also on cardiac contractility. McVeigh and colleagues[68] showed a linear relationship between circumferential shortening and electrical activation time and the ability to detect late-activating regions, using paced canines and myocardial tagging. This CMR sequence is not easy for a long time to acquisition as for analyzing the tagged images. A new sequence based on myocardial strain imaging is the cine displacement encoding with stimulated echoes (DENSE) that codify tissue displacement into the phase of the MRI signal; this method can do a rapid strain analysis but preserve accuracy and reproducibility equivalent to myocardial tagging. In the first phase cine DENSE has been validated, in canines, for quantification of mechanical dyssynchrony and later cine DENSE quantified mechanical dyssynchrony in patients with HF, shown to be predictive of CRT response. Using cine DENSE, the presence of delayed activation at the CRT LV pacing site is strongly associated to CRT response.[69]

CMR can be helpful also in follow-up of patients who receive CRT; in fact the new model was MRI conditional, and the same sequences used to select patients can be used to evaluated CRT response.

Role of nuclear imaging

Radionuclide imaging also represents an attractive option because of the comprehensive evaluation of LVEF and degree of myocardial scar, in addition to mechanical dyssynchrony. Abnormalities of resting perfusion have been associated with reduced improvement of functional and ventricular parameters after CRT.[70] Gated myocardial perfusion SPECT (GMPS) evaluates ventricular activation patterns by determining regional LV counts during the cardiac cycle. An increase in counts seems to correlate with regional LV wall thickening and may be used to assess the pattern of systolic contraction. Phase distribution maps may be generated. GMPS-assessed dyssynchrony correlated with response to CRT in a study conducted on 42 patients with severe LV dysfunction.[71]

Left Ventricular Lead Position

During implantation the location of the LV lead also can improve the response to therapy. The REVERSE study showed that a lateral LV lead position was associated with better outcomes, in comparison with other locations.[72] Moreover, data from the MADIT-CRT trial demonstrated that an LV lead location in basal or midventricular positions was superior to apical positions.[73] The recent development of LV leads with different diameters and shapes may facilitate the placement of the lead. The *quadripolar leads*, with 4 independent electrodes that allow the programming of additional vectors for LV pacing, reduces phrenic nerve stimulation, unstable lead position, or high-pacing threshold.[74,75] *Multipoint pacing*, creating a larger activation wavefront, is another new option to enhance resynchronization and CRT response, even if with a higher battery use. Several studies have shown an improved acute hemodynamic response of multipoint pacing compared with conventional one,[76,77] and a large prospective Italian registry suggests a greater improvement in clinical composite score and LVEF.[78] *Multisite pacing* is an alternative to multipoint. Using 2 bipolar LV leads in addition to the conventional RV apical and right atrial lead, different LV sites can be stimulated simultaneously. Small studies have suggested that multisite can increase CRT response[79] but was associated with a higher periprocedural complication rate.[80] The *His-bundle pacing* can overcome BBB-induced dyssynchrony.[81] In the last years, CRT using HBP (His-CRT) becomes widespread and has been described as a primary strategy to achieve CRT as first approach (before trying an LV lead) or as rescue strategy in patients in whom LV lead placement is unsuccessful. The data from observational studies suggest ventricular resynchronization with His-CRT is related to an improvement in clinical outcomes such as symptoms and LV contractile function[82] (**Table 2**).

Another point is the increasing interest in advanced multimodality imaging in identifying the optimal segment for LV pacing and in guiding LV catheter delivery. The current strategy is to place LV lead in the lateral or posterolateral branch of the coronary sinus. However, considerable evidence suggests that targeting optimal LV pacing sites may improve CRT response rate.

Table 2
Outcome of His-cardiac resynchronization therapy patients

Study	Study Population	Improvement in NYHA Class	Improvement in LVEF	Improvement in LV Dimension	Improvement in QRS Duration
Barba-Pichardo et al,[83] 2013	HBP in patients with failed LV leads	☑	☑	☑	
Lustgarten et al,[84] 2015	HBP and LV leads in all patients undergoing CRT		☑		
Ajijola et al,[85] 2017	HBP in patients with failed LV leads		☑	☑	
Sharma et al,[81] 2018	All-comers for CRT. Group 1: failed LV lead placement (rescue CRT); group 2: primary HBP	☑	☑		
Huang et al,[86] 2019	HBP in patients with LBBB and indication for CRT	☑	☑	☑	
Sharma et al,[87] 2018	HBP in patients with RBBB and indication for CRT: primary or rescue strategy	☑	☑		
Shan et al,[88] 2018	HBP for CRT in patients with chronic RV pacing		☑		☑
Vijayaraman et al,[89] 2019	HBP for CRT in patients with chronic RV pacing		☑		☑

Resynchronization may be optimally improved by LV pacing at the most delayed site, avoiding myocardial scar.[90] The TARGET (Targeted Left Ventricular Lead Placement to Guide Cardiac Resynchronization Therapy) study is the first randomized controlled study to demonstrate the benefit of a targeted approach to LV lead placement in CRT. LV lead targeting using speckle-tracking radial strain imaging demonstrated superiority versus nontargeted approach to achieve the primary endpoint of LVESV reduction.[91] The STARTER trial confirmed these data.[92] Bertini and colleagues support the superiority of combined use of MRI and longitudinal strain in identifying target area: CMR recognizes transmural scar and also identifies subepicardial fibrosis, which cannot be detected by 2D-STE radial strain. Stimulation of subepicardial scar tissue could be mechanically ineffective and also potentially proarrhythmogenic. Also, longitudinal strain assessment offers several advantages over the radial strain; especially it allows a comprehensive assessment of the left ventricle and not only of the midventricle portion.[93] Salden and colleagues recently performed an elegant study to evaluate the feasibility of intraprocedural visualization of optimal pacing sites and image-guided LV lead placement. It foresaw 4 steps. During steps from 1 to 3, scars, delayed mechanical activation, left phrenic nerve (LPN), and coronary sinus ostium were identified on a preprocedural CMR and computed tomography scan. Accordingly, the target area for LV lead delivery was chosen. In a target group, all tissue characteristics were displayed in conjunction with live fluoroscopy during LV lead implantation, enabling the implanting cardiologist to perform image-guided LV lead placement. Thus, in the target group, real-time image-guided LV lead placement was successfully executed. LV leads were positioned closer than in patients without real-time image-guided lead placement, away from scarred myocardium and the LPN, without consuming time. Target group patients gained marked LVRR at 6-month follow-up with a mean LVESV change of $-30 \pm 10\%$ and a mean LVEF improvement of $15 \pm 5\%$.[94] Optimal LV pacing site is not the same for all patients, and it seems necessary to adapt LV lead placement to individual morphofunctional features.

Stolfo and colleagues analyzed early hemodynamic effects of CRT in the immediate postimplantation in patients with dilated cardiomyopathy and mitral regurgitation. They identified a positive correlation between early hemodynamic changes (RV function and systolic pulmonary artery pressure, consequences of decrease filling pressures, improved biventricular interaction, contractile efficiency) and late stable mitral regurgitation reduction. Besides, it might be helpful to early identify nonresponders to CRT that may undergo other invasive strategies for the mitral regurgitation correction.[95]

Device Optimization

The issue of device optimization is very debated: current literature suggests that routine AV and VV delay optimization has no effect on CRT outcomes,[96] but it is well known that suboptimal programming of the *AV and/or VV delays* may limit the response to CRT. It is recommended to correct suboptimal device settings. Early CRT devices simply allowed AV delay programming, whereas modern systems allow programming of both the individual AV and VV intervals. In the last years we observed an increase of complexity of CRT programming due to additional variables and algorithms (such as rate-adaptive AV and AV delay modulation). Despite these limitations, AV and VV optimization are a useful tool to improve the response to CRT.

However, several studies of LV lead placement in areas of late electrical or mechanical delay have shown the importance of lead position on CRT clinical outcomes.[92,97,98] In particular, it has been shown that LV pacing at sites of late electrical activation, as assessed by interventricular (RV-LV) electrical delay, is associated with improved CRT response in terms of reverse remodeling, HF hospitalization, and death.[99,100] These results support a strategy of evaluating interventricular electrical delay at the time of LV lead implantation and consider repositioning or, in the case of a quadripolar lead, using a different site/electrode to achieve an RV-LV interval greater than 67 ms. Arbelo and colleagues[101] described a simple and new method to optimize AV and VV intervals in CRT, based on obtaining the narrowest QRS using fusion with intrinsic conduction (*fusion-optimized intervals* [FOI]) to create 3 activation fronts instead of 2 during pure biventricular pacing. One recent study demonstrates that device optimization based on FOI achieves greater LV remodeling, compared with nominal settings.[102] A key issue, well described also in Guidelines, is to achieve *biventricular stimulation* as close to 100% as possible. Several studies have shown that biventricular stimulation between 92% and 98% is associated with decreased mortality and HF hospitalization.[103,104] The most common cause of loss of biventricular pacing is inadequate AV delay programming or the presence of arrhythmias. In case of AF, AV junctional ablation should strongly be considered.

Despite all modern techniques and technologies, we do not forget to consider our patients with an holistic approach: an adequate *pharmacologic therapy* associate with a counseling for a tailored *physical activity* is necessary to achieve the best effects of CRT.

SUMMARY

CRT is a fundamental tool in our fight against HF. However, the last European guidelines for CRT implantation gave very stringent indication, as they require low LVEF, symptomatic patients, and the presence of significant electrical dyssynchrony on ECG (LBBB and wide QRS). This has been driven prevalently by MADIT-CRT results, which identified these parameters as powerful predictors to CRT response. However, as stated, a significant portion of CRT candidates do not experience the expected results from this invasive and expensive procedure. Moreover, the rate of nonresponders is not significantly changed from the previous guideline to the last updated despite a more rigorous selection criterion. Nonetheless, the extensive research done in the last years and presented in this review, based on an accurate analysis of patients and available technologies, seems promising to further improve patient benefit from CRT.

AUTHOR CONTRIBUTIONS

Conceptualization, Resources, and Writing—Original Draft Preparation, G. Palmiero; V. Russo, M.T. Florio, M. Rubino; Writing—Review & Editing, G. Palmiero & V. Russo; Supervision, G. Palmiero & V. Russo.

CONFLICTS OF INTERESTS

The authors declare no conflicts of interest.

REFERENCES

1. Kashani A, Barold SS. Significance of QRS complex duration in patients with heart failure. J Am Coll Cardiol 2005;46:2183–92.
2. Abraham WT, Fisher WG, Smith AL, et al. Cardiac resynchronization in chronic heart failure. N Engl J Med 2002;346(24):1845–53.
3. Cleland JG, Daubert JC, Erdmann E, et al. The effect of cardiac resynchronization on morbidity and mortality in heart failure. N Engl J Med 2005; 352(15):1539–49.
4. Moss AJ, Hall WJ, Cannom DS, et al. Cardiac-resynchronization therapy for the prevention of heart-failure events. N Engl J Med 2009;361(14): 1329–38.
5. Tang AS, Wells GA, Talajic M, et al. Cardiac-resynchronization therapy for mild-to-moderate heart failure. N Engl J Med 2010;363(25):2385–95.
6. Daubert C, Behar N, Martins RP, et al. Avoiding non-responders to cardiac resynchronization therapy: a practical guide. Eur Heart J 2017;38: 1463–72.
7. Ponikowski P, Voors AA, Anker SD, et al. 2016 ESC Guidelines for the diagnosis and treatment of acute and chronic heart failure: the task force for the diagnosis and treatment of acute and chronic heart failure of the European Society of Cardiology (ESC). Developed with the special contribution of the Heart Failure Association (HFA) of the ESC. Eur J Heart Fail 2016;18:891–975.
8. Brignole M, Auricchio A, Baron-Esquivias G, et al. 2013 ESC Guidelines on cardiac pacing and cardiac resynchronization therapy: the Task Force on cardiac pacing and resynchronization therapy of the European Society of Cardiology (ESC). Developed in collaboration with the European Heart Rhythm Association (EHRA). Eur Heart J 2013; 34(29):2281–329.
9. Ruschitzka F, Abraham WT, Singh JP, et al, EchoCRT Study Group. Cardiac-resynchronization therapy in heart failure with a narrow QRS complex. N Engl J Med 2013;369(15):1395–405.
10. Smiseth OA, Russell K, Skulstad H. The role of echocardiography in quantification of left ventricular dyssynchrony: state of the art and future directions. Eur Heart J Cardiovasc Imaging 2012;13(1): 61–8.
11. van Bommel RJ, Tanaka H, Delgado V, et al. Association of intraventricular mechanical dyssynchrony with response to cardiac resynchronization therapy in heart failure patients with a narrow QRS complex. Eur Heart J 2010;31(24):3054–62.
12. Delgado V, Tops LF, Trines SA, et al. Acute effects of right ventricular apical pacing on left ventricular synchrony and mechanics. Circ Arrhythm Electrophysiol 2009;2:135–45.
13. Sweeney MO, Hellkamp AS, Ellenbogen KA, et al. Adverse effect of ventricular pacing on heart failure and atrial fibrillation among patients with normal baseline QRS duration in a clinical trial of pacemaker therapy for sinus node dysfunction. Circulation 2003;107:2932–7.
14. Blanc JJ. BIOPACE (Biventricular pacing for atrIo-ventricular BlOck to Prevent cArdiaC dE-synchronization) Trial Preliminary Results. Presented at the 2014 Annual Meeting of the European Society of Cardiology (Hotline Session), Barcelona, September 1, 2014.
15. Wilton SB, Leung AA, Ghali WA, et al. Outcomes of cardiac resynchronization therapy in patients with versus those without atrial fibrillation: a systematic review and meta-analysis. Heart Rhythm 2011;8: 1088–94.
16. Maron BJ, Spirito P. Implications of left ventricular remodeling in hypertrophic cardiomyopathy. Am J Cardiol 1998;81:1339–44.
17. Ashrafian H, Mason MJ, Mitchell AG. Regression of dilated-hypokinetic hypertrophic cardiomyopathy by biventricular cardiac pacing. Europace 2007; 9:50–4.
18. Pezzulich B, Montagna L, Lucchina PG. Successful treatment of end-stage hypertrophic cardiomyopathy with biventricular cardiac pacing. Europace 2005;7:388–91.
19. Rinaldi CA, Bucknall CA, Gill JS. Beneficial effects of biventricular pacing in a patient with hypertrophic cardiomyopathy and intraventricular conduction delay. Heart 2002;87:e6.
20. Rogers DP, Marazia S, Chow AW, et al. Effect of biventricular pacing on symptoms and cardiac remodelling in patients with end-stage hypertrophic cardiomyopathy. Eur J Heart Fail 2008;10:507–13.
21. Lenarczyk R, Wozniak A, Kowalski O, et al. Effect of cardiac resynchronization on gradient reduction in patients with obstructive hypertrophic cardiomyopathy: preliminary study. Pacing Clin Electrophysiol 2011;34:1544–52.
22. Rinaldi CA, Kirubakaran S, Bucknall CA, et al. Initial experience of a cohort of patients with hypertrophic cardiomyopathy undergoing biventricular pacing. Indian Pacing Electrophysiol J 2011;11: 5–14.
23. Palladino A, Papa AA, Morra S, et al. Are there real benefits to implanting cardiac devices in patients with end-stage dilated dystrophinopathic cardiomyopathy? Review of literature and personal results. Acta Myol 2019;38(1):1–7.
24. Russo V, Papa AA, Williams EA, et al. ACE inhibition to slow progression of myocardial fibrosis in muscular dystrophies. Trends Cardiovasc Med 2018;28(5):330–7.
25. Russo V, Sperlongano S, Gallinoro E, et al. Prevalence of Left Ventricular Systolic Dysfunction in

Myotonic Dystrophy Type 1: A Systematic Review. J Card Fail 2020;26:849–56.

26. Feingold B, Mahle WT, Auerbach S, et al, American Heart Association Pediatric Heart Failure Committee of the Council on Cardiovascular Disease in the Young, Council on Clinical Cardiology, Council on Cardiovascular Radiology and Intervention, Council on Functional Genomics and Translational Biology, Stroke Council. Management of Cardiac Involvement Associated With Neuromuscular Diseases: A Scientific Statement From the American Heart Association. Circulation 2017;136(13): e200–31.
27. Fayssoil A, Nardi O, Annane D, et al. Successful cardiac resynchronization therapy in Duchenne muscular dystrophy: a 5-year follow-up. Presse Med 2014;43:330–1.
28. Andrikopoulos G, Kourouklis S, Trika C, et al. Cardiac resynchronization therapy in Becker muscular dystrophy. Hellenic J Cardiol 2013;54:227–9.
29. Russo V, Rago A, Papa AA, et al. Cardiac resynchronization improves heart failure in one patient with myotonic dystrophy type 1. A case report. Acta Myol 2012;31(2):154–5.
30. Russo V, Rago A, D'Andrea A, et al. Early onset "electrical" heart failure in myotonic dystrophy type 1 patient: the role of ICD biventricular pacing. Anadolu Kardiyol Derg 2012;12:517–9.
31. Penn J, Goldenberg I, Moss AJ, et al. MADIT-CRT Trial investigators. Improved outcome with preventive cardiac resynchronization therapy in the elderly: a MADIT-CRT substudy. J Cardiovasc Electrophysiol 2011;22(8):892–7.
32. Christie S, Hiebert B, Seifer CM, et al. Clinical outcomes of cardiac resynchronization therapy with and without a defibrillator in elderly patients with heart failure. J Arrhythm 2018;35(1):61–9.
33. Killu AM, Wu JH, Friedman PA, et al. Outcomes of cardiac resynchronization therapy in the elderly. Pacing Clin Electrophysiol 2013;36(6):664–72.
34. Martens P, Verbrugge FH, Nijst P, et al. Mode of death in octogenarians treated with cardiac resynchronization therapy. J Card Fail 2016;22: 970–7.
35. Martinez-Naharro A, Hawkins PN, Fontana M. Cardiac amyloidosis. Clin Med (Lond) 2018;18(Suppl 2):s30–5.
36. Seferović PM, Polovina M, Bauersachs J, et al. Heart failure in cardiomyopathies: a position paper from the Heart Failure Association of the European Society of Cardiology. Eur J Heart Fail 2019;21(5): 553–76.
37. Donnellan E, Wazni OM, Hanna M, et al. Cardiac Resynchronization Therapy for Transthyretin Cardiac Amyloidosis. J Am Heart Assoc 2020;9(14): e017335.
38. Slotwiner D, Varma N, Akar JG, et al. HRS Expert Consensus Statement on remote interrogation and monitoring for cardiovascular implantable electronic devices. Heart Rhythm 2015;12(7): e69–100.
39. Hindricks G, Varma N, Kacet S, et al. Daily remote monitoring of implantable cardioverter-defibrillators: insights from the pooled patient-level data from three randomized controlled trials (IN-TIME, ECOST, TRUST). Eur Heart J 2017; 38(22):1749–55.
40. Mullens W, Grimm RA, Verga T, et al. Insights from a cardiac resynchronization optimization clinic as part of a heart failure disease management program. J Am Coll Cardiol 2009;53:765–73.
41. Menet A, Guyomar Y, Ennezat PV, et al. Prognostic value of left ventricular reverse remodeling and performance improvement after cardiac resynchronization therapy: A prospective study. Int J Cardiol 2016;204:6–11.
42. Emerek K, Friedman DJ, Sørensen PL, et al. Vectorcardiographic QRS area is associated with long-term outcome after cardiac resynchronization therapy. Heart Rhythm 2019;16(2):213–9.
43. Sieniewicz BJ, Jackson T, Claridge S, et al. Optimization of CRT programming using non-invasive electrocardiographic imaging to assess the acute electrical effects of multipoint pacing. J Arrhythm 2019;35(2):267–75.
44. Cazeau S, Bordacher P, Jauvert G, et al. Echocardiographic modeling of cardiac dyssynchrony before and during multisite stimulation; a prospective study. Pacing Clin Electrophysiol 2003;26: 137–43.
45. Cleland JG, Daubert JC, Erdmann E, et al. CARE-HF study Steering Committee and Investigators. The CARE-HF study (CArdiac REsynchronization in Heart Failure study): rational, design and endpints. Eur J Heart Fail 2001;3(4):481–9.
46. Penicka M, Bartunek J, De Bruyne B, et al. Improvement of left ventricular function after cardiac resynchronization therapy is predicted by tissue Doppler imaging echocardiography. Circulation 2004;109(8):978–83.
47. Pitzalis MV, Iacoviello M, Romito R, et al. Cardiac resynchronization therapy tailored by echocardiographic evaluation of ventricular asynchrony. J Am Coll Cardiol 2002;40(9):1615–22.
48. Mele D, Toselli T, Capasso F, et al. Comparison of myocardial deformation and velocity dyssynchrony for identification of responders to cardiac resynchronization therapy. Eur J Heart Fail 2009;11(4): 391–9.
49. Knebel F, Schattke S, Bondke H, et al. Circumferential 2D-strain imaging for the prediction of long term response to cardiac resynchronization therapy. Cardiovasc Ultrasound 2008;6:28.

50. Sade LE, Demir O, Atar I, et al. Effect of mechanical dyssynchrony and cardiac resynchronization therapy on left ventricular rotational mechanics. Am J Cardiol 2008;101(8):1163–9.
51. Chung ES, Leon AR, Tavazzi L, et al. Results of the Predictors of Response to CRT (PROSPECT) trial. Circulation 2008;117(20):2608–16.
52. Ypenburg C, Schalij MJ, Bleeker GB, et al. Impact of viability and scar tissue on response to cardiac resynchronization therapy in ischaemic heart failure patients. Eur Heart J 2007;28(1):33–41.
53. Adelstein EC, Saba S. Scar burden by myocardial perfusion imaging predicts echocardiographic response to cardiac resynchronization therapy in ischemic cardiomyopathy. Am Heart J 2007; 153(1):105–12.
54. Bani R, Checchi L, Cartei S, et al. Simplified Selvester Score: a practical electrocardiographic instrument to predict response to CRT. J Electrocardiol 2015;48(1):62–8.
55. Nesti M, Paoletti Perini A, Bani R, et al. Myocardial Scar on Surface ECG: Selvester Score, but Not Fragmentation, Predicts Response to CRT. Cardiol Res Pract 2020;2020:9. Article ID 2036545.
56. Stankovic I, Prinz C, Ciarka A, et al. Relationship of visually assessed apical rocking and septal flash to response and long-term survival following cardiac resynchronization therapy (PREDICT-CRT). Eur Heart J Cardiovasc Imaging 2016;17(3):262–9.
57. Ghani A, Delnoy PP, Ottervanger JP, et al. Apical rocking is predictive of response to cardiac resynchronization therapy. Int J Cardiovasc Imaging 2015;31(4):717–25.
58. Risum N, Jons C, Olsen NT, et al. Simple regional strain pattern analysis to predict response to cardiac resynchronization therapy: rationale, initial results, and advantages. Am Heart J 2012;163(4): 697–704.
59. Marechaux S, Menet A, Guyomar Y, et al. Role of echocardiography before cardiac resynchronization therapy: new advances and current developments. Echocardiography 2016;33(11):1745–52.
60. Lim P, Donal E, Lafitte S, et al. Multicentre study using strain delay index for predicting response to cardiac resynchronization therapy (MUSIC study). Eur J Heart Fail 2011;13(9):984–91.
61. Yu CM, Lin H, Zhang Q, et al. High prevalence of left ventricular systolic and diastolic asynchrony in patients with congestive heart failure and normal QRS duration. Heart 2003;89(1):54–60.
62. Yu CM, Hayes DL. Cardiac resynchronization therapy: state of the art 2013. Eur Heart J 2013;34(19): 1396–403.
63. Zhu M, Chen H, Fulati Z, et al. The value of left ventricular strain-volume loops in predicting response to cardiac resynchronization therapy. Cardiovasc Ultrasound 2019;17(1):3.
64. Heydari B, Jerosch-Herold M, Kwong RY. Imaging for planning of cardiac resynchronization therapy. JACC Cardiovasc Imaging 2012;5(1):93–110.
65. Galli E, Hubert A, Le Rolle V, et al. Myocardial constructive work and cardiac mortality in resynchronization therapy candidates. Am Heart J 2019; 212:53–63.
66. Jablonowski R, Chaudhry U, van der Pals J, et al. Cardiovascular magnetic resonance to predict appropriate implantable cardioverter defibrillator therapy in ischemic and nonischemic cardiomyopathy patients using late gadolinium enhancement border zone: Comparison of four analysis methods. Circ Cardiovasc Imaging 2017;10:e006105.
67. Acosta J, Fernandez-Armenta J, Borra R, et al. Scar characterization to predict life-threatening arrhythmic events and sudden cardiac death in patients with cardiac resynchronization therapy. The GAUDI-CRT Study. J Am Coll Cardiol Cardiovasc Imaging 2018;11:561–72.
68. Wyman BT, Hunter WC, Prinzen FW, et al. Mapping propagation of mechanical activation in the paced heart with MRI tagging. Am J Physiol Heart Circ Physiol 1999;276:H881–91.
69. Auger DA, Bilchick KC, Gonzalez JA, et al. Imaging Left-Ventricular Mechanical Activation in Heart Failure Patients Using Cine DENSE MRI: Validation and Implications for Cardiac Resynchronization Therapy. J Magn Reson Imaging 2017;46:887–96.
70. Sciagrà R, Giaccardi M, Porciani MC, et al. Myocardial perfusion imaging using gated SPECT in heart failure patients undergoing cardiac resynchronization therapy. J Nucl Med 2004;45(2): 164–8.
71. Henneman MM, Chen J, Dibbets-Schneider P, et al. Can LV dyssynchrony as assessed with phase analysis on gated myocardial perfusion SPECT predict response to CRT? J Nucl Med 2007;48(7):1104–11.
72. Thebault C, Donal E, Meunier GR, et al, REVERSE Study Group. Sites of left and right ventricular lead implantation and response to cardiac resynchronization therapy observations from the REVERSE trial. Eur Heart J 2012;33:2662–71.
73. Singh JP, KleinHU, Huang DT Reek S, et al. Left ventricular lead position and clinical outcome in the multicenter automatic defibrillator implantation trial-cardiac resynchronization therapy (MADIT-CRT) trial. Circulation 2011;123:1159–66.
74. Dauw J, Martens P, Mullens W. CRT Optimization: What Is New? What Is Necessary? Curr Treat Options Cardiovasc Med 2019;21(9):45.
75. Turakhia MP, Cao M, Fischer A, et al. Reduced mortality associated with quadripolar compared to bipolar left ventricular leads in cardiac resynchronization therapy. JACC Clin Electrophysiol 2016;2(4):426–33.

76. Thibault B, Dubuc M, Khairy P, et al. Acute haemodynamic comparison of multisite and biventricular pacing with a quadripolar left ventricular lead. Europace 2013;15(7):984–91.
77. Rinaldi CA, Kranig W, Leclercq C, et al. Acute effects of multisite left ventricular pacing on mechanical dyssynchrony in patients receiving cardiac resynchronization therapy. J Card Fail 2013; 19(11):731–8.
78. Forleo GB, Santini L, Giammaria M, et al. Multipoint pacing via a quadripolar left-ventricular lead: preliminary results 51. from the Italian registry on multipoint left-ventricular pacing in cardiac resynchronization therapy (IRON-MPP). Europace 2017;19(7):1170–7.
79. Lenarczyk R, Kowalski O, Kukulski T, et al. Triple-site biventricular pacing in patients undergoing cardiac resynchronization therapy: a feasibility study. Europace 2007;9(9):762–7.
80. Bordachar P, Gras D, Clementy N, et al. Clinical impact of an additional left ventricular lead in cardiac resynchronization therapy nonresponders: the V(3) trial. Heart Rhythm 2018;15(6):870–6.
81. Sharma PS, Dandamudi G, Herweg B, et al. Permanent His-bundle pacing as an alternative to biventricular pacing for cardiac resynchronization therapy: a multicenter experience. Heart Rhythm 2018;15:413–20.
82. Ali N, Shin MS, Whinnett Z. The Emerging Role of Cardiac Conduction System Pacing as a Treatment for Heart Failure. Curr Heart Fail Rep 2020;17(5): 288–98.
83. Barba-Pichardo R, Manovel Sánchez A, Fernández-Gómez JM, et al. Ventricular resynchronization therapy by direct His-bundle pacing using an internal cardioverter defibrillator. Europace 2013;15: 83–8.
84. Lustgarten DL, Crespo EM, Arkhipova-Jenkins I, et al. His-bundle pacing versus biventricular pacing in cardiac resynchronization therapy patients: a crossover design comparison. Heart Rhythm 2015;12:1548–57.
85. Ajijola OA, Upadhyay GA, Macias C, et al. Permanent His-bundle pacing for cardiac resynchronization therapy: initial feasibility study in lieu of left ventricular lead. Heart Rhythm 2017;14:1353–61.
86. Huang W, Su L, Wu S, et al. Long-term outcomes of His bundle pacing in patients with heart failure with left bundle branch block. Heart 2019;105:137–43.
87. Sharma PS, Naperkowski A, Bauch TD, et al. Permanent His bundle pacingfor cardiac resynchronization therapy in patients with heart failure and right bundle branch block. Circ Arrhythm Electrophysiol 2018;11:e006613.
88. Shan P, Su L, Zhou X, et al. Beneficial effects of upgrading to His bundle pacing in chronically paced patients with left ventricular ejection fraction <50. Heart Rhythm 2018;15:405–12.
89. Vijayaraman P, Herweg B, Dandamudi G, et al. Outcomes of His bundle pacing upgrade after long-term right ventricular pacing and/or pacing-induced cardiomyopathy: insights into disease progression. Heart Rhythm 2019. https://doi.org/10.1016/j.hrthm.2019.03.026.
90. Derval N, Steendijk P, Gula LJ, et al. Optimizing hemodynamics in heart failure patients by systematic screening of left ventricular pacing sites: the lateral left ventricular wall and the coronary sinus are rarely the best sites. J Am Coll Cardiol 2010; 55(6):566–75.
91. Khan FZ, Virdee MS, Palmer CR, et al. Targeted left ventricular lead placement to guide cardiac resynchronization therapy: the TARGET study: a randomized, controlled trial. J Am Coll Cardiol 2012; 59(17):1509–18.
92. Saba S, Marek J, Schwartzman D, et al. Echocardiography-guided left ventricular lead placement for cardiac resynchronization therapy: results of the Speckle Tracking Assisted Resynchronization Therapy for Electrode Region trial. Circ Heart Fail 2013; 6(3):427–34.
93. Bertini M, Mele D, Malagù M, et al. Cardiac resynchronization therapy guided by multimodality cardiac imaging. Eur J Heart Fail 2016;18(11): 1375–82.
94. Salden OAE, van den Broek HT, van Everdingen WM, et al. Multimodality imaging for real-time image-guided left ventricular lead placement during cardiac resynchronization therapy implantations. Int J Cardiovasc Imaging 2019;35(7): 1327–37.
95. Stolfo D, Tonet E, Barbati G, et al. Acute Hemodynamic Response to Cardiac Resynchronization in Dilated Cardiomyopathy: Effect on Late Mitral Regurgitation. Pacing Clin Electrophysiol 2015; 38(11):1287–96.
96. Auger D, Hoke U, Bax JJ, et al. Effect of atrioventricular and ventriculoventricular delay optimization on clinical and echocardiographic outcomes of patients treated with cardiac resynchronization therapy: a meta-analysis. Am Heart J 2013;166(1): 20–9.
97. Gold MR, Singh JP, Ellenbogen KA, et al. Interventricular electrical delay is predictive of response to cardiac resynchronization therapy. JACC Clin Electrophysiol 2016;2:438–47.
98. D'Onofrio A, Botto G, Mantica M, et al. The interventricular conduction time is associated with response to cardiac resynchronization therapy: Interventricular electrical delay. Int J Cardiol 2013; 168:5067–8.
99. D'Onofrio A, Botto G, Mantica M, et al. Incremental value of larger interventricular conduction time in

improving cardiac resynchronization therapy outcome in patients with different QRS duration. J Cardiovasc Electrophysiol 2014;25:500–6.

100. Gold MR, Yu Y, Wold N, et al. The role of interventricular conduction delay to predict clinical response with cardiac resynchronization therapy. Heart Rhythm 2017;14:1748–55.

101. Arbelo E, Tolosana JM, Trucco E, et al. Fusion-optimized intervals (FOI): A new method to achieve the narrowest QRS for optimization of the AV and VV intervals in patients undergoing cardiac resynchronization therapy. J Cardiovas Elctrophysiol 2014;25: 283–92.

102. Trucco E, Tolosana JM, Arbelo E, et al. Improvement of Reverse Remodeling Using Electrocardiogram Fusion-Optimized Intervals in Cardiac Resynchronization Therapy: A Randomized Study. JACC Clin Electrophysiol 2018;4(2):181–9.

103. Hayes DL, Boehmer JP, Day JD, et al. Cardiac resynchronization therapy and the relationship of per- cent biventricular pacing to symptoms and survival. Heart Rhythm 2011;8(9):1469–75.

104. Koplan BA, Kaplan AJ, Weiner S, et al. Heart failure decompensation and all- cause mortality in relation to percent biventricular pacing in patients with heart failure: is a goal of 100% biventricular pacing necessary? J Am Coll Cardiol 2009;53(4):355–60.

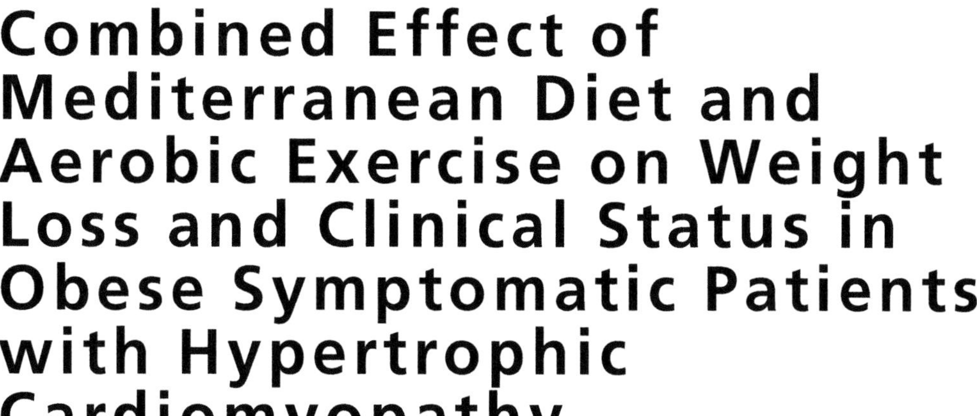

Combined Effect of Mediterranean Diet and Aerobic Exercise on Weight Loss and Clinical Status in Obese Symptomatic Patients with Hypertrophic Cardiomyopathy

Giuseppe Limongelli, MD, PhD, FESC[a,b,*,1], Emanuele Monda, MD[a,1], Antonello D'Aponte, MD[c], Martina Caiazza, MD[a], Marta Rubino, MD[a], Augusto Esposito, MD[a], Giuseppe Palmiero, MD[a], Elisabetta Moscarella, MD[a], Giovanni Messina, MD, PhD[c], Paolo Calabro', MD, PhD[a], Olga Scudiero, MD, PhD[d,e,f], Giuseppe Pacileo, MD[a], Marcellino Monda, MD, PhD[c], Eduardo Bossone, MD, PhD, FCCP, FESC, FACC[g], Sharlene M. Day, MD, PhD[h,2], Iacopo Olivotto, MD, PhD[i,2]

KEYWORDS

• Hypertrophic cardiomyopathy • Obesity • Mediterranean diet • Aerobic exercise

KEY POINTS

- Weight loss by a combined protocol of Mediterranean diet and aerobic exercise is associated with clinical-hemodynamic improvement in obese symptomatic Patients with HCM.
- 25% of patients were considered responders (weight loss $\geq$10%) and in those patients clinical-hemodynamic improvement was particularly evident.
- Body mass index changes from baseline correlated with reduction in left atrial diameter, left atrial volume index, E/E'average, pulmonary artery systolic pressure, and increase of $V_{O_{2max}}$ and peak workload.

[a] Department of Translational Medical Sciences, University of Campania "Luigi Vanvitelli", Via L. Bianchi, 80131 Naples, Italy; [b] Institute of Cardiovascular Sciences, University College of London and St. Bartholomew's Hospital, Grower Street, London WC1E 6DD, UK; [c] Department of Experimental Medicine, Section of Human Physiology and Unit of Dietetics and Sports Medicine, University of Campania "Luigi Vanvitelli", Via Santa Maria di Costantinopoli, 80138 Naples, Italy; [d] Department of Molecular Medicine and Medical Biotechnology, University of Naples "Federico II", Via G. Salvatore, 80138 Naples, Italy; [e] CEINGE Advanced Biotechnologies, Via G. Salvatore, 80138 Naples, Italy; [f] Task Force on Microbiome Studies, University of Naples "Federico II", Via G. Salvatore, 80138 Naples, Italy; [g] Division of Cardiology, Antonio Cardarelli Hospital, Via A. Cardarelli, 80131 Naples, Italy; [h] Department of Internal Medicine, University of Michigan, 500 S. State Street, Ann Arbor, MI 48109, USA; [i] Cardiomyopathy Unit and Genetic Unit, Careggi University Hospital, Largo Brambrilla, 50134 Florence, Italy

[1] These authors shared the first name.

[2] These authors shared the last name.

* Corresponding author. Inherited and Rare Cardiovascular Diseases, Department of Translational Medical Sciences, University of Campania "Luigi Vanvitelli", AO Colli - Monaldi Hospital - ERN Guard Heart Member, Naples 80131, Italy.

E-mail address: limongelligiuseppe@libero.it

Heart Failure Clin 17 (2021) 303–313
https://doi.org/10.1016/j.hfc.2021.01.003

INTRODUCTION

Hypertrophic cardiomyopathy (HCM) is a disease of the heart muscle characterized by an unexplained left ventricular wall thickness, not solely explained by abnormal loading conditions.[1–4] In more than half of cases the disease is inherited as an autosomal dominant genetic trait caused by mutations in genes encoding sarcomeric proteins.[1,2,5–7] Many patients with HCM remain asymptomatic most of their lives, although a considerable subset experience progressive symptoms (ie, dyspnea, angina) or syncope due to the complex disease pathophysiology (diastolic dysfunction, left ventricular outflow tract obstruction, hypokinetic-end stage evolution).[8–10]

Obesity is among the principal concomitant causes of dyspnea in patients with HCM, in whom it represents an important comorbidity.[11] Obesity is associated with reduced exercise tolerance and hence to sedentary lifestyle. Conversely, moderate-intensity exercise results in a significant increase in exercise capacity of patients with HCM at 16 weeks of follow-up, compared with usual activity.[12] Thus, a comprehensive nonpharmacological approach pursuing weight loss (WL) by a combined, standard protocol of aerobic exercise and appropriate dietary regime may have the potential to improve clinical profile in HCM.[13]

Therefore, we sought to investigate the impact of WL, on a Mediterranean diet and a mild-to-moderate–intensity aerobic exercise program, on clinical status of obese, symptomatic patients with HCM.

METHODS

Study Population

We studied 20 consecutive patients with HCM (45.3 $\pm$ 12.1 years of age; 65% men) with mass index (BMI) >30 kg/m^2. HCM was defined as unexplained ventricular wall thickness, not solely explained by abnormal loading conditions.[1] Patients with HCM associated with specific disease (ie, infiltrative or storage disease, genetic syndromes, metabolic and neuromuscular disorders)[14] were excluded.

Patients enrolled followed a common protocol designed by GL and EM (Monaldi Hospital, AORN Colli, University of Campania “Luigi Vanvitelli”) and AD, MM, and FML (Sport Medicine, University of Campania “Luigi Vanvitelli”). The Weight loSs and Exercise in Hypertrophic Cardiomyopathy (WISE-HCM) study protocol was approved, and written informed consent was obtained from each subject, according to the procedure established by the Ethic Committee of our institution.

Study Protocol

Patients enrolled underwent a basal evaluation, which consisted of a comprehensive cardiovascular assessment, including family and personal history, physical examination, blood tests, including N-terminal prohormone of brain natriuretic peptide (NT-proBNP) measurement, 12-lead electrocardiogram (ECG) at rest, conventional M-mode, 2-dimensional and Doppler echocardiography, 24-hour Holter ECG, treadmill or cardiopulmonary exercise testing (CPET), and cardiac magnetic resonance, following a previously described protocol.[15–17] All patients were offered participation in a dedicated program focused on WL. Specific dietary and physical activity training sessions were held by specialists (ADP) at the baseline visit and at 3-month intervals, using a tailored questionnaire to assess adherence to the protocol (**Table 1**).

Diet Protocol

All patients followed a Mediterranean diet, from dietary analysis software, prepared meals that contained 25% to 30% of calories from fat, 10% to 15% of calories from protein, and 50% to 60% of calories from primarily unrefined carbohydrate, high in dietary fiber.

In particular, patients were instructed to follow a diet composed of whole grains such as bread, pasta, and rice, olive oil (EVO), vegetables, fresh fruits, cereals, and 1 glass of milk every day; legumes for 2 days per week; white meat 2 days per week; fish and sea food for 3 days per week; 2 eggs for 1 day per week; 1 glass of red wine per day was recommended as the main source of alcohol. Furthermore, it was recommended to select white meats (poultry without skin) instead of red meats or processed meats; to limit consumption of red meat (remove all visible fat), cured ham, and chocolate to $\leq$1 serving per week; to use exclusively EVO for cooking and dressing vegetables and salad; and also, to eliminate or limit the consumption of cream, butter, margarine, carbonated and/or sugared beverages, pastries, commercial bakery products (cakes, donuts, cookies), desserts (puddings), French fries, potato crisps, sweets.

Exercise Protocol

All patients followed an aerobic exercise protocol. In the first 6 months of training protocol, it was recommended to accumulate at least 30 minutes of light physical activity during most days (4/5) of the week consisting of walking briskly (<3 METS). In a second part of physical activity protocol, for 18 months, the patients followed a moderate physical activity program consisting in 60 minutes

Table 1
Questionnaire of Adherence: Mediterranean diet and exercise training protocol

Adherence to diet protocol	Y/N/Other
(motivations)	
Use of olive oil (according to protocol)	Y/N/Other
(motivations)	
Use of vegetables (according to protocol)	Y/N/Other
(motivations)	
Use of fruits (according to protocol)	Y/N/Other
(motivations)	
Use of tomatoes (according to protocol)	Y/N/Other
(motivations)	
Use of cereals (according to protocol)	Y/N/Other
(motivations)	
Use of legumes (according to protocol)	Y/N/Other
(motivations)	
Use of white meat (according to protocol)	Y/N/Other
(motivations)	
Use of fish (according to protocol)	Y/N/Other
(motivations)	
Use of seafood (according to protocol)	Y/N/Other
(motivations)	
Use of red wine (according to protocol)	Y/N/Other
(motivations)	
Other	
(motivations)	
Adherence to exercise protocol	Y/N/Other
(motivations)	
Do you practice aerobic exercise?	Y/N/Other
(motivations)	
Have you practiced light physical exercise (<3METS) for the first 6 months?	Y/N/Other
(motivations)	
Have you practiced moderate physical exercise (>3, <6 METS) for the following months?	Y/N/Other
(motivations)	

per day for 3 sessions per week. The protocol provided 20 minutes on bicycling (60%–80% of Vo_{2max}) following by resistance exercise (65% of 1 RM): transverse thrust movements, frontal traction movements of the upper limbs, distension of the lower limbs, trunk flexions for the abdominals, and 3 stretching positions (>3 and <6 METS).

Follow-up Evaluation and Identification of Responders

At 12 and 24 months, a reevaluation of BMI and repeated cardiovascular investigations were performed. WL groups were divided as follows: less than 10% WL or weight gain (nonresponders), ≥10% WL (responders).

Cardiovascular Evaluation

Standard echocardiography was performed in all the patients at baseline and follow-up (12 and 24 months). Left ventricular (LV) chamber dimension and wall thickness was obtained according to recommendations of the American Society of Echocardiography.[18] Maximal extent of ventricular hypertrophy (maximal wall thickness [MWT]) was assessed in end-diastole by parasternal short axis view. LV end-diastolic and end-systolic volumes and LV ejection fraction (LVEF) were calculated from apical views, using the biplane method of discs (modified Simpson's rule). An LVEF less than 50% was considered abnormal. Left atrial (LA) volume index (LAVI) was measured using the biplane area-length method.[19] Systolic intraventricular gradients were assessed using continuous wave Doppler. LV outflow tract (LVOT) obstruction was defined as an instantaneous peak Doppler LVOT pressure gradient $\geq$ 30 mm Hg at rest or after a Valsalva maneuver. LV diastolic function was assessed by pulsed Doppler at the level of mitral tips. Peak flow velocity in early diastole and during atrial contraction, and E/A ratio were measured, as well as deceleration time of early diastolic flow velocity. The pattern of LV filling was classified as follows: restrictive if deceleration time less than 120 ms or E/A $\geq$2 associated with deceleration time $\leq$ 150 ms; abnormal relaxation if E/A <1 associated with deceleration time $\geq$220 ms; normal (or "pseudonormal") filling in presence of intermediate patterns.[20] In patients with atrial fibrillation, only E wave and deceleration time were measured. Systolic, early diastolic (E′), and late diastolic tissue Doppler velocities were measured at the lateral mitral and septal walls and subsequently averaged over 3 cardiac cycles in accordance with previously reported methods.[21] Trans-mitral E/E′ ratios (lateral, septal, average) were calculated for each patient. E/E′ average ratio was considered increased if higher than 15. Exercise testing was performed on a cycle-ergometer in an upright position following the Bruce protocol. The cardiovascular response was evaluated by cardiopulmonary exercise test (CPET) and expressed as maximal oxygen uptake (Vo_2max), defined as the highest Vo_2 achieved during exercise; ventilatory response to exercise, evaluated by analyzing minute ventilation expressed as absolute value; ventilatory equivalents for carbon (VE/VCO2) dioxide, measured plotting VE versus VCO2 (abnormal: >30).[22]

Clinical Outcome and Definitions

Heart failure was defined as the presence of signs or symptoms of heart failure, in presence of a preserved or reduced LVEF (>50% or <50%, respectively).[23] New York Heart Association (NYHA) class based on the degree of dyspnea and/or exercise limitation, was evaluated to define the severity of symptoms and heart failure. According to our laboratory protocol, and the specific population evaluated (obese), we considered 3 different cutoffs for NT-proBNP: less than 300 pg/mL; 300 to 900 pg/mL; greater than 900 pg/mL.[24] LVOT greater than 30 mm Hg at rest or with provocation maneuvers was defined as a severe obstruction. Systolic dysfunction was defined as an LV dysfunction with LVEF less than 50%. Diastolic dysfunction was defined as a various degree of abnormal filling and/or LV compliance (type I: abnormal relaxation; type II: pseudonormal pattern; type III: restrictive filling), with LVEF greater than 50%. Atrial fibrillation (AF) was defined as paroxysmal, permanent, or persistent AF detected on ECG, Holter monitoring, or device interrogation.[25]

Statistical Analysis

Data are shown as either mean and standard deviation in the case of continuous variables, and number and percentage for categorical variables. Differences across groups were assessed using the Student *t*-test or Wilcoxon-Mann Whitney test in case of continuous variables and the χ^2 or Fisher exact test in case of categorical data. We applied a multivariable linear regression model to evaluate the association of BMI changes at follow-up with cardiac ultrasound and exercise testing. The final multivariable model included the following covariates: age, systolic blood pressure, diastolic blood pressure, heart rate, and BMI at baseline values as continuous variables; sex and NYHA class as categorical variables. The analyses were done using SPSS Statistics, version 25.0 (IBM SPSS Statistics, Armonk, NY).

RESULTS

Baseline Clinical Characteristics

Table 2 reports basal characteristics of the patients. All the patients studied were symptomatic, including 8 patients in NYHA class III (HCM2, HCM3, HCM6, HCM10, HCM13, HCM17, HCM19, HCM20). Fourteen patients (70%) had an NT-pro-BNP greater than 300 ng/mL (including 2 patients with NT-pro-BNP >900 ng/mL: HCM 13, HCM 15). Six patients (20%) had systolic dysfunction, all protected by an implantable cardioverter-defibrillator (ICD) (HCM2, HCM4, HCM11, HCM13, HCM15, HCM20). In addition, 6 patients (20%) had obstructive HCM (HOCM), with fixed and/or latent gradient, including 3 patients (15%) with refractory symptoms despite optimal medical therapy (beta blockers and disopyramide), who were being considered for surgical myectomy (HCM 6, HCM 12, HCM 18). Three patients (15%) had paroxysmal AF (HCM 2, HCM 6, HCM 20) and nonsustained ventricular tachycardia (NSVT) (HCM 2, HCM 15, HCM19), respectively. Three patients (15%; HCM 10, HCM 13, and HCM 20) were listed for cardiac transplantation.

Table 2
Clinical characteristics of study population at baseline and at 12-month and 24-month follow-up

Clinical Features	Baseline (n = 20)	12-mo Follow-up (n = 20)	*P* value	24-mo Follow-up (n = 20)	*P* value
Weight, kg	92.5 ± 12.19	86.8 ± 11.3	<.001*	84.7 ± 10.8	<.001*
BMI, kg/m^2	32.4 ± 2.8	30.4 ± 2.8	<.001*	29.7 ± 2.9	<.001*
NYHA, Class					
I, n (%)	0 (0)	3 (15)	.072	3 (15)	.072
II, n (%)	12 (60)	12 (60)	-	12 (60)	-
III, n (%)	8 (20)	5 (25)	.311	5 (25)	.311
MWT, mm	21.0 ± 6.1	20.7 ± 6.1	.029*	20.5 ± 6.2	.003*
LA AP diameter, mm	47.9 ± 6.3	47.1 ± 5.7	.056	46.5 ± 5.7	.069
LAVI, mL/m^2	44.9 ± 10.1	44.2 ± 9.9	.054	42.7 ± 10.1	.028*
LVOTG, mm Hg	18.8 ± 23.8	16.9 ± 21.3	.037*	14.5 ± 15.2	.074
LVEF, %	57.7 ± 9.6	55.7 ± 8.3	.020*	50.6 ± 8.3	<.001*
Diastolic disfunction, stage					
I, n (%)	6 (30)	7 (35)	.736	10 (50)	.197
II, n (%)	11 (55)	10 (50)	.752	8 (40)	.342
III, n (%)	3 (15)	3 (15)	-	2 (10)	.633
E/E′ average	11.1 ± 4.8	10.9 ± 4.4	.538	10.1 ± 4.8	.175
PASP, mm Hg	34.8 ± 9.4	33.5 ± 8.3	.027*	32.0 ± 7.7	.047*
NT-proBNP, pg/mL	468.8 ± 269.5	477.9 ± 296.2	.501	418.1 ± 290.9	.010*
Vo_{2max}, mL/kg/min	16.9 ± 4.6	17.2 ± 4.4	.309	17.7 ± 4.4	.029*
Vo_{2max}, %	57.4 ± 15.1	58.6 ± 13.4	.201	60.1 ± 13.6	.032*
VE/VCO^2 slope	30.5 ± 3.6	29.3 ± 2.8	.005*	29.0 ± 2.6	.010*
Peak workload, watts	101.9 ± 30.2	107.9 ± 26.0	.005*	111.5 ± 26.0	<.001*

* p-values <0.05 were considered statistically significant.

Abbreviations: AP, antero-posterior; BMI, body mass index; LA, left atrium; LAVI, left atrium volume index; LVOTG, left ventricular outflow tract gradient; MWT, maximal wall thickness; PASP, pulmonary artery systolic pressure; VE/VCO2, minute ventilation/carbon dioxide production; Vo_{2max}, maximal oxygen uptake.

Compliance with the Study Protocol and Level of Exercise Attained

According to the questionnaire results, adherence to the protocol at 12 months was complete in 70% and incomplete in 30% of the patients; at 24 months, adherence to the protocol was complete in 90% and incomplete in 10% of the patients. Particularly, compliance to diet regimen was complete in 85% of patients, whereas compliance to exercise protocol was complete in 95%.

Overall Variations at 12 and 24 Months

Differences in clinical characteristics between basal,12-month and 24-month evaluations are reported in **Table 1**. **Fig. 1** reports changes in BMI and other principal parameters at 24 months.

At the end of the study period 5 patients were classified as responders, due to a WL ≥10% (average 12.8% ± 2.2%) and 15 as nonresponders (WL <10%, average 6.1% ± 3.0%).

Comparison of Imaging and Functional Parameters in Responders Versus Nonresponders

Table 3 shows the effect of WL on clinical, echocardiographic, and cardiopulmonary parameters, according to response to aerobic exercise and Mediterranean diet. At baseline no significant difference for age, gender, weight, or NYHA class was evidenced between the 2 groups.

Compared with nonresponders (<10% WL), responders (≥10% WL) showed a significant reduction in LA antero-posterior (AP) diameter (−4.8 ± 4.3 vs −0.3 ± 2.2 mm; *P* = .006), LAVI

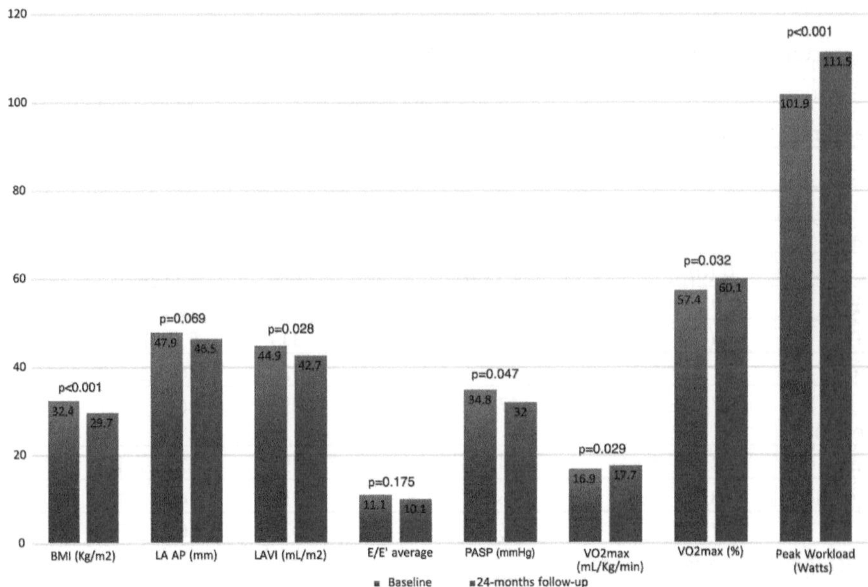

Fig. 1. Clinical, echocardiographic, and cardiopulmonary parameters changes from baseline at 24-month follow-up in the overall cohort.

(-7.0 ± 3.8 vs -0.6 ± 2.8 mL/m^2; P<.001), E/E′ average (-3.8 ± 2.9 vs 0.0 ± 2.6; P = .014), pulmonary artery systolic pressure (PASP) (-8.6 ± 7.6 vs -0.8 ± 3.5 mm Hg; P = .005), and a significant increase in Vo_{2max} (%) ($+7.4 \pm 2.4$ vs $+1.1 \pm 5.0$%; P = .015) and peak workload ($+22.6 \pm 12.8$ vs $+5.3 \pm 5.0$W; P<.001).

Correlations Between Body Mass Index and Clinical Parameters

Table 4 reports quartiles of BMI reduction in relation to other clinical, echocardiographic, and cardiopulmonary parameters changes from baseline. **Table 5** shows the results of multivariate linear regression analysis. BMI changes from

Table 3
Clinical, echocardiographic and cardiopulmonary parameters changes from baseline according to response to aerobic exercise and Mediterranean diet

Clinical Features	Responders (n = 5)	Nonresponders (n = 15)	*P* value
Weight, kg	-12.8 ± 2.2	-6.1 ± 3.0	<.001*
BMI, kg/m^2	-4.3 ± 0.6	-2.2 ± 1.1	<.001*
MWT, mm	-0.7 ± 0.4	-0.5 ± 0.8	.532
LA AP diameter, mm	-4.8 ± 4.3	-0.3 ± 2.2	.006*
LAVI, mL/m^2	-7.0 ± 3.8	-0.6 ± 2.8	<.001*
LVOTG, mm Hg	-6.8 ± 14.2	-3.5 ± 9.0	.541
LVEF, %	-7.6 ± 6.0	-6.9 ± 5.9	.830
E/E′ average	-3.8 ± 2.9	0.0 ± 2.6	.014*
PASP, mm Hg	-8.6 ± 7.6	-0.8 ± 3.5	.005*
NT-proBNP, pg/mL	-84.4 ± 64.9	-39.5 ± 81.8	.282
Vo_{2max}, mL/kg/min	$+1.8 \pm 0.7$	$+0.5 \pm 1.6$	.112
Vo_{2max}, %	$+7.4 \pm 2.4$	$+1.1 \pm 5.0$	.015*
VE/VCO2 slope	-2.2 ± 1.8	-1.3 ± 2.5	.455
Peak workload, watts	$+22.6 \pm 12.8$	$+5.3 \pm 5.0$	<.001*

* p-values <0.05 were considered statistically significant.

Abbreviations: AP, antero-posterior; LA, left atrium; LAVI, left atrium volume index; LVOTG, left ventricular outflow tract gradient; MWT, maximal wall thickness; PASP, pulmonary artery systolic pressure; VE/VCO2, minute ventilation/carbon dioxide production; Vo_{2max}, maximal oxygen uptake.

Table 4
Clinical, echocardiographic and cardiopulmonary parameters changes from baseline according to quartiles of BMI reduction

Clinical Features	Q1: BMI <0.9, ≥−2.1 (n = 5)	Q2: BMI <−2.1, ≥−2.6 (n = 5)	*P* value Q2 vs Q1	Q3: BMI <−2.6, ≥−3.4 (n = 5)	*P* value Q3 vs Q1	Q4: BMI <−3.4, ≥−4.9 (n = 5)	*P* value Q4 vs Q1
Weight, kg	−3.1 ± 3.5	−7.2 ± 1.1	0.034*	−7.9 ± 0.8	0.016*	−12.8 ± 2.2	<.001*
MWT, mm	−0.5 ± 0.7	−0.2 ± 0.4	0.446	−0.7 ± 1.1	0.740	−0.7 ± 0.4	.608
LA AP diameter, mm	−0.2 ± 1.3	−0.2 ± 1.9	1.000	−1.4 ± 3.0	0.302	−4.8 ± 4.3	.038*
LAVI, mL/m^2	−0.0 ± 1.4	−1.0 ± 1.2	0.266	−2.8 ± 3.9	0.170	−7.0 ± 3.8	.005*
LVOTG, mm Hg	−0.6 ± 1.5	−1.8 ± 3.1	0.461	8.0 ± 15.1	0.309	−6.8 ± 14.2	.360
LVEF, %	−5.0 ± 5.0	−4.4 ± 5.8	0.866	−11.4 ± 5.0	0.077	−7.6 ± 6.0	.479
E/E′ average	1.6 ± 0.9	0.1 ± 1.7	0.115	−1.8 ± 3.6	0.077	−3.8 ± 2.8	.004*
PASP, mm Hg	1.8 ± 1.8	−1.0 ± 2.9	0.105	−3.2 ± 4.0	0.035*	−8.6 ± 7.6	.018*
NT-proBNP, pg/mL	−4.8 ± 50.8	−77.4 ± 102.8	0.195	−36.4 ± 83.4	0.490	−84.4 ± 64.9	.063
Vo_{2max}, mL/kg/min	0.1 ± 1.4	0.1 ± 1.9	0.985	1.3 ± 1.5	0.239	1.8 ± 0.7	.050*
Vo_{2max}, %	0.4 ± 3.8	−0.4 ± 7.1	0.829	3.4 ± 3.4	0.222	7.4 ± 2.4	.008*
VE/VCO2 slope	−0.1 ± 2.3	−2.2 ± 2.6	0.222	−1.5 ± 2.8	0.418	−2.2 ± 1.8	.148
Peak workload, watts	4.2 ± 4.6	5.0 ± 5.8	0.815	6.6 ± 5.3	0.465	22.6 ± 12.7	.016*

* p-values <0.05 were considered statistically significant.

Abbreviations: AP, antero-posterior; BMI, body mass index; LA, left atrium; LAVI, left atrium volume index; LVOTG, left ventricular outflow tract gradient; MWT, maximal wall thickness; PASP, pulmonary artery systolic pressure; VE/VCO2, minute ventilation/carbon dioxide production; Vo_{2max}, maximal oxygen uptake.

Table 5
Multivariate linear regression of BMI reduction with clinical, echocardiographic and cardiopulmonary parameters

Dependent Variable	Coefficient Beta	(95% CI)	*P* value
MWT, mm	0.162	(−0.256 to 0.422)	.599
LA AP diameter, mm	0.656	(0.590 to 2.655)	.005*
LAVI, mL/m^2	0.831	(1.332 to 3.724)	.001*
LVEF, %	0.182	(−1.062 to 4.950)	.182
LVOTG, mm Hg	0.279	(−2.666 to 6.853)	.354
E/E′ average	0.792	(0.965 to 2.641)	.001*
PASP, mm Hg	0.766	(1.925 to 4.593)	<.001*
NT-proBNP, pg/mL	−0.246	(−24.089 to 52.578)	.431
Vo_{2max}, mL/Kg/min	−0.526	(−1.130 to −0.059)	.033*
Vo_{2max}, %	−0.684	(−4.282 to −0.951)	.005*
VE/VCO^2 slope	0.271	(−0.696 to 1.635)	.394
Peak workload, watts	−0.647	(−9.453 to −0.595)	.030*

* p-values <0.05 were considered statistically significant.

The multivariable model included the following covariates: age, systolic blood pressure, diastolic blood pressure, heart rate, and BMI at baseline values as continuous variables; sex and New York Heart Association class as categorical variables.

Abbreviations: AP, antero-posterior; BMI, body mass index; LA, left atrium; LAVI, left atrium volume index; LVOTG, left ventricular outflow tract gradient; MWT, maximal wall thickness; PASP, pulmonary artery systolic pressure; VE/VCO^2, minute ventilation/carbon dioxide production; Vo_{2max}, maximal oxygen uptake.

baseline correlated with reduction of LA AP diameter (beta 0.66; *P* = .005), LAVI (beta 0.83; *P* = .001), E/E′ average (beta 0.79; *P* = .001), PASP (beta 0.77; *P*<.001), and increase of Vo_{2max} (mL/kg per minute) (beta −0.53; *P* = .033), Vo_{2max} (%) (beta −0.68; *P* = .005), peak workload (beta −0.65; *P* = .030).

Variation in Clinical Status and Outcome

At last follow-up, 6 patients (30%) improved their NYHA class symptoms: 3 patients from class III to class II (HCM2, HCM 3, HCM20); 3 patients from NYHA class II to class I (HCM7, HCM 8, HCM11). Fourteen patients (70%) were clinically stable in class III (HCM 6, HCM 10, HCM 13, HCM 17, HCM 19) and class II (HCM 1, HCM 4, HCM5, HCM9, HCM12, HCM14, HCM15, HCM16, HCM18). At last evaluation, 11 patients (55%) had an NT-pro-BNP greater than 300 ng/mL (including 5 patients with NT-pro-BNP >900 ng/mL: HCM 9, HCM 10, HCM 15, HCM 19, HCM 20). Three patients developed systolic dysfunction (HCM 7, HCM 9, HCM 10), and underwent ICD implantation. Diastolic function improved in 4 patients (20%), including 3 patients improving from dysfunction type II to I (HCM 2, HCM 3, HCM 20), and 1 from type III to II (HCM 13). Four patients (20%; HCM 10, HCM 13, HCM15, HCM 20) had incidental AF that became permanent in 2 patients (HCM 15, HCM 20; ie, AF already observed at 6-month evaluation). Five patients (25%) showed NSVT at 24 months (HCM 6, HCM13, HCM 14, HCM15, HCM 19; NSVT was also present at the 6-month evaluation in patient HCM 19).

Of the 3 patients being considered for myectomy, 1 patient underwent myectomy (HCM 18), whereas 2 (HCM 6 and HCM 12) showed significant improvement of clinical and hemodynamic status (left ventricular outflow tract gradient [LVOTG] lowered from 75 and 80 mm Hg to 40 mm Hg and 48 mm Hg, respectively) and did not require surgery. Similarly, of the 3 patients being evaluated for transplantation, 1 patient (HCM 20) was not listed for transplantation because of clinical (NYHA class III to II) and functional capacity improvement (Vo_{2max} 10.7–12.7 mg/Kg/min; Vo_2% 59%–69%).

DISCUSSION

Obesity, defined by a BMI greater than 30 kg/m^2, represents an epidemic health problem, particularly in Western countries.[26] It affects approximately 300 million people worldwide, and it is associated with increased risk of death due to comorbidities, such as type 2 diabetes mellitus, dyslipidemia, hypertension, obstructive sleep apnea, and certain types of cancer.[27] It is well-known that morbidity and mortality are per se related to progressive BMI increase in obese patients.[27] Nevertheless, obesity represents an important comorbidity in patients affected by cardiac disease, including HCM, and combined dietary and lifestyle interventions have been advocated in this setting.

In the present pilot study, we assessed the effect of the combination of Mediterranean diet and anaerobic exercise on WL and clinical status in 20 obese, symptomatic patients with HCM. Notably, the level of adherence was high at 24 months (90%). Although only one-quarter of the participants could be defined as responders according to the predefined WL cutoff of greater than 10%, reflecting the challenges of weight reduction in the presence of limiting symptoms, there was a positive and consistent overall trend in several functional and structural parameters, associated with clinical benefit. In our cohort, we observed a significant reverse remodeling of the LA, an improvement of wedge and systolic pulmonary pressure, and improvement of exercise capacity (significant increase of Vo_{2max} (%) and peak workload). Although this general trend occurred in the overall population, improvements were particularly evident in responders (>10% WL). At last follow-up, we observed an improvement of clinical status, in term of symptoms (NYHA class) and indications to surgical procedures (ie, myectomy and transplant list). Because LA size is a major determinant of symptoms, diastolic function, wedge pressure, exercise capacity, risk of arrhythmias, and a determinant of patient clinical course,[1,2,28,29] LA remodeling decrease per se the risk of adverse outcome.

In recent years, interest on clinical significance of comorbidities in HCM is growing.[30–33] A recent study from the SHARE registry investigated the clinical impact of obesity in a very large cohort of patients with HCM (n = 3282), followed for a median of 6.8 (3.3–13.3) years.[11] The investigators report a dramatic prevalence of excess body weight in HCM cohort (70%, including 39% with pre-obesity and 32% with obesity), disproportionate compared with the general population, and may be linked to dietary and lifestyle habit (ie, less time spent in recreational and/or sport activities). Furthermore, obese patients were more symptomatic for dyspnea, were more often obstructive and had greater incidence of AF and adverse outcome due to developing HF, irrespective of age, sex, left atrium diameter, obstruction, and genetic status. The investigators conclude suggesting the need for specific exercise programs and lifestyle interventions in patients with HCM, often quite capable of exercising regularly without arrhythmic events.

Indeed, the beneficial effects of physical activity have been studied in a preclinical HCM mouse model (showing the tolerability of exercise in mutant myosin heavy chain mice, and even the ability to reverse hypertrophic phenotype)[33] and in a randomized clinical trial involving 136 patients with HCM. Patients were randomly assigned to 16 weeks of moderate-intensity exercise training or usual activity.[12] The investigators found that moderate-intensity exercise was safe and resulted in a small but significant increase in exercise capacity at 16 weeks.

Clinical Implications

Lifestyle optimization is recommended in all patients with HCM, regardless of symptoms and clinical status.[34] This includes avoidance of excess alcohol, drugs, stimulants, dehydration, and prolonged exposure to extreme temperature (eg, saunas and hot tubs), particularly in patients with obstructive disease.

American College of Cardiology Foundation/American Heart Association[2] and European Society of Cardiology[1] guideline recommendations discourage competitive sport and encourage low-intensity aerobic activities to maintain and healthy lifestyle; however, the European Association of Preventive Cardiology recommended that low-risk patients with HCM may selectively be allowed to participate in all competitive sport.[35]

Emerging data suggest the safety and potential effect of moderate-intensity exercise on clinical status, although new prospective study for further evidence (LIVE-HCM [Exercise in Genetic Cardiovascular Conditions]; NCT02549664) is still ongoing. Beyond exercise, obesity is well recognized as cause of symptoms and major determinant of outcome.[11] WL is hard to attain (only 25% of our patients were responders at 2 years), but had a favorable effect on LA, diastolic function, exercise capacity, and clinical status in obese, symptomatic patients with HCM. Thus, WL, by combined diet and low-to-moderate exercise training, should be encouraged in patients with HCM to control symptoms and clinical status. The role of more aggressive strategies, such as bariatric surgery, needs to be specifically assessed in morbidly obese patients, balancing surgical risk versus long-term benefits.

STUDY LIMITATIONS

The principal limitations of the study are represented by the small cohort analyzed and the generality (ie, absence of a specific objective to assess adherence) of the WL protocol.

SUMMARY

In obese, symptomatic patients with HCM, WL due to a combined protocol of Mediterranean diet and low-to-moderate exercise training, had a favorable effect on LA remodeling, diastolic function, exercise capacity, and clinical status.

CLINICS CARE POINTS

- In the present pilot study, we assessed for the first time the effect of the combination of a Mediterranean diet and an aerobic exercise program on WL and clinical status in obese, symptomatic patients with HCM.
- The results of the study have important implications in clinical practice for lifestyle optimization.
- The principal limitation of the study is represented by the small cohort analyzed.

CONTRIBUTORS

G. Limongelli and A. D'Aponte contributed to the conception and design of the work. E. Monda, M. Caiazza, M. Rubino, A. Esposito, G. Messina, P. Calabro, M. Monda, E. Bossone, S.M. Day, and I. Olivotto contributed to the acquisition, analysis, or interpretation of data for the work. G. Limongelli, E. Monda, E. Bossone, S.M. Day, and I. Olivotto drafted the article. All the authors critically revised the article. All gave final approval and agree to be accountable for all aspects of work ensuring integrity and accuracy.

FUNDING

The authors have not declared a specific grant for this research from any funding agency in the public, commercial or not-for-profit sectors.

COMPETING INTERESTS

None declared.

ACKNOWLEDGMENTS

This article is dedicated to the memory of Francesco Mario Limongelli, with whom we started to approach this work. The authors acknowledge our nurses (Giuseppina Cacciuottolo and Giuseppina Tabasco) for their precious support.

DISCLOSURE

The authors have nothing to disclose.

REFERENCES

1. Authors/Task Force members, Elliott PM, Anastasakis A, et al. 2014 ESC Guidelines on diagnosis and management of hypertrophic cardiomyopathy: the Task Force for the Diagnosis and Management of Hypertrophic Cardiomyopathy of the European Society of Cardiology (ESC). Eur Heart J 2014;35(39):2733–79.
2. Gersh BJ, Maron BJ, Bonow RO, et al. 2011 ACCF/AHA guideline for the diagnosis and treatment of hypertrophic cardiomyopathy: a report of the American College of Cardiology Foundation/American Heart Association Task Force on Practice Guidelines. Circulation 2011;124(24):e783–831.
3. Lorenzini M, Anastasiou Z, O'Mahony C, et al. Mortality among referral patients with hypertrophic cardiomyopathy vs the general European population. JAMA Cardiol 2020;5(1):73–80.
4. Eberly LA, Day SM, Ashley EA, et al. Association of race with disease expression and clinical outcomes among patients with hypertrophic cardiomyopathy. JAMA Cardiol 2020;5(1):83–91.
5. Barretta F, Mirra B, Monda E, et al. The hidden fragility in the heart of the athletes: a review of genetic biomarkers. Int J Mol Sci 2020;21(18):6682.
6. Limongelli G, Nunziato M, D'Argenio V, et al. Yield and clinical significance of genetic screening in elite and amateur athletes. Eur J Prev Cardiol 2020. https://doi.org/10.1177/2047487320934265. 2047487320934265.
7. Caiazza M, Rubino M, Monda E, et al. Combined PTPN11 and MYBPC3 gene mutations in an adult patient with noonan syndrome and hypertrophic cardiomyopathy. Genes (Basel) 2020;11(8):947.
8. Maron BJ. Clinical course and management of hypertrophic cardiomyopathy. N Engl J Med 2018; 379(7):655–68.
9. Monda E, Palmiero G, Rubino M, et al. Molecular basis of inflammation in the pathogenesis of cardiomyopathies. Int J Mol Sci 2020;21(18):6462.
10. Monda E, Limongelli G. The hospitalizations in hypertrophic cardiomyopathy: "The dark side of the moon. Int J Cardiol 2020;318:101–2.
11. Fumagalli C, Maurizi N, Day SM, et al. Association of obesity with adverse long-term outcomes in hypertrophic cardiomyopathy. JAMA Cardiol 2019;5(1): 65–72.
12. Saberi S, Wheeler M, Bragg-Gresham J, et al. Effect of moderate-intensity exercise training on peak

oxygen consumption in patients with hypertrophic cardiomyopathy: a randomized clinical trial. JAMA 2017;317(13):1349–57.
13. Estruch R, Ros E, Salas-Salvadó J, et al. Primary prevention of cardiovascular disease with a Mediterranean diet supplemented with extra-virgin olive oil or nuts. N Engl J Med 2018;378(25):e34.
14. Limongelli G, Monda E, Tramonte S, et al. Prevalence and clinical significance of red flags in patients with hypertrophic cardiomyopathy. Int J Cardiol 2020;299:186–91.
15. Frisso G, Limongelli G, Pacileo G, et al. A child cohort study from southern Italy enlarges the genetic spectrum of hypertrophic cardiomyopathy. Clin Genet 2009;76(1):91–101.
16. Limongelli G, Nunziato M, Mazzaccara C, et al. Genotype-phenotype correlation: a triple DNA mutational event in a boy entering sport conveys an additional pathogenicity risk. Genes (Basel) 2020; 11(5):524.
17. Lombardo B, D'Argenio V, Monda E, et al. Genetic analysis resolves differential diagnosis of a familial syndromic dilated cardiomyopathy: A new case of Alström syndrome. Mol Genet Genomic Med 2020; 8:e1260.
18. Mitchell C, Rahko PS, Blauwet LA, et al. Guidelines for performing a comprehensive transthoracic echocardiographic examination in adults: recommendations from the American Society of Echocardiography. J Am Soc Echocardiogr 2019; 32(1):1–64.
19. Limongelli G, Fioretti V, Di Maio M, et al. Left atrial volume during stress is associated with increased risk of arrhythmias in patients with hypertrophic cardiomyopathy. J Cardiovasc Echogr 2019;29(1):1–6.
20. Nagueh SF, Smiseth OA, Appleton CP, et al. Recommendations for the evaluation of left ventricular diastolic function by echocardiography: an update from the American Society of Echocardiography and the European Association of Cardiovascular Imaging. J Am Soc Echocardiogr 2016;29(4):277–314.
21. Hill JC, Palma RA. Doppler tissue imaging for the assessment of left ventricular diastolic function: a systematic approach for the sonographer. J Am Soc Echocardiogr 2005;18(1):80–8 [quiz: 89].
22. Guazzi M, Bandera F, Ozemek C, et al. Cardiopulmonary exercise testing: what is its value? J Am Coll Cardiol 2017;70(13):1618–36.
23. Maron BJ, Rowin EJ, Udelson JE, et al. Clinical spectrum and management of heart failure in hypertrophic cardiomyopathy. JACC Heart Fail 2018;6(5): 353–63.
24. Januzzi JL, van Kimmenade R, Lainchbury J, et al. NT-proBNP testing for diagnosis and short-term prognosis in acute destabilized heart failure: an international pooled analysis of 1256 patients: the International Collaborative of NT-proBNP Study. Eur Heart J 2006;27(3):330–7.
25. Kirchhof P, Benussi S, Kotecha D, et al. 2016 ESC Guidelines for the management of atrial fibrillation developed in collaboration with EACTS. Eur Heart J 2016;37(38):2893–962.
26. GBD 2015 Obesity Collaborators, Afshin A, Forouzanfar MH, et al. Health effects of overweight and obesity in 195 countries over 25 years. N Engl J Med 2017;377(1):13–27.
27. Abdelaal M, le Roux CW, Docherty NG. Morbidity and mortality associated with obesity. Ann Transl Med 2017;5(7):161.
28. Cardim N, Galderisi M, Edvardsen T, et al. Role of multimodality cardiac imaging in the management of patients with hypertrophic cardiomyopathy: an expert consensus of the European Association of Cardiovascular Imaging Endorsed by the Saudi Heart Association. Eur Heart J Cardiovasc Imaging 2015;16(3):280.
29. Losi MA, Betocchi S, Barbati G, et al. Prognostic significance of left atrial volume dilatation in patients with hypertrophic cardiomyopathy. J Am Soc Echocardiogr 2009;22(1):76–81.
30. Wasserstrum Y, Barriales-Villa R, Fernández-Fernández X, et al. The impact of diabetes mellitus on the clinical phenotype of hypertrophic cardiomyopathy. Eur Heart J 2019;40(21):1671–7.
31. Wang S, Cui H, Song C, et al. Obstructive sleep apnea is associated with nonsustained ventricular tachycardia in patients with hypertrophic obstructive cardiomyopathy. Heart Rhythm 2019;16(5):694–701.
32. Esposito A, Monda E, Gragnano F, et al. Prevalence and clinical implications of hyperhomocysteinaemia in patients with hypertrophic cardiomyopathy and MTHFR C6777T polymorphism. Eur J Prev Cardiol 2020;27(17):1906–8.
33. Konhilas JP, Watson PA, Maass A, et al. Exercise can prevent and reverse the severity of hypertrophic cardiomyopathy. Circ Res 2006;98(4):540–8.
34. Geske JB, Ommen SR, Gersh BJ. Hypertrophic cardiomyopathy: clinical update. JACC Heart Fail 2018; 6(5):364–75.
35. Pelliccia A, Solberg EE, Papadakis M, et al. Recommendations for participation in competitive and leisure time sport in athletes with cardiomyopathies, myocarditis, and pericarditis: position statement of the Sport Cardiology Section of the European Association of Preventive Cardiology (EAPC). Eur Heart J 2019;40(1):19–33.

Printed and bound by CPI Group (UK) Ltd, Croydon, CR0 4YY
03/10/2024
01040372-0014